1978

THE ACQUISIT
OF DISTINCTIVE
FEATURES

THE ACQUISITION OF DISTINCTIVE FEATURES

by
Stephen E. Blache, Ph.D.
Assistant Professor
Department of Speech Pathology and Audiology
Southern Illinois University

University Park Press
Baltimore

UNIVERSITY PARK PRESS
International Publishers in Science and Medicine
233 East Redwood Street
Baltimore, Maryland 21202

Typeset by The Composing Room of Michigan, Inc.
Manufactured in the United States of America by The Maple Press Company

Library of Congress Cataloging in Publication Data
Blache, Stephen E
    The acquisition of distinctive features.

    Bibliography: p.
    Includes index.
    1. Children—Language.   2.   Distinctive features
(Linguistics)   3.   Speech disorders in children.
4.   Jakobson, Roman, 1896–   I.   Title.
[DNLM: 1.   Language Development. WS105.5.C8 B627a]
P118.B58   401   77-29056
ISBN 0-8391-1208-4

To those who wrote with love,
To those who taught with love,
To those I love: Vic, Louise, Ian, Nathan, (especially) Donna Lee

Contents

Foreword

Distinctive feature theory is currently at an important stage. It is being used to predict (generate) the phonological acquisition, speech perception, and speech production of the normal language user. It is also being used to predict the delays and deviations in the acquisition of phonology and the distortions and deviations in the speech perception and speech production of the non-normal language user.

It is important, therefore, to question the validity of the theory itself and its power to explain data. To do so, obviously the theory must be fully understood. It is here that the history of the theory becomes of value. The history of this or any other theory provides an important perspective on the theory's construction and application. It illuminates the philosophical and theoretical origins of the theory and situates them within their broader historical framework. Apparent ambiguities, internal inconsistencies, and inadequate data support may be explained and possibly resolved. The connection between the intent of the theory's constructors and the theory's subsequent application becomes clearer.

In this volume, Dr. Blache presents history, theory, and philosophy as the foundation for distinctive feature theory. He traces the work of the theory's constructors, focusing on Jakobson, and relates the theory to its larger historical context. To further probe the validity of distinctive feature theory and its explanatory power, Dr. Blache examines the theory to see first if it fits the scientific criteria for any theory. He then goes on to emphasize the application of the theory in generating acquisition, perception, production, and acoustics of speech—the theory's power as a theory of language.

The relationship between theory and reality is one test for the appropriateness of the theory. The greater the breadth and the depth of the reality of a theory, the more stable the theory's foundation. Dr. Blache discusses the feature hypothesis in light of both theory and application. He makes a unique contribution in establishing distinctive feature theory's historical and theoretical bases and in applying the theory to explain feature components and their articulatory and acoustic correlates within the framework of phonological acquisition. Although the primary emphasis in this book is on acquisition, Dr. Blache has made a remarkable contribution in the area of diagnosis and treatment of phonological deviations.

According to the twentieth-century Danish philosopher, Hjelmslev, a theory of language has three prerequisites: consistency, exhaustiveness, and simplicity.[1] In *Prolegomena to a Theory of Language* (1943; quoted in Lamb, 1966) Hjelmslev wrote that a "linguistic theory must be of use for describing and predicting not only any possible text composed in any language whatsoever... [T]he linguistic theoretician... must take the precaution to foresee all conceivable possibilities... and to admit them into his theory so that it will be applicable even to texts and languages that have not appeared in his practice, or to languages that have perhaps never been realized."

Hjelmslev, however, hoped for a theory of language that would attain a level of abstraction "whose science of the expression is not phonetics and whose science of the content is not semantics. Such a science would be an algebra of language, operating with unnamed entities, i.e., arbitrarily named entities without natural designation, which would receive a motivated designation only on being confronted with the substance."[1] This hope for the attainment of the utmost level of abstraction for a theory of language resounds the zeal of an Indian school of philosophy of language, स्फोटवाद , or शब्दब्रह्मवाद whose translation in English is that the sounds of a language are (have a basis) as abstract as Brahma. Modern linguistic theory's quest for the universality hypothesis can be shown to have a link with this very early school of the philosophy of language as well as with the language theory of Hjemslev.

Modern linguistic theories have emphasized the species specificity and universality of language in man. Language is a highly organized system, unique to this species; all people use a small set of universal linguistic features and patterns. These universals are universal characteristics of man's neurological system, as demonstrated by the known neurological correlates of language development and use.

Distinctive feature theory contains elements that Hjemslev proposed as "algebra of language" on the one hand, and models for what he called "motivated designation" when "being confronted with the substance" on the other. Chomsky's and Halle's *The Sound Pattern of English* (1968) demonstrated the algebraic representations and transformations of phonological rules and "substantive designation" in the form of articulatory manifestations. They examined the phonological universals within the framework of adult English-language users. Dr. Blache, on the other hand, investigates the potential of these universals in the acquisition of linguistic features. One of the highlights of this book is its search for detailed acoustic correlates whose basis is in features.

Sadanand Singh, Ph.D.
Professor of Speech and Hearing Sciences
University of Texas Health Science
Center at Houston

[1]Lamb, S. M. Epilegomena to a Theory of Language. Romance Philology 19(4): 531–573, 1966.

[2]Hjelmslev, L. Prolegomena to a Theory of Language (F. J. Whitfield, trans.). 1961. Revised English edition: The University of Wisconsin Press, Madison. pp. v, 144. (Originally published, 1943.)

Preface

One of the most exciting aspects of the early childhood years is the acquisition of the speech sound system. Until recently,however, we have been unable to study phonemic growth because of the lack of a strong analytical orientation and a precise vocabulary. Distinctive feature theory, which has its roots in the phonemic acquisition process, has begun to provide the necessary tools for appreciating the young child who begins to acquire the sounds of speech.

This book provides, in as simple a manner as possible, the basic structural linguistic orientation commonly referred to as distinctive feature theory. The analytical orientation and vocabulary of structural linguistic analysis have great power in that they provide a unique perspective to view the sounds of speech and their significance as they are introduced into the child's cognitive phonemic structures. Whereas traditional approaches to speech sound acquisition have viewed the acquisition process as a form of simplistic learning of some forty physiological gestures, modern thought is beginning to view the process as more subtle and, subsequently, much more interesting.

Any attempt to explain the manner in which children acquire the sounds of speech is highly dependent upon the works of Roman Jakobson, as the subsequent narrative will make clear. Jakobson, in his attempt to wed the disciplines of historical and comparative linguistics, developed a synthesizing rationale that centered upon the evolution of man in general and the child in particular. This system of thought, like other accidental and brilliant discoveries, is beginning to shape disciplines far beyond child development. Distinctive feature theory is currently being used to revolutionize techniques for analyzing anthropological kinship arrangements, psychoperceptual visual arrays, literary folk tale structures, modern forms of biblical exegesis, and psychoanalytical techniques, particularly in France. Furthermore, a careful examination of the growth and development of the modern theories of syntax will reveal a great deal of dependence upon the works of this one scholar.

This book presents the essentials of Jakobsonian thought. Chapters 1 through 5 are structured as a running historical narrative of the growth and development of the structural linguistic theory. This has the advantage of presenting the simplest ideas in their proper order—first! The student of the theory can then build upon this foundation to understand the more complex aspects presented in later chapters. Whereas the first five chapters tend to be philosophically oriented, as food for thought, so to speak, the later chapters are more specific and technical. Chapters 6 through 8 establish the parameters of the first major organization of the theory. These three chapters present the heart of Jakobson's theory, which deals with the integration of the former philosophical principles into the acquisition process.

The initial theory serves as the large brush strokes into which the refined details are introduced, to create the full distinctive feature picture. Once the reader is familiar with the tenets of the structural linguistic philosophy of the Prague School and the subsequent Jakobsonian perspective, there is a brief interlude. Although prelinguistic behavior is not incorporated into distinctive feature theory, any attempt to discuss acquisition would be remiss without some comment concerning the first year of life. For this reason, the classical thought concerning early physiological and social growth is detailed for the full theory.

The next nine chapters, Chapters 10 through Chapter 18, deal with the sequential acquisition process. These chapters are constructed in such a way that the acoustic, physiological, cognitive, and sociocultural aspects of the theory are integrated into a synthetic didactic format. Whereas the former chapters depend to a large extent upon Jakobsonian writings, the latter chapters are a culmination of attempts to communicate Jakobsonian theory in the classroom. Although rooted in Jakobsonian theory, the overall character of these latter chapters is shaped by the interpretation of the implications of the basic theory, and, therefore, is my responsibility.

Chapter 19, one of the longer chapters, is difficult to characterize. In this chapter, I have attempted to crystallize the abstract theory into a testable format for research and application. This chapter, which is based upon eight years of sustained research and examination, details a twenty-two stage theory of development, with initial supportive evidence. The inspiration for this theoretical revision is definitely Jakobsonian, but the details and the sustaining postulates are my own invention.

Although the basic format of the book is in the direction of more abstract to more detailed, a collateral development may be noted from Jakobsonian reportage to personal interpretation and elaboration. Chapter 20, the final chapter, applies the theory in the clinical setting. Several specific techniques are offered to workers in the fields of speech pathology, child development, and education of deaf people, to apply the revised theory in everyday practice. A theory, in and of itself, is created to explain behavior. If the theory is a successful tool for appreciating, examining, and predicting behavior, it will have a lasting effect regardless of its elegance. Although commentary concerning a theory may generate thought and excitement, the specific success a theory has in transforming itself into a body of law is the ultimate assessment guideline.

In all, this book is meant to be read as a whole. Although the initial chapters may serve as the focus of a seminar, the middle chapters as the supplementary substance of undergraduate courses in speech science, physiological phonetics, or child development, and the final chapters as therapeutic tools; the entire work is meant to serve as an orientation to the acquisition process. The ultimate goal has been to entertain. Knowledge cannot, and should not, be force fed, even under the finest sauces.

Henry Fielding, in a much more charming and witty manner than I can muster, set forth his sentiments as follows:

> My reader then is not to be surprised, if, in the course of this work, he shall find some chapters very short, and others altogether as long. . . . For all which I shall not look on myself as accountable to any court of critical jurisdiction whatever; for as I am, in reality, the founder of a new province of writing, so I am at liberty to make what laws I please therein. And these laws, my readers, whom I consider as my subjects, are bound to believe in and to obey; with which that they may readily and cheerfully comply, I do hereby assure them that I shall principally regard their ease and advantage in all such institutions; for I do not, like a *jure divino* tyrant, imagine that they are my slaves or my commodity. I am, indeed, set over them for their own good only, and was created for their use and not they for mine. Nor do I doubt, while I make their interest the great rule of my writing, they will unanimously concur in supporting my dignity, and in rendering me all the honor I shall deserve or desire.

Many are deserving of thanks in terms of the creation of the present book. I would like to thank in particular Janet S. Hankin, who repeatedly attempted to get the surface structure of my syntax to match my deep structural intent; Nancy Hager, Helen Kammlade, and Donna Olson, who supervised the Southern Illinois articulatory survey that serves as the foundation of Chapter 19; Cheryl Keaveney, who diligently pursued the logistical problems of securing permission for the acknowledged sources; and last, but above all not least, Donna Lee Blache, who repeatedly proofread the manuscript through its many revisions. I would further like to take this opportunity to thank Drs. James Hardy, Leija McReynolds, Sadanand Singh, and Ralph Shelton for their suggestion and encouragement to expand the original manuscript into its full form.

Credits and Acknowledgments

Excerpt from C. Baltaxe, N. S. TRUBETZKOY: PRINCIPLES OF PHONOLOGY, Copyright © 1969 by The Regents of the University of California; reprinted by permission of the University of California Press.

Excerpt from L. Carmichael, in E. Lenneberg (ed.), NEW DIRECTIONS IN THE STUDY OF LANGUAGE, reprinted by permission of the MIT Press.

Excerpt from STRUCTURALISM edited by Jacques Ehrmann. Copyright © 1966 by Yale French Studies. Reprinted by permission of Doubleday & Company, Inc.

Excerpt from W. Nelson Francis, THE STRUCTURE OF AMERICAN ENGLISH. Copyright © 1958, The Ronald Press Company, New York.

Excerpt from D. Fry, in F. Smith and G. Miller (eds.), THE GENESIS OF LANGUAGE. Reprinted with permission from the MIT Press.

Excerpt from Edna Heidbreder, SEVEN PSYCHOLOGIES, © 1933 renewed 1961, pp. 65–66. Reprinted by permission of Prentice-Hall, Inc., Englewood Cliffs, N.J.

Excerpt from R. Jakobson, MAIN TRENDS IN THE SCIENCE OF LANGUAGE, reprinted by permission of George Allen & Unwin Ltd.

Excerpts from D. Jones, THE PHONEME, reprinted by permission of Cambridge University Press, New York.

Figure from W. Koenig, H. Dunn, and L. Lacy reprinted by permission of the Acoustical Society of America and Mrs. H. Dunn.

Excerpts from M. Marx (ed.), THEORIES IN CONTEMPORARY PSYCHOLOGY, copyright 1963, reprinted by permission of the Macmillan Publishing Company.

Excerpt from D. McNeill, in Mussen (ed.), CARMICHAEL'S MANUAL OF CHILD PSYCHOLOGY, 3rd Ed. Reprinted by permission of John Wiley & Sons, Inc.

Excerpt from THE PSYCHOLOGY OF COMMUNICATION: Seven Essays, by George A. Miller, © 1967 by Basic Books, Inc., Publishers, New York.

Excerpt from A. Moskowitz reprinted by permission of the Linguistic Society of America.

Excerpt from THE TACIT DIMENSION by Michael Polanyi. Copyright © 1966 by Michael Polanyi. Reprinted by permission of Doubleday & Company, Inc.

Table from M.C. Templin reprinted by permission of the University of Minnesota Press.

Excerpt from Charles Van Riper, SPEECH CORRECTION: Principles and Methods, 4th Ed., © 1963. Reprinted by permission of Prentice-Hall Inc., Englewood Cliffs, N.J.

Excerpt from Harris Winitz, ARTICULATORY ACQUISITION AND BEHAVIOR, © 1969, p. 62. Reprinted by permission of Prentice-Hall, Inc., Englewood Cliffs, N.J.

The author acknowledges the following for granting permission to reprint their material in the appendices: the MIT Press (Appendix A); the American Mathematical Society (Appendix B); Harper & Row (Appendix C); the Acoustical Society of America (Appendix E); S. Singh (Appendix F); W. Wickelgren (Appendix G); and Cambridge University Press (Appendix H).

The author also thanks the following for permission to reprint, adapt, or otherwise cite their material: L. Brosnahan; J. R. Crocker; J. L. Flanagan; O. C. Irwin; R. Jakobson; W. Leopold; A. M. Liberman; G. Miller; F. Minifie; E. K. Sander; the Acoustical Society of America; the American Psychological Association; ASHA; the Bell Laboratories; Johns Hopkins Neurocommunications Laboratory; Mouton Publishers, the Hague; the Philosophical Library; and Springer Verlag, Heidelberg.

CREDITS ADDED IN PROOF

Excerpt from E. Lenneberg (ed.), NEW DIRECTIONS IN THE STUDY OF LANGUAGE. Reprinted by permission of the MIT Press.
Excerpt from George A. Miller, THE PSYCHOLOGY OF COMMUNICATION. Reprinted by permission of Penguin Books Ltd.

The author additonally thanks P. Lieberman, R. Plomp, and R. K. Potter for permission to reprint their material.

chapter 1

Introduction

The process by which children acquire the sounds of language has been the object of conjecture and examination for almost two centuries. Since the 1787 publication of Dietrich Tiedemann's observations, students of phonemic acquisition have been unable to answer the most basic questions of speech sound development. For instance, little definitive information is available to specify when specific speech sounds are, or should be, acquired. Sander (1972) designated the problem as follows:

> When do children acquire the various speech sounds of our language? Considering the wealth of schedules in such areas as motor behavior, physical growth, and cognitive skill, the question might be assumed to be an easy one for the student of child behavior to answer. Surprisingly, however, *a concise reply to the question is difficult to provide* [emphasis mine], for reasons that have only partly to do with the available research knowledge. (p. 55)

THE PROBLEM

Three major cross-sectional studies have examined the question, "When are speech sounds learned?". In 1931, Wellman et al. examined 204 children in the midwestern United States. Three years later, as part of a dissertation project, Poole (1934) studied a similar group of 141 children in the Michigan area. These two studies, based upon children enrolled in university laboratory schools, remained the major source of normative data until 1957. In that year, Templin (1957) presented a detailed examination of 480 children from the Minneapolis and St. Paul, Minnesota, public school systems. The interpolated results of these three studies were presented in tabular form in *Certain Language Skills in Children* (Templin, 1957, p. 53). This table (see Table 1) still serves as the basic normative guideline for acquisition in contemporary textbooks (Singh, 1976, pp. 157–161; Winitz, 1969, p. 59).

1

Table 1.   Comparison of ages at which 75% of subjects correctly produced specific consonant sounds in the Templin, the Wellman et al., and the Poole studies

	Age correctly produced				Age correctly produced		
Sound	Templin	Wellman et al.	Poole	Sound	Templin	Wellman et al.	Poole
m	3	3	3.5	r	4	5	7.5
n	3	3	4.5	s	4.5	5	7.5[c]
ng	3	—[a]	4.5	sh	4.5	—[b]	6.5
p	3	4	3.5	ch	4.5	5	—[b]
f	3	3	5.5	t	6	5	4.5
h	3	3	3.5	th	6	—[a]	7.5[c]
w	3	3	3.5	v	6	5	6.5[c]
y	3.5	4	4.5	l	6	4	6.5
k	4	4	4.5	~~th~~	7	—[b]	6.5
b	4	3	3.5	z	7	5	7.5[c]
d	4	5	4.5	zh	7	—[b]	6.5
g	4	4	4.5	j	7	6	—[b]
				hw	—[a]	—[a]	7.5

Source: Templin, 1957.

[a]Sound was tested but was not produced correctly by 75% of the subjects at the oldest age tested. In the Wellman data the "hw" reached the percentage criterion at 5 but not at 6 years, the medial "ng" reached it at 3, and the initial and medial "th" at 5 years.

[b]Poole, in an unpublished study of 20,000 preschool and school-age children reports the following shifts: "s" and "z" appear at 5.5 years, then disappear and return later at 7.5 years or above; "th" appears at 6.5 years and "v" at 5.5 years.

[c]Sound not tested or not reported.

Upon close scrutiny, the results of these studies reveal few answers as to when specific sounds are learned. The [t] sound is stipulated as "acquired" at 4.5 years of age by Poole, 5 years of age by Wellman et al., and 6 years of age by Templin. The [f] sound is given at 3 years of age by Templin and by Wellman et al., but 5.5 years of age by Poole. A 3½-year spread is found for the [r] sound: Templin indicates 4 years of age for acquisition, Poole indicates 7.5 years of age. In all, there is an average range variation for the 24 sounds tested by two or more experimenters of 1.35 years. Given that speech sounds are acquired in the age period from 1.5 to 8 years, the period under study is only 6.5 years long (Templin, 1957, p. 6). Considering this, the variation of 1.35 years represents a 20.8% error for the estimates.

A major reason posited for the variation among the three studies is the different percentage estimates for acquisition. Templin and

Wellman et al. used a 75% group criterion, Poole a 100% criterion. This difference does account for some of the variation. The error between the Templin and Wellman et al. data, which used the same criterion, is 10.1%. Sander (1972), in an attempt to reduce the variability and make the numbers more meaningful, suggested that the 50% level of group

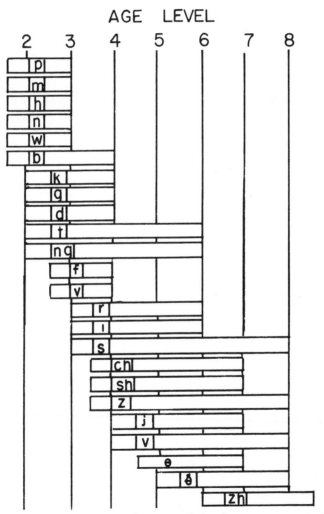

Figure 1.   Average age estimates and upper age limits of customary consonant production. The solid bar corresponding to each sound starts at the median age of customary articulation; it stops at an age level at which 90 percent of all children are customarily producing the sound. (Based on Sander, 1972, p. 62.)

attainment (customary production level) and the 90% level of group attainment be used as range estimates for each sound (see Figure 1). This procedure reduces the importance of the point estimates. However, as will be noted, the 50–90% range estimates create extremely broad standards of measurement with a range of 2.7 years on the average. The shortest range is 1.5 years; the longest range is 5 years. It is generally conceded that certain sound classes are acquired early, [p, m, h, n, w] or [k, g, d], but within the classes little differentiation in terms of age can be made. In reviewing data of this type Leopold (1953) concluded:

> The crushing bulk of data amassed in the thousands of studies from many lands and many fields of scholarship threatened to overwhelm the student who tried to discover great lines of development in child language. It looked as if every child went its own way in mastering the language of its environment. One scholar after another tried to establish a generally valid sequence in the acquisition of sounds, for example. *But no two lists agreed sufficiently to show a consistent line of development* [emphasis mine], ... Cross sections of group observations, often based on the speech of thousands of children of a certain age, did their share in reducing the weight of the less common features and in establishing averages. But even in the results of such studies, the variations within each category remained large. (pp. 1–2)

The lack of a consistent line of development in phonological data still remains a problem. As recently as 1969, Winitz echoed the sentiments of Leopold:

> We know that a child turns over before he sits up, sits up before he crawls, crawls before he walks. Although early motor acts have been established as essential for later motor acts, the developmental sequence is fairly orderly. No comparable sequence of orderly development is apparent for phonemes. (p. 62)

The inability to determine the sequential order of phonemic acquisition has remained a problem for nearly 200 years. The gross estimates of the Templin, Wellman et al., and Poole studies provide important information, but they offer vague parameters for building an explanatory theory of the acquisition process. The keys to such problems of such long-standing periods have often been found among the presumptions of the questions at hand. The question, "When and in what order are phonemes learned?", as well as, "Why are the sounds of speech acquired in a specific order?", may be inappropriate questions. In fact, the "phoneme" or "speech sound" may not even be the basic unit of acquisition.

CHILD LANGUAGE, APHASIA AND PHONOLOGICAL UNIVERSALS

In 1939 a new theory proposed that the basic unit of speech is not the phoneme, but its constituent properties. This shift in emphasis, from the speech sound to its phonetic components, commonly referred to as distinctive feature theory, represented a radical reorientation to the acquisition process. Unfortunately, for many years this theory had little impact in the United States because it was originally published in German. In 1941, the work that pioneered distinctive feature theory, *Kindersprache, Aphasie und allgemeine Lautgesetze,* written by Roman Jakobson, appeared in Germany. It was finally translated into English by Allan Keiler in 1968. *Child Language, Aphasia and Phonological Universals* presented distinctive feature theory to the non-German-speaking public for the first time in its full scope. This one work remains the basic point of departure for modern discussion, research, and theory (Edwards, 1974; Ferguson & Farwell, 1975; Ingram, 1974a, 1974b, 1976a; Menn, 1971, 1975; Moskowitz, 1970; Oller et al., 1976; Olney & Scholnick, 1976; Rūķe-Draviņa, 1976; Stampe, 1969, 1972).

The importance of Jakobson's text, *Child Language, Aphasia and Phonological Universals,* to modern discussion should not be underestimated. This one book shook, and continues to shape, the various fields related to the study of child language. Moskowitz (1970) succinctly summarized current thinking as follows:

> For many decades, those interested in the acquisition of phonology have collected data about the order in which different children acquired phones or phonemes. The comparison of such data has caused despair, as almost no two children acquired such units in the same order, and no patterns could be found.
>
> In 1941 the study of child phonology took a great leap forward as Jakobson's highly significant work integrating the studies of phonology acquisition, sound change, and aphasia switched the emphasis from the units of sound to distinctive features. Although subsequent workers have found that some of Jakobson's proposals concerning the order of acquisition of distinctive features are inaccurate, and others are not explicit enough to be tested, the framework has become available for many of the regularities of phonology acquisition to be discussed. It is interesting and significant that, despite the considerable changes and advances in the theory of distinctive features, and the long-standing knowledge that Jakobson's theory is not completely accurate, no advances in the theory of phonology acquisition have been made. (p. 439)

Many might argue that since the time of Moskowitz's writing, Stampe's theory of natural phonology (1969, 1972) has become an alternative to the Jakobsonian viewpoint (Ingram, 1976a; Oller & Kelly, 1975). However, a careful and detailed examination of natural phonology, undertaken in Chapters 7 and 8, will reveal that Stampe's position is an extension of Halle's theory of distinctive features and markedness. Stampe's viewpoint will be shown to be a counter-hypothesis rather than a counter-theory. Once the Jakobsonian viewpoint is understood in detail, it can be shown that Stampe's "theory" is an extension in the phonotactic component of a much larger theory. Whereas Jakobson has created a macrotheory, Stampe's natural phonology may be seen as a microtheory for language-specific idiosyncratic phenomena. As has been pointed out by Menn (1975):

> The pervasive difficulty that seems to crop up in almost every reference to the Jakobson (1968) schema has arisen here [Commenting on an article by Ingram, 1974a]. Jakobson's examples lead one to believe that he is making much stronger claims than he actually did (see Menn 1973a). His predictions deal only with *phonemic oppositions,* not with *phonetic properties* [emphasis mine], up to the level of interpretation of the distinctive features. (p. 295)

PRELIMINARIES TO SPEECH ANALYSIS

The distinction between phonemic versus phonetic approaches has long been a difficulty for distinctive feature theory. This problem has arisen through a historical accident peculiar to the United States. The fact that *Child Language, Aphasia and Phonological Universals* was not published in English until 1968 facilitated another text, *Preliminaries to Speech Analysis: The Distinctive Features and Their Correlates* (Jakobson, Fant, & Halle, 1952) to be viewed as the major source of distinctive feature theory. Unfortunately, this book was not the theory, nor was it meant to be. The authors point out specifically in their preface that this book was devoted to a heuristic discussion of the acoustic and physiological properties (i.e., phonetic aspects) of the distinctive features. Furthermore, their discussion was to be viewed as tentative at best. They said:

> We regard the present list of distinctive features, particularly their definition on different levels, as a provisional sketch which is open to discussion and which requires experimental verification and further elaboration. (Jakobson, Fant, & Halle, 1952/1967, p. v)

The presentation of the phonetic aspects of the distinctive feature, prior to the presentation of the underlying linguistic assumptions of the theory, set the course for a phonetic rather than a phonemic reception in many circles in the United States.

FUNDAMENTALS OF LANGUAGE

The first discussion of the acquisition theory was presented in 1956, in a monograph Jakobson co-authored with Morris Halle. This work, *Fundamentals of Language,* contains a brief 15-page outline of the theory originally presented in *Kindersprache.* This discussion utilized an expression, "phonemic patterning," which capsulized the theory into an idiom rather than a full explanation. This synopsis served as the basic presentation of the theory for 12 years. By 1968, Jakobson's co-author, Halle, had become a national expert in distinctive feature theory. The precepts underlying the theory were virtually unknown to most American scholars. In the same year that *Child Language, Aphasia and Phonological Universals* appeared in print, Noam Chomsky and Morris Halle, inspired by Jakobson, published *The Sound Patterns of English.* This comprehensive attempt to explain the diachronic evolution of the English phonemic system, at the segmental and suprasegmental levels, overshadowed the newly translated foundation text. The modifications and revisions of the basic theory, introduced by Chomsky and Halle, have gone virtually unnoticed due to a lack of familiarity with the original theory.

PROSPECTUS

This book comprehensively reviews the Jakobsonian approach to distinctive features. It first traces the inception, formulation, and revision of the theory from 1917, when it began, through 1939. At that juncture, the Jakobsonian viewpoint is contrasted to that of Halle, in order to pinpoint the basic theoretical differences between the two approaches. By concentrating on these differences, the reader should be able to distinguish the essential differences between a phonemic versus a phonetic theory.

This presentation of the early history of distinctive feature theory is followed by a detailed discussion of the Jakobsonian acquisition model. Modern-day theories of phonemic and/or phonetic acquisition are then discussed as alternatives or extensions of the basic theory. The works of Ferguson and his colleagues (1973, 1975), Ingram (1974a, 1974b, 1975, 1976a, 1976b), Menn, 1971, 1975), Olmsted (1971), Smith (1973), Stampe (1969, 1972), and Waterson (1971) are reviewed in detail for the development of a formal syncretistic theory of phonological acquisition. After that, one aspect of Jakobsonian phonology is revised because of a possible inherent contradiction, and this revision in turn integrates two diffuse areas of contemporary writing, psychoperceptual research and the current contemporary diary studies of phonological acquisition.

Finally, the voluminous writings pertaining to deviant phonological acquisition are examined in detail. In general, this discussion begins with the most abstract aspects of the theory, its basic assumptions and terminology, and proceeds to a step-by-step analysis of the specific theory. The theory is then revised, and its practical implications are examined primarily for the field of clinical rehabilitation and child development.

THE HISTORY
OF DISTINCTIVE
FEATURE THEORY

chapter 2

Structural Philosophy

THE EPISTEMOLOGICAL PROCESS
THE USE OF MODELS
THE IMPORTANCE OF MODELS
PARSIMONY
THE ORGANIZING PRINCIPLE
THE METAMORPHOSIS FROM ART TO SCIENCE
THE DERIVATION OF THE LATENT STRUCTURE
A BROAD PERSPECTIVE
BASIC ASSUMPTIONS

The origin of distinctive feature theory can be traced to a linguistic philosophy commonly referred to as structuralism (Ferguson & Garnica, 1975, p. 153). Structuralism can be defined as a scientific viewpoint devoted to "discovering and describing as concisely and accurately as possible the interrelationships and patterns which make up the intricate structure of language" (Francis, 1958, p. 26). Each language, the object of study, is viewed as a "coherent, homogeneous entity with inter-relation of pattern and changes" (Pei, 1966, p. 262). The structural linguist, in the process of attempting to discover the latent principles of linguistic growth and differentiation, is constantly formulating hypotheses to explain the specific object of study. The fact that language—the object of study—is ordered, is axiomatic and not subject to proof. The basic question for the structural linguist is to determine *how* language is structured.

THE EPISTEMOLOGICAL PROCESS

The manner in which the structuralist formulates the underlying inter-relationships and patterns of language is reminiscent of Kant's understanding of the epistemological process. Philosophically, *a priori* knowledge, that which is formulated as a hypothetical construct, is viewed as the basic realm of human knowledge and higher thought. This knowledge, which is derived from *a posteriori* knowledge, that which is directly observable from nature, is the constant cultural extension of man. The synthetic interaction between what is presumed to

11

be and what is borne out in reality sets up the basic paradigm for the learning process. Kant (1781/1973) explains this as follows:

> But though all our knowledge begins with experience, it does not follow that it all arises out of experience. For it may well be that even our empirical knowledge is made up of what we receive through impressions and of what our own faculty of knowledge (sensible impressions serving merely as the occasion) supplies from itself. If our faculty of knowledge makes any such addition, it may be that we are not in a position to distinguish it from the raw material, until with long practice of attention we have become skilled in separating it.
>
> This then, is a question which at least calls for closer examination and does not allow any off-hand answer: whether there is any knowledge that is thus independent of experience and even of all impressions of the senses. Such knowledge is entitled *a priori,* and distinguished from the *empirical* which has as its sources *a posteriori,* that is, experience. (pp. 686–687)

A simple dichotomy between conjecture and hidden reality sets up a prototype to be seen over and over in structural linguistic philosophy.

THE USE OF MODELS

The formal presentation of the conjectures of man, whether it be verbal, symbolic, geometric, mathematical, or pictorial, is referred to as modeling. The model is the basic tool of the structuralist. Linguistic study is seen as a form of model building to explain the underlying patterns of organization, growth, and change. Martinet (1970), in his essay on structuralism, summarized the process as follows:

> To sum up, the model is not the structure, for the structure is always in the object, latent as it were but only if latent is not opposed to real. The best that can be expected of a model is that it represent the structure exactly, and it will do so if the scholar has succeeded in correctly disentangling the latencies involved and has not tried to force them into a prefabricated model founded on a set of a priori ideas currently in fashion. (p. 4)

To date, models have been developed for the structure of language and its various subcomponent sciences. The subsciences of phonology, morphology, lexicology, and syntax have formal models of varying degrees of sophistication. Furthermore, the various objects of study—the phoneme, the morpheme, the lexeme, and the syntactic structure rule—have now received extensive hypothetical discussion. The model, in and of itself, may be as restricted as a verbal hypothesis concerning an object of study, or as intricate as a theory of organization of these elements. This potential variation in the size of the model is only restricted by the goals of the constructor.

THE IMPORTANCE OF MODELS

Chapanis (1963) pointed out that the use of models has many advantages, as well as dangers. From a positive viewpoint models help us to:

1. Understand complex systems or events
2. Learn complex skills
3. Provide a framework for experimentation
4. See new relationships
5. Predict when experimentation is impossible

On the other hand, models are too often not validated and may divert useful energy into nonproductive activity. Because models may explain only a small part of the behavior, the theoretician should be on guard against overgeneralization and should constantly remember the possibility that the elements of the model may not be all-inclusive or ideally arranged. With this in mind, the model builder works for a specific goal—practicality. In general, the more intricate the model, the more difficult it is to use.

By implication, the goals of a good model should tend to simplify the behavior at hand. The reduction of the complexity of systems, events, and skills points toward the value of parsimony.

PARSIMONY

As M. Marx (1963) has pointed out, when two possible models are available to explain a particular phenomena, the simpler explanation will prevail:

> This [the problem of testing models] is the role of the law of parsimony, sometimes called William of Occam's razor (in animal psychology, Lloyd Morgan's cannon). Essentially, this says that the simplest of alternative explanatory propositions should be accepted. (p. 20)

Basing his position on that of Conant (1947), Marx (1963) pointed out that theories are not displaced by contradictory fact but only by simpler theories. He notes, "The necessity of parsimony must be impressed particularly on all those who mourn the destruction of the 'beautiful theory' by the 'ugly fact'." (Marx, 1963, p. 21)

THE ORGANIZING PRINCIPLE

Returning to Marx's proposition concerning the advantages of models, we may note a strong emphasis on the organizational goal. The creation of a framework to see new relationships for experimentation has long been the work of scientific method. Francis (1958), in his text, *The Structure of American English,* develops in detail the idea that linguistics is truly a science. As we will see in the next few pages, he notes that a science is marked by a five-step process:

> 1. A science directs its attention to a coherent body of facts, entities or events which can be separated from the rest of the universe by consistent and clearly statable definitions. This is its *subject matter.* (p. 15)

Structural linguistic scientists have directed their attention to subject matter as broad as language, as narrow as phonotactics, or as finite as the [r] sound. The models created to deal with these various areas have been as complex as the generative-transformational frame of Chomsky (1965) in the area of grammar, or as simple as the International Phonetic Association (IPA) alphabet in the area of phonetics.

The second step in the formulation of a science is devoted to the reliability component. Once the limits of the science are defined, the labels, or tools of thought, must be shown to be recognizable to the public at large. As Francis (1958) points out:

> 2. A science directs upon its subject matter a close and unprejudiced scrutiny and attempts to record the results of the scrutiny in such a manner that they can be verified by any competent observer. It produces, in short, *careful objective descriptions.* (p. 15)

Child phonologists have had to rely on trained transcription skills to meet the verifiability criterion when dealing with their subject matter. The quality of the observations is directly related to the quality of the phonetic training. Lynip (1951), for instance, insists that the study of speech utterances in young children must be "devoid of the fallibility of the human ear" and "analyzed in an objective manner" (p. 227). This suggestion is, of course, ideal. The major tool of objective measurement in the area of phonetics is the sound spectrograph. However, the information derived from this instrument is still under active investigation (Fant, 1961, 1968, 1973). As Winitz (1969) points out, the interpretations from the sonogram are just as susceptible to error as the interpretations of the acoustic signal from the transcription process. The nuances of the sound spectrograph have only been under study for three decades. Martin Joos was the first linguist to study this area in depth. In his monograph, "Acoustic phonetics" (Joos, 1948), he writes:

> The author of this book had no part in the development of the key instrument—the acoustic spectrograph—but accidentally became the first linguist permitted to use it extensively, beginning over two years before

the public disclosure of November 9, 1945 (in *Science, Life, Time,* and other publications). (p. 5)

The classified nature of the instrument and the subsequent research is well known. Thus, the suppression of Jakobson's *Kindersprache* was not the only historical factor in the development of distinctive feature theory. World War II repeatedly affected the basic sequence of events as child phonology was transformed from a descriptive art to an explanatory science.

THE METAMORPHOSIS FROM ART TO SCIENCE

The difference between a rock collector and a chemist is, in one sense, a drastic one. In another sense, the difference is small. A rock collector assembles the various objects of the earth's crust and applies labels. The reason for inclusion is aesthetic appeal: this or that rock is desirable. The chemist works with the same subject matter, the earth's crust, but *orders* the elements in certain ways. The use of specific gravity or crystal shape indicates a higher order perspective of the task at hand. This ordering is a key component of the scientific method. As Francis (1958) goes on to state:

> 3. A science further attempts to put together the results of its descriptions in such a way that they form orderly and systematic patterns which display the relationships that exist within its subject matter. In brief it *makes generalizations*. (p. 15)

The orderly arrangement of the subject matter constitutes the creation of the formal model. The types of arrangements in child phonology are few. The objects of study, the sounds of speech, have been classified for the purposes of identification. This was done in hope of developing a sequence of acquisition, among other things. The manner, place, and voicing format of the IPA is just one example. This chart, as well as the distinctive feature matrix, shares much in common with the table of periodic elements in chemistry. Each model identifies the subject matter at hand. Each model orders the elements according to a certain strategy. Each arrangement has as its goal an orderly display of the relationships in order to make predictions. Thus we have Francis' (1958) fourth criterion of a science:

> 4. A science tests its generalizations by applying them to parts of its subject matter not used in forming the generalizations. In other words, it *makes predictions*. (p. 15)

In structural linguistics this modeling process is an ongoing activity because of the relative newness of the science.

THE DERIVATION OF THE LATENT STRUCTURE

The experimental process is the major way in which models are accepted or rejected. The hypothetical construct of the latent underlying patterns of the subject matter must be validated. Constructs that are so vague or so complex as to defy testing should be avoided. If no potential exists to test the idea, either directly or indirectly, the theory is subject to question. In modern times, phonology is being challenged to maintain a scientific rigor in its explanations and models. Akhmanova (1971) notes that:

> It is deplorable that linguistics (the scientific study of natural human languages) should have so often been confounded with "... intellectual pastimes consisting of elegant rearrangement of symbols" [quoting Fant]. Unless the two are kept strictly apart much harm will be done (has already been done in fact) to linguistic research in general and the training of phonologists, in particular. When there is no 'feedback' between the particular kind of speculation and the intricate realities of linguistics, all the 'pastimes' can do is give aesthetic satisfaction (provided, of course, the Scientific Hedonist succeeds in discovering the 'most elegant' rules for the description and grouping together of the imaginary entities he is playing with). (p. 13)

This position is, of course, strongly worded. It may be an overstatement of the case at hand. But it does crystalize a sentiment of dissatisfaction that is held by many people today.

Chapanis (1963) has warned that models tend to encourage overgeneralization and logical fallacies. But most important, he points out that models too often are not validated:

> Another serious criticism which can be leveled against many models is that they cannot be validated, or, if attempts are made to validate them, the procedures used are scientifically valueless. This is not so much a criticism of the models themselves but the model builders. I am sometimes frankly appalled by the faith which some model builders have in their powers of analytical and synthetic reasoning when it comes to making models of human behavior. (p. 126)

If it seems that the structural viewpoint is fraught with such dangers, it should be remembered that there are adequate safeguards. In general, the safeguards are of two types, formative and concurrent. First, the model or theory should be extensively founded in the current facts at hand. In other words, the model must be founded on data. Second, the model or theory must be constantly under test until the predictive power of its tentative hypotheses are confirmed. In other words, there must be experimental validation of any theory. Without this twofold effort, structural theories will not be transformed into scientific systems. As Francis (1958) notes:

> 5. Finally, a science examines the outcomes of its predictions and in the light of their success or failure corroborates or revises its generalizations. If the corroboration is satisfactory, it may call its generalizations *laws,* which are simply statements of predictable behavior. (p. 15)

The ultimate goal of the structural linguist is to discover the basic laws of language. By a concerted effort to design and revise the explanatory models of linguistic behavior, the theoretician transforms hypothetical conjecture into well-formed and consistent systems of explanation. In all, we are dealing with a five step process:

1. Defining the area of study
2. Learning to label the objects of study   ← Model level 1
3. Learning to arrange the objects of study ← Model level 2
4. Making predictions   ← Model level 3
5. Establishing laws   *Latent structure*

The evolution from a descriptive science that labels its subject matter to a predictive science that organizes data is a key element in the transition from an art to a science. An interesting aside is that good Art may be, conversely, the application of these very same principles.

A BROAD PERSPECTIVE

The analogy between the principles of the deductive scientific method and the use of models in structural linguistics is too strong to ignore. The structural point of view is really, as in the time of Francis Bacon, just the scientific method in operation. In the words of DeGeorge and DeGeorge (1972):

> 'Structuralism' is a term used to reflect a variety of different types of endeavors, all more or less, interrelated. It cuts across traditional disciplinary boundaries, and bibliographies on structuralism can be virtually endless if one succumbs to the temptation to include everything related to the topic.... Both the term 'structure' and many basic ideas behind structuralism are not new to Western intellectual thought. Marx, Freud, and Saussure are clearly precursors of present day structuralism. (p. vi).

If, then, structuralism is so broad a topic and so abstract an area as to be an epistemological perspective, what implications are there for the student of distinctive feature theory at the outset? The following basic assumptions should be readily apparent.

BASIC ASSUMPTIONS

Axiomatic Assumption (A)

The phenomena of the world have a latent structure.

Corollaries A-1: The *language system* has a latent structure.
A-2: The *phoneme* has a latent structure.
A-3: The *phonemic system* has a latent structure.
A-4: The *development* of the phonemic system has a latent structure.

Axiomatic Assumption (B)

The latent structure of the world can be modeled.

Corollaries B-1: The *phoneme* can be modeled.
B-2: The *phonemic system* can be modeled.
B-3: The *development* of the phonemic system can be modeled.

Axiomatic Assumption (C)

The model of the world must eventually match the latent structure of the world.

Corollaries C-1: The model of the *phoneme* must eventually match the latent structure of the phoneme.
C-2: The model of the *phonemic system* must eventually match the latent structure of the phonemic system.
C-3: The model of the *development* of the phonemic system must eventually match the latent structure of the acquisition process.

The constant revision of the model is really the application of scientific method. The use of models, therefore, simply constitutes the commitment to apply the scientific approach to the phonemic system and its subsequent development in the mind of the child.

chapter 3

The Phoneme

Scholars generally agree that the philosophical movement referred to as structural linguistics began between 1920 and 1935, depending upon the place of reference (Blache, 1970, p. 8). Fischer-Jørgensen (1956) has isolated four centers of growth for the structural analysis of language, three European and one American. She states, "If one goes by printed evidence, the beginning for Prague was 1928, for London, 1929, for the United States, 1921 (Sapir) or perhaps 1933 (Bloomfield) and for Copenhagen, 1935" (Fischer-Jørgensen, 1956, p. 140). In reference to phonology, the topic at hand, Malmberg (1963) synthesizes these centers into two broad linguistic movements:

> Taken in this sense, phonology was founded at Prague about thirty-five years ago [1928] by a group of linguists (Trubetzkoy, Jakobson, and others) whence the name *Prague School*. A similar development took place in the United States (Sapir, Bloomfield, etc.), perhaps independently of the European movement. (p. 97)

For ease of presentation, the grouping of Malmberg will be used as a broad outline for the exposition of the basic philosophical ideas underlying the conceptualization of distinctive features. The European and American approaches to distinctive features, although they share much in common, do differ significantly on many basic points. Proponents of distinctive feature theory are often grouped into one class, but a full understanding of the basic assumptions of both philosophical schools will reveal that they are dealing with two totally different subject matters (Menn, 1975, p. 295).

THE EUROPEAN MOVEMENT: THE PRAGUE SCHOOL

One of the central figures in the development and growth of the structural linguistic movement in Europe was Roman Jakobson. Jakobson helped found the European structural point of view, generally referred to as the Prague School. In the 50-year period from 1912 to 1962, he wrote and published in excess of 287 articles which revised and redefined the basic tenets of the Prague School. It is from this school of thought that the distinctive feature concept arose, evolved, and gained its initial logical formulation.

ROMAN JAKOBSON

The Early Years: 1912–1927

The methodology by which speech is analyzed by distinctive features was an outgrowth of the interest in the definition of the phoneme and poetic analysis. As a freshman linguistic student, in 1912, Jakobson submitted a reading list to his teacher, D. N. Ušakov. One article, a monograph on Russian vowels by L. V. Ščerba, caught the teacher's eye. Ušakov insisted that Jakobson have nothing to do with the article and had him remove it from the list. This, of course, just whetted the appetite of a young student (Jakobson, 1962, p. 637).

Defining the Phoneme (A)

It is Lepschy (1970) who fills in the details of the significance of this interaction. Jakobson was a student of Ušakov at the University of Moscow. The Moscow School, that of Ušakov, and the Leningrad School, that of Ščerba, differed in their approaches to the phoneme. Whereas the former program ascribed to a traditional orientation, the latter championed a psycholinguistic philosophy. It was the approach of the Leningrad School that first influenced Jakobson.

Ščerba (1912/1970) defined the phoneme as follows:

> a phoneme is "the *shortest* general *sound image* of a *given language*
>   [1]   [4]   [6]
> which can be associated with *meaning images*, and can *differentiate*
>   [5]   [2]
> *words*" (cited in Lepschy, 1970, p. 62; italics and numerals mine)

This definition was an extensive refinement of a related definition that had appeared 31 years earlier. In 1881, J. Baudouin de Courtenay, Ščerba's predecessor in the chair of linguistics at the University of Leningrad, in *Versuch einer Theorie phonetischer Alternationen* had defined the phoneme as:

a *unitary* image, *belonging to the phonetic world,* which *originates in the*
  [1]   [6]   [5]
soul by means of psychic fusion of the impressions *preserved through the*
                                                                    [3]
pronunciation of the same sound (cited in Lepschy, 1970, p. 60; italics and

numerals mine)

A close examination of these two definitions reveals the six basic properties of the phoneme. The phoneme is the:

1. shortest, unitary image   (Ščerba, Baudouin)
2. which can differentiate words,   (Ščerba)
3. having a physiological component   (Baudouin)
4. and an acoustic component   (Ščerba)
5. which are psychologically perceived   (Ščerba, Baudouin)
6. and are culturally defined.   (Ščerba, Baudouin)

Both Ščerba and Baudouin de Courtenay emphasize that the phoneme
is the most basic element of the speech signal. Furthermore, both
authors stress the psychological aspects of the phoneme. Whereas
Baudouin de Courtenay emphasizes the importance of the physiological component, Ščerba emphasizes the acoustic or auditory component. Ščerba specifies the function of the phoneme: it differentiates
words. The emphasis on this one aspect on the part of Jakobson, in
later years, causes him to be labeled a structural-functionalist
(Lepschy, 1970, p. 92). In reviewing these six requirements and comparing them to later Jakobsonian thought, it is apparent that he does
not reject either definition. He absorbs both men's points of view.

The Eclectic Tendency

The key to understanding Jakobson's model-building strategy begins
with an appreciation that he discards little and works at a highly
abstract and integrative level. This ability to select and organize various viewpoints into a consistent theory, the eclectic approach, is the
basic strength of the Jakobsonian position. Commenting on the anti-
nomy between those who hold that a phoneme is totally psychological,
the "inner" approach, as opposed to those who feel that the phoneme
exists as an exterior acoustic entity, the "outer" approach, he notes:

> The search for the ultimate discrete differential constituents of language
> can be traced back to *sphota*-doctrine of the Sanskrit grammarians and to
> Plato's conception of στοιχεῖον, but the actual linguistic study of these
> invariants started only in the 1870's and developed intensively after World
> War I, side by side with the gradual expansion of the principle of invar-

iance in science.... The subsequent theoretical and practical achieve-
ments in the structural analysis of language required even more adequate
and consistent incorporation of speech sounds into the fields of linguistics
with its stringent methodology; the principles and techniques of phonology improve and its scope becomes even wider. (Jakobson & Halle,
1956a, pp. 7–8)

Jakobson criticizes the "mentalistic" position of Baudouin de Courtenay as being too extreme: "In the oldest of these approaches going
back to Baudouin de Courtenay, and still surviving, the phoneme is a
sound imagined or intended, opposed to the emitted sounds as a
'psychophonetic' phenomena to the 'physiophonetic' fact. It is the
mental equivalent of an exteriorized sound" (Jakobson & Halle, 1956a,
p. 11). Only by tempering Baudouin de Courtenay's position with that
of Ščerba's insistence on the importance of the acoustic component,
the cultural influence, and the differential function, is the equation
balanced.

The Differential Component

The emphasis on the importance of the phoneme as a differential unit is
the most important concept in the Jakobsonian position. He repeats,
over and over again, this basic idea:

> La théorie phonologique, fidèle aux suggestions de F. de Saussure, a
> toujours insisté sur le fait que ce n'est pas le phonème, mais *l'opposition*,
> et par conséquent la *qualité différentielle*, qui est l'élément du système
> ["Phonological theory, faithful to the suggestions of F. de Saussure, has
> always insisted on the fact that it is not the phoneme, but the *opposition*,
> and consequently the *differential property*, which is the primary element
> of the system"]. (Jakobson, 1939b/1962, p. 279)

Or again:

> A phoneme, as Sapir remarked, 'has no singleness of reference.' All
> phonemes denote nothing but mere otherness. The lack of individual de-
> notation sets apart the distinctive features, and their combinations into
> phonemes, from all other linguistic units. (Jakobson & Halle, 1956a, p. 11)

Both *Preliminaries to Speech Analysis* (Jakobson, Fant, & Halle,
1952/1967) and *Fundamentals of Language* (Jakobson & Halle, 1956a)
begin with an extensive discussion of the importance of the *minimal
pair*. A minimal pair is two words that differ by only one phonemic
contrast. Both words are totally identical except for one phoneme in
one position. (This definition will later be revised and narrowed.) For
example:

[pi]	pea		[eɪp]	ape
↕			↕	
[bi]	bee		[eɪb]	Abe

[pɪt]	pit		[tæp]	tap
↕			↕	
[bɪt]	bit		[tæb]	tab

[pɛst]	pest		[kræp]	crap
↕			↕	
[bɛst]	best		[kræb]	crab

The Physiological and Acoustic Components

Not only does Jakobson follow the integrated assumptions of Ščerba and Baudouin de Courtenay for the differential criterion, he consistently maintains the importance of both the physiological aspects and the acoustical aspects of the phoneme. Neither component is missing from his conceptualization:

> Phonemic entities draw on the gross sound matter but readjust this extrinsic stuff dissecting and classifying it along its own lines. Above all, the procedure is one of selection. Among a multitude of *acoustico-motor* possibilities [emphasis mine], there is a restricted number upon which language chooses to set a value. (Jakobson, 1949/1962, p. 423)

Sound properties or features are always defined acoustically and physiologically. In *Preliminaries to Speech Analysis,* each property is defined as "stimulus" (acoustic) and "production" (physiological). In *Fundamentals of Language,* and its subsequent numerous revisions, we find the same balance. Each property is discussed "acoustically" and "genetically." The latter term is used, of course, to mean origin or genesis, as of the acoustic product. It is incorrect to assume that a distinctive feature or sound property is merely an acoustic definition. An emphasis on the importance of the acoustic component is readily observable:

> And since not the motor act but the acoustical aspect of speech sounds, aimed at by the speaker, has a social value, the teleological conception of sound problems increases the relevance of the acoustical analysis in comparison with the physiology of speech. (Jakobson, 1928a/1962, p. 2)

However, the tendency to work with acoustic labels should not tend to obscure the importance of the articulatory or physiological component of the phoneme. Sometimes the choice of labels for specific sound properties is a matter of tutorial convenience rather than bias:

> In so far as the feature we define has a traditional term, we use the latter regardless of the stage of the speech event to which it relates.... A traditional articulatory term is retained as long as it points to an important criterion of division with respect to the sound transmitted, perceived, and decoded. In several cases, however, there is no current phonetic term to cover the feature we define. For such features we take over terms from physical acoustics or psycho-acoustics. But since each of these features is definable and has actually been defined *both* on the *acoustic* and on the *motor level* [emphasis mine], any of them could with equal right bear a newly coined articulatory designation.... We are not concerned with substituting an acoustic classification for an articulatory one but solely in uncovering the most productive criteria of division valid for both aspects. (Jakobson & Halle, 1956a, p. 36)

The Psychological and Cultural Components

Just as Jakobson retains the acoustic and motor components in the definition of the phoneme, he balances the importance of the individual and the society. The psychological perception of the individual, the "nature" component, is integrated with the cultural data that nurture man. The nature/nurture dichotomy is avoided by retaining both aspects in the phonemic frame:

> Where nature presents nothing but an indefinite number of contingent varieties, the intervention of culture extracts pairs of opposite terms. The gross sound matter knows no oppositions. It is human thought, conscious or unconscious, which draws from this sound matter the binary oppositions for their phonemic use (Jakobson, 1949/1962, p. 423)

Summary

The overall influence of the writings of the Leningrad School must be distilled and incorporated into any explanation of distinctive feature theory. Because these influences are assumptions, they must be treated axiomatically. For convenience, a sequential code is used, but this is not to imply a hierarchy. The distillation below is merely a listing.

BASIC ASSUMPTIONS

Axiomatic Assumption (D)
The phoneme is the *smallest unit* of the speech chain. (To be revised.)

Axiomatic Assumption (E)
The phoneme has a *differential* function.

Axiomatic Assumption (F)
The phoneme has a *physiological* component.

Axiomatic Assumption (G)
The phoneme has an *acoustic* component.

Axiomatic Assumption (H)
The phoneme has a *psychological* component.

Axiomatic Assumption (I)
The phoneme is *culturally defined.*

These six assumptions are, of course, ways of defining the latent structure of the phoneme initially presented in axiomatic assumption A, corollary A-1 ("The language system has a latent structure"). By implication each aspect described above—1) segmentation, 2) differential function, 3) physiological component, 4) acoustical component, 5) psychological component, and 6) cultural component—can be modeled. In fact, if one ascribes to a Jakobsonian position it would seem essential that each of these six aspects be included in any explanation of the theory at hand.

chapter 4

The Structure
of Language

THE RETURN OF KARCEVSKIJ
FERDINAND DE SAUSSURE
  The Saussurian Phoneme
  The Two Levels of Language
  Semiology
THE IMPORTANCE OF THE SYSTEM
SUMMARY
BASIC SAUSSURIAN ASSUMPTIONS

THE RETURN OF KARCEVSKIJ

Whereas a forbidden monograph introduced a young student of linguistics to the discussion of the phoneme, a second seemingly insignificant event opened the topic to its widest realm, language. The event, the return of Karcevskij, is reported by Jakobson in his biographical sketch "Retrospect" (Jakobson, 1962). He tells the story this way:

> When, as a freshman, I asked my teacher, D. N. Ušakov, to go over my reading list in linguistics, he approved all the many titles except the 1912 monograph on Russian vowels by L. V. Ščerba, a work which grew from the quest of Baudouin de Courtenay and followed a trend quite alien to the orthodox disciples of the Moscow linguistic school. Naturally it was just this forbidden book which I read first, and I was captivated at once by its challenging introductory glosses to the concept of the phoneme. Somewhat later, in 1917, S. J. Karcevskij returned to Moscow after years of study in Geneva and acquainted us with the essentials of the Saussurian doctrine. (Jakobson, 1962, p. 631)

As the ideas of Ščerba and Baudouin de Courtenay became a reference for phonological concepts, the ideas of Ferdinand de Saussure (the Geneva School), introduced to Jakobson by his friend Karcevskij, became canonical in the area of language. Saussurian doctrine was to become a reference point for all aspects of language; its structure, its history, and its changes.

The use of Saussure as a reference should not be underestimated. Beginning in 1927 and continuing to the present, Jakobson's works are replete with references to Saussure.[1] These references are not casual citations. Most references are strongly worded and respectful in character. For example:

> La thèse de F. de Saussure definessant ["Saussure's position states"] ... (1928b/1962, p. 4)
> La doctrine de F. de Saussure contamine ["Saussurian doctrine contaminated by"] ... (ibid., p. 5)
> F. de Saussure and his school broke a new trail ... (1928a/1962, p. I)
> The first foundations of phonology were laid by Baudouin de Courtenay, F. de Saussure, and their disciples. (1932/1962, p. 232)
> Le grand révélateur des antinomies linguistiques, Ferdinand de Saussure, a fait valoir ["The great discovery of linguistic oppositions which Ferdinand de Saussure strongly emphasized"] ... (1938/1962, p. 237)
> On ne pourrait mieux définer la thèse fondamentale de la phonologie qu'en citant la formule classique de Ferd. de Saussure ["One will not be able to define in a better fashion the fundamental theory of phonology than that of the classical formula of Ferd. de Saussure"] ... (1939b/1962, p. 272)
> La théorie phonologique, fidèle aux suggestions de F. de Saussure, a toujours insisté sur le fait ["Phonological theory, faithful to the suggestions of F. de Saussure, has always insisted on the fact" ...](ibid., p. 279)
> Overcoming the one-track mind of the neogrammarian bias, F. de Saussure pointed out ... (1949/1962, p. 419)
> Ferdinand de Saussure pointed out its fundamental role ... (1951/1962, p. 442)
> Ferdinand de Saussure realized half a century ago ... (1964, p. 22)

As can be seen, the precepts of Saussure are in most instances considered "cardinal" (1949/1962, p. 421; 1973, p. 18). In *Kindersprache,* Jakobson does not even mention Saussure by name; he simply refers to him as "the great Genevan scholar" (1941/1968, p. 16) and assumes the reader is aware of the referent. Evidence is obtained from "rereading the *Cours* of Ferdinand de Saussure, the man..." (1958/1962, p. 525).

In 1973, Jakobson succinctly stated his assessment of Saussure in the *Main Trends in the Science of Language:*

> The late nineteenth and very early twentieth centuries were marked by a continuous upsurge of comparative historical studies. At the same time, however, tentative writings of lone seekers in different countries reveal the first precursory inklings of a prospective, structural approach to languages. These anticipations and efforts culminate in Ferdinand de Saus-

---

[1]Jakobson, 1928a/1962, p. 2; 1928b/1962, pp. 4, 5; 1929/1962, p. 7; 1932/1962, p. 232; 1937/1962, p. 267; 1938/1962, pp. 237, 239; 1939a/1962, p. 312; 1939b/1962, pp. 272, 279; 1941/1968, pp. 16, 25; 1949/1962, pp. 418, 419, 421; 1951/1962, p. 442(2); 1958/1962, pp. 525, 529; 1962, pp. 631, 636, 637, 656; 1964, p. 22; 1972, p. 73; 1973, pp. 18, 19, 20, 21, 22, 28(2).

sure's *Cours de Linguistique generale* [*"Course in General Linguistics"*: see Saussure, 1915/1966)], a posthumous edition of 1916 arranged by Ch. Bally and A. Sechehaye on the basis of students' records. The five subsequent decades have witnessed an unprecedented, strenuous rise and capital revision of the linguistic science, and the clearest way to point out the essential innovation will be to confront them with the Saussurian doctrine, which has been viewed as the start of a new era in the science of language. (Jakobson, 1973, p. 18)

Because Saussure's position is so central to Jakobson's theory of distinctive features, certain points should be reviewed.

FERDINAND DE SAUSSURE

Jakobson's strong support for Saussure can be traced to three sources. First, Saussure's concept of the phoneme totally complemented the position of the Leningrad School. Second, Saussure's view of language permitted the integration of phonology into a larger philosophical and abstract science, semiology. Third, and most important, Saussure stressed the importance of the "system" over the "constituent element." Each of these aspects of Saussure's philosophy appealed to Jakobson and found ready acceptance in his eclectic frame. At a subtle level, Saussure tended to think in terms of dichotomies in all aspects of phonology and language. As we will see, in the hands of Jakobson this tendency to frame discussions into bipolar attributes will generate the basic distinctive feature conceptual model.

The Saussurian Phoneme

Saussure strongly maintains that a phoneme has an acoustic as well as a motoric aspect. This position, the syncretistic position for Ščerba and Baudouin de Courtenay, complemented the original leanings of Jakobson in 1912:

> Articulated syllables are acoustical impressions perceived by the ear, but the sounds would not exist without the vocal organs; ... We simply cannot reduce language to sound or detach sound from oral articulation; reciprocally, we cannot define the movements of the vocal organs without taking into account the acoustic impression. (Saussure, 1915/1966, p. 8)

> Many phonologists limit themselves almost exclusively to the phonational act, i.e., the production of sound by the vocal organs (larynx, mouth, etc.) and neglect the auditory side. Their method is wrong. Not only does the auditory impression come to us just as directly as the image of the moving vocal organs, but it is also the basis of any theory. (Saussure, ibid., p. 38)

Not only is Saussure's position compatible with the Leningrad School's concept of the phoneme, the motoric aspect and the acoustic aspect, it incorporates the psychological component as a hierarchal axiom:

> But suppose the sound were a simple thing: would it constitute speech?
> No, it is only the instrument of thought; by itself, it has no existence. At
> this point a new and redoubtable relationship arises: a sound, a complex
> acoustical-vocal unit, combines in turn with an idea to form a complex
> *physiological-psychological unit* [emphasis mine]. (Saussure, ibid., p. 8)

Furthermore, Saussure not only embedded the motoric/acoustic aspects of the phoneme into the perceptual aspect, he, in turn, placed the process into its cultural context. This is Saussure's second major hierarchal axiom:

> But that [the physiological-psychological unit] is not the complete picture.
>   Speech has both an individual and a social side, and we can not
> conceive of one without the other. (Saussure, ibid., p. 8)

These three bipolar aspects of the phoneme—the motoric/acoustic dichotomy, the phonetic/phonemic dichotomy, and the psychological/ sociological dichotomy—not only complemented Jakobson's earlier thought, it tended to organize it along certain lines:

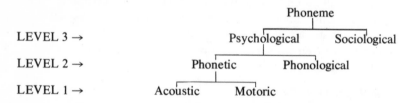

This three-ranked bifidity tends to be transformed into an oppositional frame. The psychological process involved at the psychocultural level of operation (level 3) is clearly specified as differential in nature. Lexical differentiation is seen as the basic function of phonemes.

> Every language forms its words on the basis of a system of sonorous
> elements, each element being a clearly delimited unit and one of a fixed
> number of units. Phonemes are characterized not, as one might think, by
> their own positive quality but simply by the fact that they are *distinct*.
> Phonemes are above all else *opposing, relative,* and *negative* entities
> [emphasis mine]. (Saussure, ibid., p. 119)

The motoric, acoustic, differential, psychological, and cultural aspects of the phoneme, as stipulated by the Leningrad School, were identical to the concepts of the Geneva School. Phonology as a separate area of study, however, gained most in Saussurian doctrine when it was welded to the latent structure of language with the development of a broad frame for communication. The structural linguistic discussions of the phoneme tended toward a binary solution, but the discussion of language produced the greatest dichotomy of all.

The Two Levels of Language

From its most abstract perspective the leader of the Geneva School separated language into two levels, *langue* and *parole*. Authors at times have tried to specify exactly what was intended by each term. But because only the unsigned notes of Saussure's students remain as evidence, scientific precision is not possible (Lepschy, 1970, p. 43). Fortunately, enough of Saussure's theory is intact to posit, at least, a partial explanation.

In several of his lectures, Saussure (1915/1966, pp. 22, 88–89, 110) was fond of making direct analogies between language and a game of chess. This is one of Saussure's explanatory models. (An explanatory model, as opposed to a theoretical model, is created for the purpose of heuristics or discussion rather than prediction.) Whereas, the position of the pieces and their material composition are concrete and observable, the "game" itself—the underlying rules—are abstract and more binding. The number of chessmen and the way in which they are moved, the conventions agreed upon, tend to be immutable.

Saussure saw language much as a game of chess. Each social function has an abstract conceptual level (*langue*) and a concrete tangible level (*parole*):

> Language is a system that has its own arrangement. Comparison with chess will bring out the point. In chess, what is external can be separated relatively easily from what is internal. The fact that the game has passed from Persia to Europe is external; against that, everything having to do with its system and rules is internal. If I use ivory chessmen instead of wooden ones the change has no effect on the system; but if I decrease or increase the number of chessmen, this change has a profound effect on the "grammar" of the game. (Saussure, ibid., pp. 22–23)

Semiology

The internal abstract aspect of language and the external concrete aspect of language are bonded together in one basic concept, the *linguistic sign*. The linguistic sign, most often discussed at the lexical or word level, in Jakobson's eyes, is the most significant contribution of Saussure (Jakobson, 1962, p. 631; 1964, p. 22; 1973, p. 19). Maintaining the intrinsic duality of the sign, Saussure postulated, according to Bally and Sechehaye (1966), that the sign was a two-sided psychological entity.[2] The idea is depicted as follows:

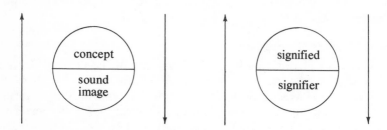

By inference, the reference was "that which was *signified*"; the sound image was "the *signifier*." It is this dichotomy that seemed so important to Jakobson in 1917:

> It was in those years, too, that students of psychology and linguistics in our university were passionately discussing the philosophers' newest attempts toward a phenomenology of language and of signs in general. We learned to sense the delicate distinction between the *signatum* (the signified) and the *denotatum* (the referred-to), hence to assign an intrinsically linguistic position, first to the *signatum* and then, by inference, to its inalienable counterpart as well—that is, to the *signans*. The necessity of establishing phonology as a new, strictly intralinguistic discipline, became ever more apparent. (Jakobson, 1962, p. 631)

According to Saussure, language was a series of ideas (signified) which were to be expressed by means of signs (signifiers). He postulated that, from a philosopher's viewpoint, a science should be developed to study the life signs of the community. Furthermore, he felt that linguistics was a part of the science of signs:

> Language is a system of signs that express ideas, and is therefore comparable to a system of writing, the alphabet of deaf mutes, symbolic rites, polite formulas, military signals, etc. But it is most important of all these systems.
>
> A *science that studies the life signs within society* is conceivable; it would be part of social psychology and consequently of general psychology; I shall call it *semiology* (from Greek *sēmeîon*, 'sign'). Semiology would show what constitutes signs, what laws govern them. Since the science does not yet exist, no one can say what it should be; but it has a right to existence, a place staked out in advance. Linguistics is only a part of the general science of semiology; the laws discovered by semiology will

---

[2]There is a controversy as to the subtleties of Saussure's position on the realm of *langue* and *parole*. See Jakobson (1962, p. 637) and Bally and Sechehaye (1966, pp. 66–67). For our purposes here, Jakobson's assumption of what Saussure intended is more important than the specifics of the case at hand.

be applicable to linguistics, and the latter will circumscribe a well defined area within the mass of anthropological fact. (Saussure, 1915/1966, p. 16)

By implication this viewpoint established the first formal statement of a world divided into a latent structure (communicative intent) and a specific model (the various life signs of the community). To illustrate this effect one need only view the intriguing interplay between equivalent sign systems and one specific idea. For instance, if one wants to transmit the idea of a small furry animal that meows and has a long tail (the signified), there are a multitude of community signs for communication. From our modern perspective, we may group signs into three basic categories: the written sign, the spoken sign, and the gestural sign. Examples of some of the numerous ways of transmitting the word for the above concept are:

Written signs:

Orthographic:	CAT	Block printing system
	cat	Cursive writing system
Pictographic:	🐱	Artistic representation
	貓	Symbolic representation (Mandarin Chinese)[3]

Spoken signs:

Pronunciation:	[kæt]	Phonetic speech production system
	[si⁺eɪ⁺ti]	Oral spelling system

Spoken signs:
Pronunciation: [kæt]   Phonetic speech production system
            [si$^+$eɪ$^+$ti]   Oral spelling system

Gestural signs:

Action:	*Imitate the actions of a cat to create impression.*	Mime
	Imitate pulling of whiskers on your face with thumb and index finger.	Signs of the Deaf[4]
	With right thumb and index finger touching nose, tilt same slightly upward indicating the size of the animal [Meaning: Flat nosed animal].	Signs of the Plains Indians[5]

Each of these potential signs or sign systems are sciences in and of themselves. No attempt has been made to be exhaustive. Specialists teach skills in each of the areas. From a productive viewpoint, the public school teacher works with the block printing system; the penmanship teacher, the cursive system; the art teacher, the pictographic representation. The speech teacher or rhetorician works with phonetic

---

[3]Wang (1973, p. 58).

[4]WSSD (1972, p. 140).

[5]Tomkins (1969, p. 19).

production; the grade school teacher works on spelling. Mime is the province of the drama coach or teacher of theater. The teacher of the deaf has his or her own signs to teach. The anthropologist or Boy Scout leader may use the signs of the Indians. In a receptive mode, as opposed to the previous productive specialties, the student of signs can see other specialists being called into play. The receptive decoding of block printing is taught in the public schools by the reading teacher. The skills of the art and theater critic are also apparent. Deviations in learning these sign systems are met culturally by the speech pathologist and therapist, the specialist in learning disabilities, and the audiologist, to mention a few. As can be seen, the breadth of the science of semiology is extremely large.

From Jakobson's viewpoint, phonology fitted easily into the larger linguistic view of Saussure. The idea of things signified naturally called to mind the abstract level of the phoneme; the idea of the "sign" integrated the motoric and acoustic levels into this higher realm. The manner in which the signification process is learned culminated in the production of *Kindersprache* (Jakobson, 1941/1968). The motoric and acoustic aspects of speech provided a sphere of investigation that reaches fruition in *Preliminaries to Speech Analysis* (Jakobson, Fant, & Halle, 1952).

THE IMPORTANCE OF THE SYSTEM

Not only did Saussurian doctrine complement the views of Ščerba and Baudouin de Courtenay, and provide a larger structural frame for phonology, it stressed the most important aspect of structural linguistics, the "system" concept. In the formative years of linguistics a traditional dichotomy between comparative and historical linguistics was established. As Saussure points out:

> I prefer to speak of *synchronic* and *diachronic* linguistics. Everything that relates to the static side of our science is synchronic; everything that has to do with evolution is diachronic. Similarly, *synchrony* and *diachrony* designate respectively a language-state and an evolutionary phase. (Saussure, 1915/1966, p. 81)

In later years this dichotomy produced optional techniques for explaining linguistic fact. At times what appeared to be true while studying language over a period of time contradicted facts that were apparent when studying specific modern languages comparatively. For example, it is true that there has been a general tendency to voice certain unvoiced sounds in the evolution from Middle English to Modern English. For example:

'absurd' = [æbzɜ˞d]

'gosling' = [gɔzlɪŋ]

'husband' = [hʌzbənd]

These are phenomena from a diachronic perspective. From a comparative or synchronic viewpoint a general tendency to devoice voiced sounds can be seen, for example:[6]

the Russian word 'muzh' (husband) = [muʃ]

the German word 'gorb' (basket) = [kɔrb]

the English word 'walked' = [wɔkt]

The contradictory views concerning the importance of voicing, by analogy, cannot be resolved. Diachronically it appears that voiceless sounds are weak and subject to change. From a synchronic viewpoint it appears that voiced sounds are the weak ones. At the turn of the century, one's opinion concerning the importance of such things as voiced versus unvoiced sounds was a matter of technique rather than broadly based, well founded conjecture.

Jakobson, in one of his first publications, "The concept of the sound law and the teleological criterion," tried to solve this problem in a new way:

> This antinomy between synchronic and diachronic linguistic studies should be overcome by a transformation of historical phonetics into the history of the phonemic system. In other words, phonetic changes must be analyzed in relation to the phonemic system which undergoes these mutations. (Jakobson, 1928a/1962, p. 2; see also Jakobson, 1929/1962, p. 3; 1931b/1962, p. 203)

This stress upon the importance of the system was not a totally new contribution from Jakobson. An archetype can be found in Saussure's *Cours*:

> Speech always implies both an established system and an evolution; at every moment it is an existing institution and a product of the past. To distinguish between the system and its history, between what it is and what it was, seems very simple at first glance; actually the two are so closely related that we can scarcely keep them apart. (Saussure, 1915/1966, p. 8)

---

[6]Those without a background in linguistics are strongly encouraged to review *The Bases of Speech* (Gray & Wise, 1959, pp. 350–379). This discussion includes an entertaining and in-depth collection of some 49 types of sound change organized into phonetic, semantic, and miscellaneous categories.

However, Jakobson's insistence upon the importance of the system has more to do with the fact that he thought and wrote within the context of a highly turbulent artistic period, rather than his noted dependence on Saussurian doctrine. Citing the stimulation of the ideas of men like Picasso, Joyce, Braque, Stravinsky, Xlebnikov, and LeCourbusier, he points out that these divergent creative artists, from literature, music, and art, were concerned with the "interaction between the parts and the whole":

> Those of us who were concerned with language learned to apply the principle of relativity in linguistic operations; we were consistently drawn in this by the spectacular development of modern physics and by the pictorial theory and practice of cubism, where everything "is based on relationship" and interaction between parts and wholes, between color and shape, between the *representations* and the *represented* [emphasis mine]. "I do not believe in things," Braque declared, "I believe only in their relationship." (Jakobson, 1962, p. 632)

This same point of emphasis, the importance of the relationship, opens *Kindersprache*: "What is truly unifying are the relationships of foundation—HUSSERL" (Jakobson, 1941/1968, p. 11).

The relationships that Jakobson saw were Saussurian dualities bound in the context of a functional linguistic system. Saussure had laid the foundation for at least 11 basic dichotomies intrinsic to language: langue/parole, signified/signifier, concept/sound image, orthographic/phonetic, motoric/acoustic, phonetic/phonemic, individual/social, structure/function, system/history, synchronic/diachronic, and the simultaneous/successive axes of speech (discussed later).

This duality was later to be called "binarism." Students and colleagues of Jakobson in later years often could not recount why things were binary as opposed to tertiary, quarternary, etc. Some, such as Halle, simply felt that "That's the way it has to be!" (personal discussion, S. Singh, Ohio University, 1969). Fant (1973) posited the idea that it is a question of "economy" (p. 153). In truth, the idea of duality is axiomatic and requires proof. If the subsequent systemization predicts reality consistently, the binary principle will be confirmed.

SUMMARY

In all, Saussurian doctrine, at the time of Karcevskij's return in 1917, reaffirmed many tenets of the Leningrad School. What was new, was a shift in emphasis from the phoneme to the language as a subject of discussion. This process, and the subsequent discussion of the sign and its domain of semiology, produced a specific organization for the axioms of the structural linguistic movement. The bipolarization of the physiological, perceptual, and linguistic levels of language linked the motoric and acoustic components, the physiological and psychological components, and the individual and cultural components of the phoneme. Further organization was seen in the realm of language. The abstract frame of semiology permitted the integration of phonology into its larger self, social communication. Precepts concerning the sign organized the phonetic and phonemic aspects of the speech sound. Once the concepts of the phoneme, language, and sign were organized, Jakobson transformed the solid state aspects of structuralism with the idea, "This is all true and, furthermore, it is all relative"!

BASIC SUASSURIAN ASSUMPTIONS

The Phoneme

Axiomatic Assumption (J)
A bipolar *phonetic continuum* exists that relates the motoric and the acoustic aspects of the phoneme.

Axiomatic Assumption (K)
A bipolar *perceptual continuum* exists that relates the phonetic (physiological) and the phonemic (psychological) aspects of the phoneme.

Axiomatic Assumption (L)
A bipolar *linguistic continuum* exists that relates the individual (psychological) and the cultural (sociological) aspects of the phoneme.

The Levels of Language

Axiomatic Assumption (M)
Social communication is a concatenated system.

Corollaries M-1: A *phoneme* is a constituent part of a system.
M-2: A *phonemic system* is a constituent part of historical development.
M-3: An *historical development* is a constituent part of language.

The Linguistic Sign

Axiomatic Assumption (N)
The "sign" (verbal model) structures the relationship between the phonetic and phonemic aspects of the phoneme.

Corollaries N-1: Culture establishes the *phonemic parameters* of the phoneme.
N-2: The *phonemic parameters* of the phoneme are defined by means of *phonetic values*.
N-3: *Phonetic values* are established in a motoric and acoustic domain.

The Jakobsonian Extension

Axiomatic Assumption (O)

Language is a system of *interrelated* elements.

Corollaries O-1: A *phoneme* is a system (collection) with interrelated elements (distinct, opposing, relative, negative entities which differentiate words).
O-2: The *phonemic system* is a system (arrangement) with interrelated elements (phonemes).
O-3: *Historical development* is a system with interrelated elements (laws of change and acquisition).

chapter 5

The Prague School

CERCLE LINGUISTIQUE DE PRAGUE

By 1926, the ideas of Baudouin de Courtenay, Ščerba, and Saussure had spread internationally. The topics of the phoneme and language were being discussed not only in Russia and Switzerland, but were spreading to Czechoslovakia, Germany, Yugoslavia, England, France, and Australia (Lepschy, 1970, p. 53). Under the influence of Victor Mathesius, an international panel of structural linguists gathered in Prague in October 1926. Daniel Jones (1957/1967), the noted phonologist and participant, notes:

> During the later 1920's impetus was given to the study of the phoneme by the group of Eastern European scholars who, on the initiative of V. MATHESIUS in 1926, formed themselves into the Cercle Linguistique de Prague. Foremost among them, in addition to MATHESIUS, were N. TRUBETZKOY (1890–1938), R. JAKOBSON, and S. KARCEWSKI [Karcevskij]. (Jones, 1957, p. 17)

These men, as well as others such as Martinet, discussed, defined, and developed the basic lines of structural thought that have reached us today in their distilled form. Although each participant maintained certain unique positions, the group in general supported a majority of the assumptions previously discussed. The motoric/acoustic aspect of speech, the phonetic/phonemic dichotomy, and the differential function of the phoneme were prominent ideas. The contrast between a physiological versus a psychological approach was well understood. A reliance on the works of the Geneva and Leningrad Schools pushed these men forward in discovering the latent aspects of the phoneme and language in general.

DANIEL JONES

Each participant had been influenced by Ščerba, Baudouin de Courtenay, and Saussure. Daniel Jones depended so much on the works of

Baudouin de Courtenay as a basic reference point that his monograph, "The history and meaning of the term 'phoneme'," contains 23 references to him. This is noteworthy considering that the entire discussion is only 20 pages long! Jones' introduction to the works of the leader of the Leningrad School is quite similar to Jakobson's:

> The idea of the phoneme is no new one. It was first introduced to me in 1911 by the late Professor L. Ščerba of Leningrad, but both the theory and the word itself date back to more than thirty years before then. According to J. R. Firth, the term "phoneme" was invented as distinct from "phone" in 1879 by a linguistic scholar named Kruszewski, a pupil of the Polish linguistician Baudouin de Courtenay. (Jones, 1967, p. vi; see also p. 257)

Not only did Jones ascribe to a motor and acoustic component for the phoneme, he maintained a "concrete" versus "abstract" level for the unit. As he notes:

> There are "concrete" sounds and "abstract" sounds. A concrete sound is a physical thing, a sound actually uttered on a particular occasion. When we speak of *hearing* a sound or *making* a sound, the reference is generally to concrete sounds. An abstract sound may be said to be that which is common to, or can be abstracted from, a number of utterances of what we call "the same sound." (Jones, 1950/1967, pp. 6–7)

The specification of "that which is common" as a component of "the same sound" illustrates a typical collection tendency of the early years of the history of phonetics. Beginning in 1886, a small group of language teachers in France, under the inspiration of Paul Passy, had attempted to create an ideal alphabet. This new alphabet was to contain separate letters for each distinctive sound of the language. Furthermore, these symbols were assigned in such a way that they would be international in character, as similar as possible to existing symbols, and few in number. This alphabet, or symbol system, originally published in 1888 has constantly undergone revision and improvement through the efforts of the founding organization, the International Phonetic Association, IPA (Jones, 1957/1967).

The creation of alphabets, a common pastime of the linguist, caused the symbols to take on the aspects of the model for certain theoreticians. Jones defines the phoneme as, "a family of sounds in a given language which are related in character" (1967, p. 10). This "family of sounds" was represented by a certain grapheme or letter symbol. This grouping or pulling together of sounds, on the basis of "that which is common," is recurrent in Jakobsonian writing. Jakobson at times used the idea of "correlation" (a mutual relationship or connection) interchangeably with the term "opposition" (a contradiction or contrast). In his paper to the First International Congress of Linguistics in Prague he stated:

> Une corrélation phonologique est constituée par une série d'oppositions binaires définies par un principe commun qui peut être pensé indépendament de chaque couple de termes opposés ["A phonological relationship is made up of a series of binary oppositions defined by a common principle which can be thought of independently of each opposing term"]. (1928b/ 1962, p. 3)

The search for a common principle to collect sounds lead Jakobson and Jones in two different directions or areas of theory. Whereas Jakobson began to investigate the sound properties themselves, Jones concentrated on the concepts of the "phoneme," "allophone," and "phone."

To the phonetician creating alphabets, the phonetic world is made up of a myriad of identifiable elements. Perhaps this is because alphabetically inclined linguists tended to be multilingual and were exposed to many different sound variants. Most college students up to recent years have been required to be proficient in at least two languages other than their native one. In an unusual sense, a polyglot—or anyone, such as a phonetician, who is exposed to a variety of phonemes—has an atypical phonological system. A layman hears approximately 42 sounds. Although 26 letters are appropriate for written work, most phoneticians agree that 41 to 44 symbols suffice for "broad" transcription. Even this number of sounds needs transcriptional training. According to Kantner and West (1960, pp. xiiiv–xix) American English contains 41 sounds; Leutenegger (1963, pp. 4–5), 41 sounds (with dialectical variants and syllabics removed); Ladefoged (1975, pp. 33, 34, 68), 41 sounds; Carrell and Tiffany (1960, p. xi), 44 sounds. A trained phonetician should probably discriminate at best 65 different consonant sounds after training (see Ladefoged, 1975, p. 294). This distinction between the natural phonemic system of the layman and the hybrid system of the polyglot or phonetician is an important one. The group of sounds that belong to the "family" are the distinct sounds the phonetician hears. These sounds are "allophones," a term coined by Whorf in 1934 (Jones, 1950/1967, p. 7). The constituent elements of the phoneme, as defined by Jones, are the sound variants. This definition is directed toward phoneticians and not perceptual theoreticians.

Jones had always insisted upon the importance of lexical differentiation as an essential aspect of the phoneme:

> It is therefore a corollary to the explanation given in §31 [the full family of sounds definition of the phoneme previously cited] that phonemes have a semantic function in languages. . . . Such an alteration may change a word

into another word. In other terms the differences between phonemes are "significant," i.e. capable of distinguishing one word from another. (Jones, 1950/1967, p. 14)

Structural phonologists, upon close examination, always seem to agree on issues of importance such as basic axioms but tend to differ on points of emphasis. The same phenomenon is found in the writings of another participant and member of the Prague School: N. S. Trubetzkoy.

N. S. TRUBETZKOY

Trubetzkoy, a friend and collaborator of Jakobson, although a Russian linguist (Jones 1957/1967; Lepschy, 1970), occupied the chair for Slavic Languages at the University of Vienna at the time of the First International Congress of Linguistics (as related by Jakobson—see Trubetzkoy, 1939/1969, p. 320). Trubetzkoy's ideas on the basic assumptions of phonology are so similar to Jakobson's that it is almost impossible to separate them. Christiane Baltaxe (1969; in press), who has translated and analyzed Trubetzkoy's work, made the following point in reference to Jakobson:

> Closely linked with the name Trubetzkoy is that of Roman Jakobson, his friend and collaborator. He was to become the principle exponent of Prague phonology in the United States. His theory of "distinctive features" in many ways parallels Trubetzkoy's theory of distinctive oppositions. A constant interchange of ideas existed between the two scholars. (Baltaxe, 1969, p. vi)

Not only are the concepts of the "distinctive feature" and the "distinctive opposition" similar, Trubetzkoy stressed the importance of the motoric and acoustic aspects of the phoneme (Trubetzkoy, 1939/1969, p. 9). He constantly maintains the phonetic/phonemic dichotomy (ibid., pp. 8, 11, 12) that emanated from the differential function of the phoneme. He stressed the importance of the system (ibid., p. 321). Finally, the importance of the precepts of the Leningrad and Geneva Schools of linguistics is constantly maintained (ibid., p. 2, 4, 5). In a letter sent in July of 1929, he wrote:

> I am moving further and further away from Baudouin's system. This is, of course, inevitable, but it seems to me that, if one disregards the later definitions by Baudouin and Ščerba, which in my opinion are often insufficient and inexact, and if one only considers the essence of their systems, in other words, how they applied these systems in practice, one would recognize that our present-day conceptions (those of Jakobson and myself) are a further development of those systems rather than a contradiction of them. (Trubetzkoy, 1939/1969, p. 322)

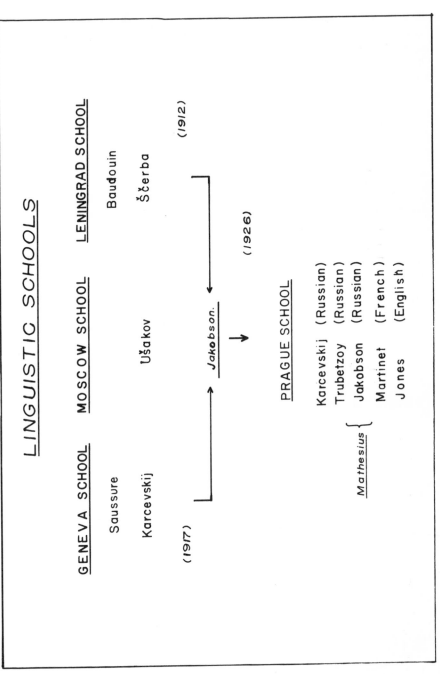

Figure 1. Schematic pattern of the evolution of the Prague School in reference to the Moscow, Leningrad, and Geneva Schools of linguistics.

The most significant development from the Jakobsonian perspective was a detailed discussion and development of the concept of opposition. Opposition, the most primitive concept of relativity, in Trubetzkoy's theory is a starting point for the full comprehension of phonology. The opposition is the one element that gives meaning to language in a unique sense:

> The concept of distinctiveness presupposes the concept of *opposition*. One thing can be distinguished only from another thing: it can be distinguished only insofar as it is contrasted with or opposed to something else, that is, insofar as a relationship of contrast or opposition exists between the two. A phonic property can therefore only be distinguished in function insofar as it is a member of an opposition of a sound. Oppositions of sounds capable of differentiating the lexical meaning of two words in a particular language are *phonological* or *phonologically distinctive* or *distinctive oppositions*. (Trubetzkoy, 1939/1969, p. 31)

Whereas Jones stressed the concept of similarity, Trubetzkoy stressed the concept of dissimilarity. The similar difficulty with the terms "correlation" and "opposition" in Jakobsonian terminology would create enough dynamic tension to produce a problem to be solved. As Jakobson developed his explanation and theoretical model in later years, he would solve this apparent contradiction in the context of the "system."

SUMMARY

Jakobson, like Jones and Trubetzkoy, retained the basic elements of the Leningrad and Geneva Schools of linguistics. These ideas lead to the creation of the Prague Linguistic Circle, or the Prague School (see Figure 1). In Jakobson's early life, from 1912 to 1927, he was exposed to the basic tenets of structural linguistic philosophy. He balanced the personal viewpoints of the leaders of each of the centers of learning. He integrated phonology into the larger Saussurian linguistic frame. Finally, he became one of the central figures of the Prague School. From an innocent monograph in 1912, to the return of an excited friend in 1917 and the stimulating intellectual milieu of 1926, we can date the beginning of distinctive feature theory.

AN HISTORICAL ASIDE

Not only did World War II postpone English translations of *Kindersprache* (1941/1968) and *Grundzüge* (1939/1969) in the United States, it cut short the life of one of the developers of distinctive feature theory. As Jakobson relates:

Hitler's occupation of Austria was disastrous for Trubetzkoy. He had never attempted to conceal his antinational-socialist views. In an article on the racial question he had subjected the racist theory to devastating criticism. He neither could nor wanted to remain at the University of Vienna. Trubetzkoy's last hope was to emigrate to America to continue his scientific work there. The Gestapo looked for him and subjected him to an impudent house search and interrogation. His files were confiscated. As a direct consequence of the visit, Trubetzkoy suffered a severe heart attack. In the hospital he still hurried to complete his book. He dictated it up to his final days. Except for a final review, the volume was almost completed. Only about twenty pages remained to be written when on June 25, 1938, Trubetzkoy suddenly died. (Baltaxe, 1969, p. 323)

Because of the devastating effects of the War on Europe, many people tend to date items, ideas, and concepts in pre- and post-War modes. Significant events in Europe that are beginning to influence thought in this country must take this into account. The emigration of a German Jew to the United States in the same time period was to have significant repercussions in later years. Albert Einstein, a student of Jost Wintler (Trubetzkoy's teacher) would apply the relativity concept to the field of physics with profound effects (Jakobson, 1972, p. 75).

THE
JAKOBSONIAN
APPROACH

chapter 6

The Jakobsonian Model

THE COMPLEX UNIT

The problem of the ambiguity between the terms "similarity" and "dissimilarity" is resolved in the evolution of the Jakobsonian model of the phoneme and the phonemic system. In 1914 Jakobson postulated his first conception or model of the phoneme in a letter to a noted poet of the period, Xlebnikov (1885–1922). In 1932 he expanded the model in the form of a definition for a Czechoslovakian encyclopedia. Subsequently, in 1949, he revised the model pictorially in collaboration with John Lotz. Finally the model was put into its most advanced form in collaboration with an acoustical engineer, C. Gunnar Fant, and an American linguist, Morris Halle. These time periods—1914, 1932, and 1952—are important milestones in the expansion of the Jakobsonian model. At each milestone significant new assumptions were added to the basic structural precepts. These principles tend to be the unique contributions of Jakobson to distinctive feature theory.

Poetry and Music

The first discussion of the model of the phoneme came in an unusual way. Jakobson dispatched a letter discussing vowel harmony to Xlebnikov, a Russian poet. In this letter he began to evolve the idea that speech sounds were simultaneous sign-units comparable to musical chords:

> Attracted by the problem of sign units, I had written to Xlebnikov in February, 1914, about the prospect of synchronism (*'odnovremennost'*) and "certain analogies to musical chords" in experimental poetry. (Jakobson, 1962, p. 635)

Although Jakobson did not expand on the musical chord concept, this is the first biographical piece of information alluding to the analogy. A musical chord is an ideal introductory model to represent the phoneme, the distinctive feature, and the sound system:

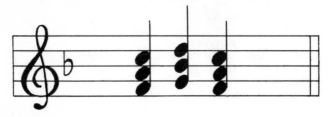

This model has the capacity to represent the phoneme as one unit (the chord itself). The chord has a variety of components (the notes). These notes are comparable to the features, a variety of motorically produced acoustic properties. A chord is heard as one element and yet is made up of other elements. This transformation, a shift in emphasis from the unit to its subcomponents, was and is a consistent goal of distinctive feature theory:

> The breaking up of correlative phonemes into their common core and differential property was obviously at variance with the definition of the phoneme as the "phonemic unit, insusceptible of being dissociated into smaller and simpler phonemic units" [from Saussure (Jakobson, 1928b/ 1962, p. 8)], which obstinately survives even to the present. (Jakobson, 1962, p. 635)

In essence, Jakobson's model illustrates that a phoneme is not a *scalar* quantity, but a *vector* quantity. *Each phoneme is a complex element.* This one assumption causes a radical revision of previous assumptions and hypotheses. Axiomatic assumption D ("the phoneme is the smallest unit of the speech chain") obviously must be revised. This is true in only certain limited conditions. Axiomatic assumption M ("social communication is a concatenated system") needs to be expanded. An additional corollary should indicate that a series of motoric/acoustic properties are constituent parts of the phoneme. This represents what is partially implied by Corollary O-1 ("a phoneme is a system with interrelated elements").

The Locke Experiment

In 1968, John A. Locke, as part of his doctoral dissertation, attempted to teach German "phones," [œ], [ç], and [χ], to English-speaking children in the southern Ohio area. This study, in essence a replication of the Winitz and Lawrence (1961) study, attempted to show that first grade children (42 males) differed from kindergarteners (18 males) in their ability to learn the production of the non-English phones. Little difference was found between the two groups, but the experimenter's conclusions are significant. Commenting on the children's ability to fully approximate the target sound (a scalar approach), Locke noted:

> The significance of this observation seems to be that some children responded to place-of-articulation features and other children mimicked manner-of-articulation characteristics or could not decide which to sacrifice. In some children the preserved feature was velarity with sacrifice of prolonged friction, in other children the product was friction with the sacrifice of place characteristics. (Locke, 1969, 190–191)

In other words, it appears that you cannot teach children "chords" because they attend to the "notes." Seven years earlier, Winitz and Lawrence (1961) had shown that simple "imitative" tasks do not effectively distinguish children with good versus poor articulation. Working with kindergarten children who scored in the upper and lower 12.5% on the screening portion of the Templin-Darley Test of Articulation, no significant differences could be found. Experiments built upon the "scalar" approximation model have to date failed to predict phonemic skills with the functional articulation population (Winitz, 1969, p. 132).

DEFINING THE PHONEME (B)

In 1932, Jakobson was asked to discuss the phoneme and phonology in the second supplementary volume to a Czech encyclopedia. In this brief article, Jakobson combined the musical chord concept with the differential property at the word level. He stated:

> [The] Phoneme is the basic concept of phonology. By this term we designate a *set* of those concurrent sound properties which are used in a given language to *distinguish words* of *unlike meaning* [emphasis mine]. (Jakobson, 1932/1962, p. 231)

First Jakobson noted that the phoneme is a "set" or vector quantity. By implication the elements of the set, the properties, distinguish words—not the phoneme itself. Cast in the form of an abstract model of "simultaneous sign units" (Jakobson, 1962, p. 635), this effect becomes apparent. The presence or absence of sound elements are the key units that make words different.

$$
[A]\quad\quad [A]\quad\quad [A]
$$

$$
\begin{bmatrix} + \\ - \\ + \\ + \end{bmatrix} \text{ or } \begin{bmatrix} yes \\ no \\ yes \\ yes \end{bmatrix} \text{ or } \begin{bmatrix} 1 \\ 0 \\ 1 \\ 1 \end{bmatrix} \text{ etc.}
$$

In his earliest writings, Jakobson had insisted that the properties were binary (1928b/1962, p. 3; 1929/1962, p. 9). It was Trubetzkoy who supplied the basic idea for the transformation of the "chord" concept to the "simultaneous-sign" concept. As Jakobson relates:

> Another fundamental discovery of Trubetzkoy in the field of phonological structure was soon to follow. This was the observation that one of the two terms of a binary opposition "is to be considered as positive, characterized by a specific mark while the other is simply to be regarded as lacking the mark." (Jakobson, in Baltaxe, 1969, p. 321.)

THE AXES OF SPEECH

In *Cours,* Saussure had insisted that speech existed in two dimensions: an instantaneous domain and a continuous domain. The Jakobsonian model was designed primarily for one axis rather than the other. Saussure labeled his axes "simultaneous" (AB) and "successive" (CD) (see Saussure, 1915/1966, p. 80).

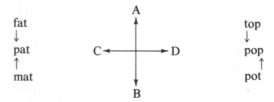

This same dichotomy is retained today but has been relabeled the "paradigmatic" (AB) and "syntagmatic" (CD) axes, respectively. It is clear that the differential function of the phoneme is best viewed in the simultaneous or paradigmatic domain. According to Martinet (1970), this axis is the one of phonemic choice. The other axis is the domain of time, the speech chain:

> To discover the structure of language, therefore, one starts from the one-dimensional object, the linear chain of speech, which unfolds along what has been called the syntagmatic axis. But at each point another dimension will be called into play, that of choices made by the speaker and which is generally designated as the paradigmatic axis. As to the possible choices at any one point, we will get our information by comparing various segments of speech which present different elements in identical contexts. This is the operation called "commutation" and is practiced by all structural schools. (Martinet, 1970, p. 6)

It is obvious from this discussion that the chord or simultaneous-sign unit exists primarily as a model along the paradigmatic axis. However, the first illustration of the vector came in a discussion of the syntagmatic dimension of the French language.

A Collaboration: 1949

The year 1949 marks the first time in which the use of the formal vector model appeared in print. In that year two separate articles appeared which contained the model. Interestingly, one article contained a paradigmatic configuration, the other a syntagmatic configuration. The syntagmatic configuration occurred in a tribute to Henri Muller on the occasion of his 70th birthday. Jakobson and John Lotz (1949) began with a simple expression in the domain of speech.

> Cher Maître, voulez-vous nous permettre de vous présenter nos hommages et nos meilleurs voeux de santé, de parfait bonheur et de tranquillité d'âme! ["Dear Teacher, would you permit us to present our respects and best wishes for good health, happiness and peace of mind!"]. (See Jakobson, 1962, p. 426)

Using this sentence, or string of phonemic segments, the authors attempted a two-fold phonemic transcription which they termed "simple" and "analytical." The initial phonemic transcription represented the simple analysis. Specifically, the IPA symbols represented a series of scalar quantities. After the phonemic string was established, the authors analyzed each scalar quantity for its vector components. They postulated that the French language could be analyzed along six features or dimensions (Table 1). Each sound (graphic symbol) is in reality a vector or complex quantity. The 'v' is: 1) not a vowel, 2) not a nasal, etc. At the same time, each dimension or property can be traced as it is seen over time. Dimension 1, vocality, or vowelness, may be traced

Table 1. Jakobson and Lotz' (1949/1962, p. 434) six-feature analysis of French

														Sound															
Dimension	ʃ	ɛ	r	m	ê	t	r	ə	v	u	l	ê	v	u	n	ʊ	p	ɛ	r	m	e	t	r	e	ə	d	e	v	u
1. Vocality vs. consonantness	−	+	±	−	+	−	±	#	−	+	±	+	−	+	−	+	−	+	±	−	+	−	±	#		−	#	−	+
2. Nasality vs. orality	−			+	−				−			−	−		+		−			+	−					−		−	
3. Saturation vs. diluteness	+	±		−	±				+	±		±	−		−		−	±		−	±					−		−	
4. Gravity vs. acuteness		−		+	−				+	+		−	+	+	−	+	+	−		+	−					−		+	+
5. Tenseness vs. laxness	+			+	+				−			+	−		−	+	+			−	+					−		−	
6. Continuousness vs. interception	+	−		−	−				+	+		+	+		−	+	−			−	−					−		+	

54

Table 2. Jakobson's (1949/1962, p. 421) identification matrix of the phonemic system of Serbo-Croation

Dimension	t	d	c	s	z	p	b	f	v	ć	đ	č	ǵ	š	ž	k	g	x	n	m	ń	r	l	l'	i	u	e	o	a
Vocality																						±	±	±	+	+	+	+	+
Nasality																			+	+	+								
Saturation		–	–	–	–	–	–	–	+	+	+	+	+	+	+	+	+	+			+		–	+	–	–	+	±	+
Gravity		–	–	–	–	+	+	+	+	–	–	–	+	–	–	+	+	+		+					–	+	+	+	
Continuousness		–	+	+	+	–	–	+	+	–	–	+	+	+	+	–	–	+				–	+	+					
Voicing	–	+	–	–	+	–	+	–	+	–	+	–	+	–	+	–	+	–											

from 'ʃ' to 'E' to 'r' to 'm,' etc., meaning that the production is "not vowel-like," "vowel-like," "not vowel-like and vowel-like" (such as a semivowel), etc. In their article Jakobson and Lotz traced the "on" and "off" characteristics for each sound in the salutation. Because the sound of the epigraph is continuous, this configuration is called a syntagmatic system. In another article published the same year, under Jakobson's name alone, a paradigmatic model can be found (Jakobson, 1949).

THE IDENTIFICATION MATRIX

In "On the identification of phonemic entities" (Jakobson, 1949/1962, pp. 418–425), Jakobson extended the ideas concerning French to Serbo-Croatian phonemes. At that time, the two phonemic systems were considered approximately equivalent (see Table 2). All features were identical with the exception of the voiced/voiceless dichotomy of Serbo-Croatian replacing the tense/lax dichotomy of French.

The purpose of this type of matrix, the identity matrix, is not to describe the chain of speech. In this configuration the object is to define or identify each sound in the entire phonemic system of the language. The former model, the syntagmatic, is open and unlimited, and may be continuous in the time domain. The latter model, the paradigmatic, is a closed system limited by the number of features and phonemes in the particular language.

THE PARADIGMATIC MODEL

The paradigmatic model, as a phonemic identification process, carries with it certain inherent assumptions that occur irrespective of the specific sound system in question. A clear understanding of these assumptions should prevent the confusion of phonetic precepts for phonemic precepts. To begin, several authors have shown that a distinctive feature is primarily a logical choice (Fant, 1973, p. 152; Greenberg, 1967; Martinet, 1970, p. 6; Singh, 1976, p. 4). Understanding the type of logic employed will clarify the true meaning of distinctive feature.

What is a Distinctive Feature?

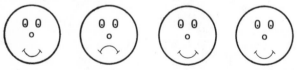

A distinctive feature is any property that separates a subset of elements from a group.

The binary process (+ versus −) or (1 versus 0) is a simple way of saying that a group of elements have or do not have a certain trait, characteristic, aspect, property, or feature upon which a decision is made. When these decisions are concatenated and organized, the identification process is systematized.

What is a Distinctive Feature System?

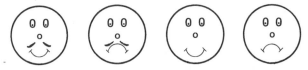

A distinctive feature system is a collection of properties that serve to separate each element of a set of elements from all other elements.

In the foregoing example no two faces are identical; therefore, each element has its own identity. This identity must be based upon a series of dimensions that produce this uniqueness. These logical properties establish the system. Furthermore, these properties may be used to generate the original elements. For example:

Properties	Elements
1. Smile (⌣)	Happy man
2. Moustache (╱ ╲)	Sad man
	Happy woman
	Sad woman

The elements and their properties are really scalars reassessed through vector dimensions. The importance of these vector dimensions was pointed out by Michael Polanyi in his lecture, *The Tacit Dimension.*

> I shall consider human knowledge by starting from the fact that *we can know more than we can tell.* This fact seems obvious enough; but it is not easy to say exactly what it means. Take an example. We know a person's face, and we can recognize it among a thousand, indeed a million. Yet we usually cannot tell how we recognize a face we know. So most of this knowledge cannot be put into words. But the police have recently introduced a method by which we communicate much of this knowledge. They have made a large collection of pictures showing a variety of noses, mouths, and other features. From these the witness selects the particulars of the face he knows, and the pieces can be put together to form a good likeness of the face. (Polanyi, 1967, pp. 4–5)

The idea that we know more than we can tell can be illustrated by a casual assessment of our previous example. If asked which face seems the most dissimilar, the happy man is contrasted to the sad woman, or the sad man is contrasted to the happy woman. The remaining combinations are seldom chosen. The reason this occurs is best seen not with the elements but by using a model of their properties. Generally this model is done in matrix form.

What is a Distinctive Feature Matrix?

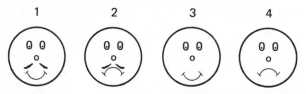

A distinctive feature matrix is a graphic representation of a distinctive feature system. It contains both the elements and the differential properties.

		Elements			
		1	2	3	4
Distinctive features:	Smile Moustache	$\begin{bmatrix} yes \\ yes \end{bmatrix}$	$\begin{bmatrix} no \\ yes \end{bmatrix}$	$\begin{bmatrix} yes \\ no \end{bmatrix}$	$\begin{bmatrix} no \\ no \end{bmatrix}$

Several phenomena can be seen at the outset. Each element, 1–4, has its own identity. No two faces are identical. This individuality is created by the series of answers to the questions of relevance for the case at hand. The code for each element is different. If there were two identical codes, there would be two identical twins. However, as can be seen, each face is different. The answers to the questions, for elements 1–4, indicate that the faces are different in two ways: Smile? (yes/no), and Moustache? (yes/no). Note that the difference between faces 1 and 4, as well as 2 and 3, involve both cognitive parameters, the smile and the moustache. When elements 1 and 2 are contrasted there is just one property difference, the presence or absence of the smile. The same relationship is found when elements 3 and 4 are contrasted. The contrast between elements 1 and 3, as well as 2 and 4, reveal a similar relationship, a single property difference but the use of a different feature, the presence or absence of a moustache.

Quantity and Quality

Before we apply these principles to the realm of phonology, we should note that the use of the matrix produces two significant types of information regarding dissimilarity (Dorf, 1969). The use of the vectors or column codes permits the specification of the *number* of differences between two elements (quantity) and the *type* of differences between two elements (quality). Two faces in the previous collection may differ by one or two differences. A comparison of faces 1 and 2 reveals a single difference, between faces 1 and 3 a double difference. Moving from the number to the type of differences, we can see that the contrast between faces 1 and 2 is a question of emotional state. The difference between faces 1 and 3 is a question of sex. Both types of information are important. The matrix itself permits the derivation of quantitative and qualitative information in the realm of dissimilarity. Knowing the degree and kind of difference is often more important than knowing which element is in error.

At the phonemic level the matrix has the same power. By using a matrix, the phonologist can determine the type and number of sound property errors when an inappropriate phone is used in the place of a target phoneme. The following discussion illustrates this concept. If one were to assume that a language had only four phonemes ([p], [b], [t], [d]) for its entire sound system, the following configuration would be appropriate to identify the sounds:

Identity matrix

	p	b	t	d
1. Made by the lips?	+	+	−	−
2. Is it voiced?	+	−	+	−

At this juncture, the number of possible comparisons between any two sounds may be determined. For instance, if one wants to compare each sound to every other sound, there are initially (4 × 4) or 4^2 (x^2) possibilities:

	p	b	t	d
[p]	*1*	*2*	*3*	*4*
[b]	*5*	*6*	*7*	*8*
[t]	*9*	*10*	*11*	*12*
[d]	*13*	*14*	*15*	*16*

However, not all these combinations are relevant. Notice that [p] equals [p] in the phonemic sense, $/[p]_1 = [p]_n/$. The same is true of $[b]_1/[b]_n$, $[t]_1/[t]_n$, and $[d]_1/[d]_n$. In other words, any phone compared to itself in a phonemic context must be equal to no (or zero number of) distinctive feature differences. Therefore, these comparisons—those of a sound with itself—must be subtracted from the total number of combinations, $(4^2 − 4)$ or $(x^2 − x)$:

	[p]	[b]	[t]	[d]
[p]	0	a	b	c
[b]	a	0	d	e
[t]	b	d	0	f
[d]	c	e	f	0

This operation is represented by the zeros in the main diagonal.

Finally, the difference of [p] being substituted for [b] equals the difference of [b] being substituted for [p]: (p/b = b/p). In a phonetic sense the laryngeal activity in either substitution is of significance from an organic viewpoint. However, the presence or absence of this activity, once structural normality has been ascertained (i.e., organic problems ruled out), points to a problem of learning, not capacity. From a learning or phonemic viewpoint, p/b is equal to b/p because the quantity and quality of difference are identical. By analogy, the distance and scenery on a trip from New York to San Francisco, in general, is the same as the distance and scenery from San Francisco to New York. A child who substitutes p/b does not understand the importance of voicing. The same is true for the child who substitutes b/p. To reduce this type of redundancy in the equation simply divide by 2:

$$N = \frac{x^2 - x}{2} \quad \text{Derived equation} \tag{1}$$

$$N = \frac{x(x - 1)}{2} \quad \text{Torgerson (1958, p. 265)} \tag{2}$$

$$2N = x(x - 1) \quad \text{Twaddel (1935, p. 53)} \tag{3}$$

where N is the number of relevant combinations, and x is the number of elements to be compared.

In effect this division extracts the comparisons of the upper righthand triangle, elements a through f, from the lower lefthand triangle, i.e., the repeated comparisons.

The Attribute Dispersion Matrix

In 1970, Blache pointed out that it was possible to specify the number of feature differences in a matrix similar to the identity matrix (p. 24). This idea, based upon a similar concept evolved in the syntagmatic axis by Saporta (1955, pp. 26–27), portrayed the phonemic differences rather than the features themselves. This matrix, termed the "attribute dispersion matrix," denotes the number and type of distinctive feature difference between each phoneme and every other phoneme in the system:

Attribute dispersion matrix

	p	b	t	d
p	0	1 (voice)	1 (place)	2 (voice) (place)
b		0	2 (voice) (place)	1 (place)
t			0	1 (voice)
d				0

The configuration of the attribute dispersion matrix may be recognized by the fact that the ordinate and abscissa are equivalent (phoneme-by-phoneme matrix). The identity matrix, however, has a feature-by-phoneme design for coordinates:

Identity matrix

	p	b	t	d
1. Place?	+	+	−	−
2. Voiced?	−	+	−	+

The initial configuration of Jakobson and Lotz (1949/1962) is merely a representation of change in the identity matrix over time. The attribute dispersion matrix merely specifies the magnitude and type of change that occur.

The Decision Process

The size of the paradigmatic or identity matrix depends upon the number of phonemes in the system. As the number of phonemes increases, the number of features must increase. The tension that causes the number of phonemes to increase would seem to be the size of the vocabulary pool. As the vocabulary increases in a certain language, more distinctions must be made. These distinctions can be made by either lengthening the number of segments in the word pool or by increasing the number of phonemes as part of the segmental stock. The former solution, a syntagmatic one, is based upon an increase in the use of features. The latter solution, a paradigmatic one, is based upon the creation of new features or feature combinations.

Considering the matrix paradigmatically, it can be seen that each new feature represents a new question or choice for the system at hand. These choices differentiate the phonemic elements. As the number of possible elements in the data pool increases (i.e., the number of end nodes) the number of questions must increase (Pierce, 1965, pp. 73–74; Singh, 1966, pp. 39–41):

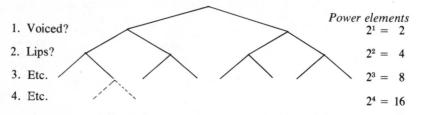

Power elements

1. Voiced? $2^1 = 2$

2. Lips? $2^2 = 4$

3. Etc. $2^3 = 8$

4. Etc. $2^4 = 16$

To determine the number of features needed for a phonemic system, the following formula is appropriate:

$$2^n = x \qquad \text{Jakobson, Cherry, \& Halle, 1953; 1962, p. 453} \qquad (4)$$

where n is the number of features required, and x is the number of elements to be coded.

Given a phonemic system such as English, with some 42 sounds, an initial estimate of the number of distinctive features needed is approximately 5½. This can be determined through a logarithmic equation:

$$2^n = x$$
$$log_2 x = x \qquad\qquad (5)$$

If x equals 42 phonemes, the equation becomes:

$$log_2 x = \frac{log_{10} x}{log_{10}{}^2} \qquad\qquad \text{Pierce, 1965, p. 286} \quad (6)$$

or:

$$log_2 42 = \frac{1.62320}{.30103} = 5.3922 \text{ features}$$

Notice that the log to the base ten of 2 is a constant in the decision process. Given any size phonemic pool, merely divide the log to the base ten of the number in question by this figure (.30103). This will produce the figure for the number of features needed for the array.

Not only is equation 6 important for estimating the number of features in the adult system, it can be used to demonstrate an important characteristic of the acquisition process itself. As the child learns the

Table 3. Comparison of proportional increase of phonemes with logarithmic increase of features for various numerical bases

Elements	Proportions	D	Logarithmic base[a]		
			2	3	4
2	0.04	0.04	*1.00000*	.63093	.50000
7	0.16	0.12	2.89735	*1.77124*	*1.40368*
12	0.28	0.12	*3.58496*	2.26186	1.79248
17	0.40	0.12	*4.08746*	2.57890	*2.04373*
22	0.52	0.12	4.45943	2.81359	2.22972
27	0.64	0.12	4.75489	*3.00000*	2.37744
32	0.76	0.12	*5.00000*	3.15465	*2.50000*
37	0.88	0.12	5.20945	3.28680	2.60473
42	1.00	0.12	5.39232	3.40217	2.69616

[a]Italicized numbers indicate the mathematical point at which a new distinctive question must be added.

first two sounds (the basic oppositional system), he or she has one distinctive feature in the linguistic repertoire. As the acquisition process unfolds, more features are learned in the early stages, whereas the later stages involve a generalization process (Table 3). Irrespective of the logarithmic base, the acquisition of features predominates over their generalization in the early years. It seems that the assumption that the phoneme is a complex variable carries with it certain implications inherent in the process of geometric progression. Irrespective of the type of decision—binary, tertiary, quarternary, etc.—more properties are learned early. These same properties are integrated in later acquisition stages. The presumption of linear acquisition, a phoneme-by-phoneme approach, has not borne a great deal of fruit. The presumption of dimensional or featural acquisition, as opposed to the linear assumption, carries with it an inherent proposition. The rules of mathematics govern the scalar and vector approaches. Once the assumption of phonemic complexity is accepted, a new mathematical scale is formulated.

Phonemic Interdistances

If one reviews the number of internal comparisons possible or available to the child as each new sound is added to the repertoire, the inadequacy of the linear speech sound scheme will become apparent. Using equation 1 for the same phonemic series, in Table 4, it will become apparent that the emphasis on features in the early years is coun-

Table 4. Comparison of the number of phonemic elements acquired, the number of interdistances, and the proportional increases in interdistances

Elements	P_1	Interdistances	P_2	Increase
2	0.04	1	0.00	0.00
7	0.16	21	0.02	0.02
12	0.28	66	0.07	0.05
17	0.40	136	0.16	0.08
22	0.52	231	0.27	0.11
27	0.64	351	0.41	0.14
32	0.76	496	0.58	0.17
37	0.88	666	0.77	0.20
42	1.00	861	1.00	0.23

teracted by a heavier concentration on the interdistances within the system.

The child who has two phonemes and adds five new speech sounds increases the internal comparisons or interdistance knowledge by 2.3%. But the same child who has 37 sounds and adds five new sounds increases his or her knowledge by 22.8%. The acquisition of new sounds implies their integration into the existing phonemic system. The larger the existing phonemic system, the greater the number of cross-comparisons to be made. To monitor the child's phonemic progress, it may be wiser to estimate the number of comparisons the child can make rather than the number of phonemes that are in use.

Similarity and Dissimilarity

The binary sign and the matrix approach reveal unusual power in another area. The matrix and sign system permits the demonstration of similarity and dissimilarity at the same time. For instance, in the reference to the minute four-phoneme system, we may convert the matrix notation into Venn diagrams:

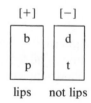

The first feature, "made by the lips?", correlates two subsets: 1) those having a labial property, [p] and [b], and 2) those not having a labial property, [t] and [d]. At the same time that these phones are correlated internally, they serve as phonemic representatives that have contrastive value across the boundaries. In other words, [p] and [b] are in free variation. No distinction is made between the two sounds, ([p] = [b]). The same relationship will be noted for [t] and [d]: ([t] = [d]). But when all the elements are combined [([p] = [b]) ≠ ([t] = [d])], a disjunctive relationship results. The two *classes* do not equal each other. Rephrasing the mathematical expressions into phonetic terms, voicing is neutralized and place of articulation has a phonemic status. Although voicing is detectable in some contexts, it is irrelevant for the case at hand. This is phonetic information with no phonemic value. Later in the book this status will be reversed.

Considering our other major property, the voicing feature, we may also develop a similarity/dissimilarity configuration:

[+] | b   d | voiced

[−] | p   t | not voiced

Now [b] and [d] are joined, as well as [p] and [t], such that the following relationship is produced: [([p] = [t]) ≠ ([b] = [d])]. In this situation, sounds with the same voicing characteristics are part of the same class. Furthermore, only the contrast, the presence or absence of the feature, is important. An excellent example of the free variation problem is often found in the cross-linguistic context. For instance, a Japanese speaker trying to learn English will often say [raripap] for 'lollypop,' i.e., r/l. In turn the same speaker will pronounce 'railroad' as [leʊlod]. In this case the /l/ appears to be replacing /r/. However, this total behavior pattern only indicates that no phonemic distinction is being made, [l] = [r]. One sound is not replacing the other, because neither sound is understood. Because this contrast is significant in English, the Japanese speaker will have to learn this cognitive disjunction. Note also in the previous example that the problem is not one of physiological incapacity, for both sounds can be produced. The problem is really one of learning, a conceptual difficulty.

Returning to the four-phoneme system, both features, voicing and place, may be used to identify each phoneme. The Venn diagram illustrates this effect:

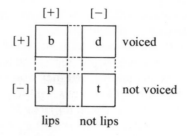

The use of both features demonstrates that each class is unique: [p] ≠ [b] ≠ [t] ≠ [d]. Therefore, /p/, /b/, /t/, and /d/ are phonemic in status. The similarity component can be seen in reference to that which is common to the various elements that are joined to the working units. The dissimilarity component is seen in reference to the working units themselves. The signs, (+ and −), are used to denote that which is phonemic, or linguistically distinctive. Those subjects joined by either sign are the basic collective categories. Sounds within these categories are nondistinctive.

THE BASIC THEME

In all, a distinctive feature is that which is truly distinctive from a logical perspective. This same concept of distinctiveness is applied to words (Chomsky, 1965, p. 83), myths (Lévi-Strauss, 1972a, p. 186; 1972b, p. 203), and objects (Greenberg, 1967, p. 215; Singh, 1976, p. 4), illustrating that the concept is an abstract one not restricted to acoustics. It is through this distinctiveness that we can know more than we can tell. From the outset, the identity matrix is a paradigmatic hypothesis about the nature of the sound system. This paradigmatic hypothesis is an arrangement of the subject matter to make predictions. These predictions relating to the magnitude and nature of speech sound differences are directly obtainable from the matrix itself, irrespective of the arrangement. The process of the arrangement is a tenet of the formulation of a science, not phonology itself. Therefore, distinctive feature theory is merely a visual manner of applying the scientific method to the acquisition process. This is true only if predictions are made and behavior is accounted for.

MODELS (A RETROSPECTIVE)

It should be noted that most of the configurations in this chapter are explanatory. Their purpose is to demonstrate the intent of the authors in question or to illustrate the implications of these same ideas. However, one configuration, the identity matrix, is not merely didactic in intent. The basic purpose of the identity matrix is to code or identify each phoneme in a system along certain hypothetical lines. The establishment of an orderly and systematic pattern, which displays the relationships within the subject matter, is a process of generalization or theory construction. The actual configuration is incidental to the fact that generalizations are formed. The use of the matrix has the power to transform a phonetic subject matter into a phonemic science. If the matrix used is fully confirmed, the full latent structure of the phonemic system will be revealed. As noted by Singh (1972):

> A theory of speech sounds has to explain the internal consistencies amongst a group of sounds of a language. Internal consistencies must be explained in terms of a finite set of invariant attributes called features. The finite set may consist of only those attributes which explain the production and perception of speech sounds.... However solid the logical basis of deduction of a feature system, modern scientists must insist on the empirical verification of a theory. (p. 1)

Attempts have been made to derive matrices experimentally. If the true intent or purpose of the matrix were fully understood, the verification process would then take precedence over the derivation and expansion process. The discussion of which matrix, how many features, and which features should not obscure the need to verify the matrix itself.

What Does the Distinctive Feature Matrix Represent?

In its abstract form, a distinctive feature matrix is a model of differential properties. A distinctive feature, from a Jakobsonian perspective, is a logical operation. From a structural viewpoint, the differential properties may be used to identify any set of elements. From a phonological perspective, it was conjectured that the phoneme and the phonemic system could be modeled (axiomatic assumptions A-2, A-3, B-1, and B-2). Because the phoneme is a constituent part of the system (axiomatic assumption M-1) and the phoneme and the system are represented in the matrix, axiomatic assumptions C-1 ("the model of the phoneme must eventually match the latent structure of the phoneme") and C-2 ("the model of the phonemic system must eventually match the latent structure of the phonemic system") can be synthesized and refined. Using the matrix as the working base, it may be said that a *matrix* must eventually match the latent structure of the phoneme and the system simultaneously. If one accepts the Jakobsonian hypothesis that a phoneme is a complex unit (axiomatic assumptions O-1 and O-2), a matrix orientation is inherent. The matrix is the classical format to relate scalar and vector quantities. Above all, it must be remembered that the matrix may be used to represent anything. It may be used to represent phonemic production, or phonemic retention, or phonemic reception. But there is no value or justification in restricting its use to phonology. A matrix may be used to systematize morphological rules, lexical items, grammatical rules, or even ideas.

In phonology, a bipolar continuum relates the psychological process of the individual, so important to Baudouin de Courtenay, to the physiological world of motoric production and reception, so important to Ščerba. This continuum begins in the realm of *langue* and ends in the realm of *parole*. In its phonemic sense, as well as the semantic sense, the organization of the perceptual process, by which groups of identifiable units are sorted, depends upon a differential or discriminative process. The essence of the distinctive feature concept is the abstract logical component:

> The gross sound matter knows no oppositions. It is human thought, conscious or unconscious, which draws from this sound matter the binary oppositions for their phonemic use. The term *opposition* (or correspondingly, *contrast*) is currently used in modern linguistic literature, but it is still opportune to recall the vital implications of this concept as, for instance, H. J. Pos neatly formulated them: "L'opposition n'est pas un fait isolé: c'est un principe de structure. Elle réunit toujours deux choises distinctes, mais qui sont liées de telle façon, que la pensée ne puisse poser l'une sans poser l'autre. L'unité des opposés est toujours formée par un concept, qui, implicitement, constient les opposés en lui et se divise en opposition explicite quand il est appliqué à la réalité concrète" ["The opposition is not an isolated fact: it is a principle of structure. It always unites two distinctive choices which are joined in such a fashion that one cannot think of one without the other. The unity of the opposition is always formed by a concept, which, implicitly, contains the opposition within itself and divides itself in the explicit opposition when it is applied to concrete reality"]. (Jakobson, 1949/1962, p. 423)

Twelve years later, in 1961, at the Conference of Language Universals at Gould House in Dobbs Ferry, New York, Jakobson reaffirmed his commitment to this position:

> The "logical operations" which H. J. Pos, the outstanding Dutch theoretician of language, apprehended in the binary opposition of distinctive features do indeed give the purely formal bases for a precise investigation of language typology and universals. (Jakobson, 1966, p. 267)

THE SMALLEST UNIT OF SPEECH

As was noted earlier, Saussure had postulated that the phoneme was the smallest unit of speech that was insusceptible of being dissociated into smaller and simpler units. Jakobson challenged this idea by positing the idea that the phoneme is a complex set of properties which implies that the feature or property is the smallest unit of speech. It would seem that there is a contradiction between the two positions, the feature versus the phoneme. However, the problem is relative. Given a phonemic arrangement of four elements:

$$[1][2][3][4]$$
$$+ + - -$$
$$+ - + -$$

it may be seen that the phoneme is the smallest unit of speech, in certain contexts. Comparing each of the four elements—1 to 2 or 3; 2 to 4 or 1; 3 to 4 or 1; and 4 to 2 or 3—it may be seen that elements 1, 2, 3, and 4 are the smallest units when (and this proviso is critical) they are in minimally distinctive feature *contexts*. In the paradigmatic domain certain contrasts will show minimal aspects of each phoneme. This observation, however, must give way to the idea that, whereas the phoneme *may* be basic, the distinctive feature itself is always basic. Saussure's position is only partially true; Jakobson's position would seem to be always true.

THE MINIMAL PAIR

As was implied earlier, all phonemic contrasts have magnitude. The degrees of difference have been given formal labels.

> A distinction is called *minimal* if it cannot be resolved into further distinctions which are used to differentiate words in a given language. We owe this term to Daniel Jones, from whom we also borrow the following definition—"wider differences may be termed *duple, triple,* etc., according to the number of minimal distinctions of which the total difference is composed." (Jakobson, Fant, & Halle, 1952/1967, p. 2)

By implication a minimal pair must be defined not only by segmental differences but by the feature differences, the paradigmatic and syntagmatic axes respectively. A minimal pair then must meet four conditions. It:

1. is composed of two words,
2. with an equal number of segments in each word,
3. in which one segment, and only one segment, in a reciprocal position can be shown to be different in the syntagmatic domain, and,
4. in which one feature, and only one feature, can be shown to be different between the two segments, i.e., the paradigmatic domain.

Each level of these conditions represents a refinement of semantic minimalness, to syllabic minimalness, to segmental minimalness, to featural minimalness. In later contexts these precepts will lead to techniques to teach the proper production of segments and features. By manipulating social contexts with varying communicative intent—which requires semantic, lexical, segmental, or featural differentiation—the remedial worker can spotlight the various requirements of the word. quirements of the word.

FURTHER ASSUMPTIONS

An Additional Saussurian Assumption

Axiomatic Assumption (P)
Language has a paradigmatic (simultaneous) axis and a syntagmatic (successive) axis.

> Corollaries P-1: The *phoneme* has a paradigmatic axis and a syntagmatic axis.
> P-2: The *phonemic system* has a paradigmatic axis and a syntagmatic axis.
> P-3: *Historical development* of the phonemic system has a paradigmatic axis and a syntagmatic axis.

An Additional Jakobsonian Assumption

Axiomatic Assumption (Q)
The matrix model represents the latent structure of the perceptual process.

SUMMARY

So far, 17 basic assumptions have been postulated to be relevant to distinctive feature theory. These hypotheses seem intrinsic to a structural phonemic orientation, especially to those ascribing to a Jakobsonian approach. Isaac Newton once observed that no great discoveries were made without bold guesses. The assumptions a scientist is willing to make are in a sense the map of research. If one experiments true to one's own axioms and fails, the map may be faulted, the map builder may be faulted, but the map-making process is never at fault. The map merely needs revision.

chapter 7

The Theory
of Acquisition

THE INITIAL ARTICLE

The manner in which children acquire speech sounds was first discussed by Jakobson (1939c/1971) in an article entitled, "Les lois phoniques du langage enfantin et leur place dans la phonologie générale" ("The sound laws of child language and their place in general phonology"). This article was written for and presented to the Fifth International Congress of Linguists, which met in Brussels in September 1939. It is a relatively short article, but contains a succinct description of the rationale and development of distinctive feature theory. From a historical perspective, however, this work had little impact because it was not published until 10 years later. It appeared in 1949 as an appendix to Trubetzkoy's posthumous publication, *Grundzüge der Phonologie*.

THE FULL THEORY

In 1941, an amplified discussion of the earlier French article appeared in German, *Kindersprache, Aphasie und allgemeine Lautgesetze* (*Child Language, Aphasia and Phonological Universals*). This three-part work discusses the interaction between phonological development in the child and phonological dissolution in the adult. Normal development and pathological dissolution in the aphasic adult are first presented as aspects of general linguistics. Subsequently the specific stages of development and dissolution are described in a step-by-step fashion. This description is mainly from a cultural point of view. The underlying implications of the parallels between aphasia and articulatory development are delineated from an evolutionary perspective of the languages of the world. Finally, the phonological acquisition sequence of the child is presented as a basic reinteration of the previous stages. These stages, and rationale for their proposal, constitute the essence of distinctive feature theory.

A SUBSEQUENT SYNOPSIS

As mentioned previously, *Child Language, Aphasia and Phonological Universals* did not appear in English until 1968. The American public's first exposure to the stages of phonological development was through a work entitled "Phonology and phonetics" (Jakobson & Halle, 1956b). This work is one of the best traveled articles of distinctive feature theory. Written in 1955, this article was first published as part I of *Fundamentals of Language* (Jakobson & Halle, 1956a, pp. 1–51). One year later, "Phonology and phonetics" was revised and shortened for L. Kaiser's (1957) *Manual of Phonetics* (pp. 215–251). This revision, entitled "Phonology in relation to phonetics," was to appear again in the subsequent edition of the same text edited by B. Malmberg (1968, pp. 411–449). Abbreviated portions of "Phonology and phonetics" have appeared in other anthologies. In 1961, parts of chapter 4 appeared in S. Saporta's text *Psycholinguistics* (pp. 346–348). In 1971, the entire article appeared in A. Bar-Adon and W. Leopold's *Child Language: A Book of Readings* (pp. 218–227). And, of course, an article so important was also included in Jakobson's own *Selected Writings* (1962, pp. 464–505). The brief initial statement of "Les lois ...", the full statement of *Kindersprache*, and the synopsis of "Phonology and phonetics," all of which explained the theory of acquisition, were preceded by another text that discussed the specifics of the theory rather than its broad linguistic realm.

THE DISTINCTIVE FEATURES

In 1952, four years before the publication of the synopsis in *Fundamentals of Language* and 16 years before the publication of *Child Language, Aphasia and Phonological Universals* in English, a technical report (#13) was published by the Acoustics Laboratory of MIT. This work, *Preliminaries to Speech Analysis: The Distinctive Features and Their Correlates*, contained an in-depth discussion of each sound property used in language. Collaborating with M. Halle and G. Fant, Jakobson defined the phonetic substance, the physiological and acoustic requirements, of the distinctive features developed previously in the acquisition model. This monograph, reissued on the average of every other year, has remained the classical presentation of distinctive feature theory. However, it is only through all three sources that the entire theory reaches its full force and scope. No one to date has integrated the basic assumptions of the structural linguistic movement with the rationale that was used to formulate the theory and the specific definitions of the features used in the theory. A thorough, comprehensive, and systematic presentation of these three aspects of the theory is needed. Whereas *Child Language* and related articles presented the abstract theory and its derivation, *Preliminaries* and *Fundamentals* added necessary details for the full appreciation of the theory. It is only through an integration of these texts that an inclusive orientation can be developed.

THE DERIVATION OF THE THEORY

Ease of Articulation

The basis of Jakobson's theory of phonological acquisition is embedded in a controversy of the late 1800's. Several theoreticians at the turn of the century had postulated that children learn speech sounds in a sequence dictated by a strong physiological principle. Some sounds were surmised to be easier than others to produce. This orientation is commonly referred to as the *principle of least effort*:

> The fact that a fixed order must be inherent in language acquisition, and in phonological acquisition in particular, has repeatedly been noticed by observers and has been explained by appealing to the principle of least effort. First mentioned by Buffon, this principle is nonetheless generally cited as Schultze's law of the succession of phonological development, since it is Fritze Schultze who, fifty years ago, energetically sought to prove that those speech sounds which require the least physiological effort for their production are learned first by children. (Jakobson, 1941/ 1968, pp. 20–21)

The idea that the order of acquisition of speech sounds is inherently physiological in nature was formulated quite clearly in Fritze Schultze's text *Die Sprache die Kindes*. This book was published in Leipzig, Germany, in 1880. In this text, Schultze sees each sound of language requiring different amounts of energy and subsequently some sounds are easier to produce than others:

> Here I believe I can, on the foundation of my observations, state the following basic law: that the speech sounds are produced by children in an order which begins with the sounds articulated with the least physiological

effort, gradually proceeds to the speech sounds produced with greater effort, and ends with the sounds which require the greatest effort for their production.

By physiological effort is meant the amount of nerve and muscle energy needed to bring about the position of the speech organs necessary for production. (Schultze, 1880/1971, p. 28)

Alternative Explanations

It should not be assumed that the physiological explanation for speech sound development was the only one available at the turn of the century. A German philosophical-psychological school of thought, beginning with Immanuel Kant, had evolved alternative hypotheses for the explanation of speech sound development. Kant, the man who laid the foundation for an abstract and dichotomous philosophical world view, was eventually succeeded at the University of Königsberg in East Prussia by Johaan Fredrich Herbart. Herbart, embedded in his own philosophical tradition, added a new factor to the thought of the times—the "apperception mass." As Heidbreder noted:

> Herbart was Kant's successor at Königsberg and as Kant's thought is a development of the critical side of British empirical philosophy, so Herbart's theories resemble the more positive side of the same movement. Like the British associationists, Herbart undertook to explain the most complex mental phenomena in terms of simple ideas. He was impressed by the thought that each idea has a certain degree of force, and emphasized the phenomena of inhibition as well as association. Some mental facts he explained in terms of ideas that form compounds or blends, but he made *inhibition,* rather than association, the key-note of his system. Every idea, according to Herbart, has the tendency to maintain itself and to drive out ideas with which it is incompatible; and ideas vary in strength. When an idea encounters a stronger idea or groups of ideas with which it is incompatible, it is thrust below the level of consciousness.... This process Herbart calls apperception, and the group of ideas into which the entering idea is introduced is known as the *apperception mass*. [all emphasis mine] (Heidbreder, 1933/1961, pp. 65–66)

The animistic concept that ideas have force or a life of their own, an idea that recurs in subsequent Jakobsonian writings as the teleological criterion, is de-emphasized by later psychologists. The mass of ideas or the person's psychological experience is viewed as a static condition rather than a changing and organized phenomena. Although the philosophers of the 19th and 20th centuries are seldom quoted in Jakobson's early phonological writings, the influence of these men is constantly seen. The direct analogies between distinctive feature opposition and cognitive inhibition, or the idea that a mass of ideas or perceptual system is a real though intangible component of scientific exploration, link Jakobson with the wider philosophical movement. Furthermore these influences are constantly seen.

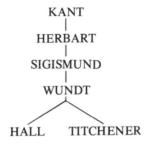

Berthold Sigismund, a German physician and follower of Herbart, passed on the psychostructural orientation of Kant to Wilhelm Wundt, a professor of philosophy and psychology at the University of Leipzig (Leopold, 1948/1971, pp. 3, 5). In 1900, in his work *Völkerpsychologie,* Wundt accepted Schultze's "principle of least effort" but emphasized that other conditions affect articulatory growth (see Bar-Adon & Leopold, 1971, p. 43). Wundt noted as early as 1900 that vision, hearing, and coarticulation are important factors for articulatory growth. Furthermore, and more important, speech sound substitutions, which he referred to as mutilations or transformations, were seen as having a linguistic explanation:

> As a matter of fact observation of the child and a closer look at the sound transformations which take place yield two conditions which make it quite understandable that more or less radical changes must take place in the imitation of sounds, although the child is capable of producing the required sounds. The first of these conditions is the imperfect acoustic and optic apperception of the sounds and the sound movements. The second is the contact effect of sounds which plays a part in coherent speech and is greatly increased in children's speech. (Wundt, 1900/1971, pp. 43–44)

From a cultural point of view, the mutilations of child language are seen by Wundt as directly analogous to questions concerning language in general. Specifically, he notes that there is a connection between the languages of the world and the language of the child:

> The child has of course very little practice of this kind [integrating thought and movement] and the conceptual movement is slower compared with normal consciousness. That explains why the language of the child is replete with these contact effects by which sounds are assimilated to or by dissimilation separated from each other or suppressed completely. The slower conceptual movement of the child explains particularly the other fact that progressive assimilations are more numerous in child language.... This preponderance of progressive assimilation is noteworthy

because in all cultural languages of Indo-European and Semitic prove-
nience, the opposite, regressive form of assimilation prevails, whereas in
other languages, for example, the Ural-Altaic, progressive assimilation,
primarily vocalic, is dominant, as in child language. (Wundt, 1900/1971,
pp. 44–45)

It is in this intellectual milieu that Jakobson's theory gets its impetus. Whereas Schultze, and, earlier, Buffon, according to Jakobson
(1941/1968, p. 21), had posited a strict physiological explanation for the
acquisition of speech sounds, Jakobson's style would be to seek balance following the tenets of the structural linguists and philosophers of
Russia, Germany, and Switzerland. In essence, in 1939, Jakobson reit-
erated in his own mind a discussion that had occurred some 40 years
earlier.

THE WILD SOUNDS OF BABBLING

Whereas Wundt accepted the idea of "least effort" as being partially
relevant, Jakobson rejected the idea that certain sounds are easier to
produce than others. To Jakobson, all sounds are equally *possible* in
the babbling period, and the specific sounds that do occur are "wild"
in nature (Jakobson, 1941/1968, p. 25). In a review of the writers of this
period, Jakobson concluded that no sound is impossible to produce for
the young child:

> The actual beginning stages of language, as is known, are preceded by the
> so-called babbling period, which brings to light in many children an as-
> tonishing quantity and diversity of sound productions. A child, during his
> babbling period, can accumulate articulations which are never found
> within a single language or even a group of languages ... According to
> findings of phonetically trained observers and to the summarizing state-
> ment of Gregoire [author of the classical study, L'Apprentissage du lan-
> gage, 1937](β101), the child at the height of his babbling period "is capable
> of producing all conceivable sounds." (Jakobson, 1941/1968, p. 21)

From Jakobson's viewpoint all sounds are possible in a prelinguistic
period. Oller et al. (1976) have interpreted this position to mean that all
sounds are random or equiprobable in a natural context (pp. 1–2, 9).
However, a careful reading of the Jakobsonian position reveals that
Jakobson never denies that some sounds are more *probable* than others. In fact Jakobson specifically states that imitation is a necessary
component of the natural setting of the theory itself (Jakobson, 1941/
1968, pp. 13–14, 16, 24). The role of the environment is seen as a
necessary aspect of phonemic growth:

> It is easy to understand that those articulations which are lacking in the
> language of the child's environment easily disappear from his inventory.

> But it is striking that, in addition, many other sounds which are common to the child's babbling and to the adult language of his environment are in the same way disposed of, in spite of this environmental model that he depends on. (Jakobson, 1941/1968, pp. 21–22)

Wundt had noted in 1900 that, in the babbling period, it is the *capacity* of production and not the performance which is of essence. The competence of *langue* should not be confused with the performance of *parole,* so to speak.

> I am inclined on the contrary, to grant a certain validity to the rule postulated by Schultze.... On the other hand I do not think it is possible to maintain the rather generally accepted theory that the child substitutes other sounds whenever required ones are impossible or difficult for him. It seems to me this assumption is invalidated simply by the fact that the child is usually *in full possession of all the articulations which are needed* [emphasis mine] for the various sound formations from the beginning of his imitative speech movements and uses them constantly in the emotive sounds which precede real speech. (Wundt, 1900/1971, p. 43)

Jakobson objects to the use of the principle of least effort not to explain or characterize babbling but to raise the rhetorical question, "If one sound is not easier to produce than another, how are we to explain the vague patterns of sequential development that are exhibited?". It is generally conceded that bilabial stops and nasals precede the sibilant classes, although the specifics of the total phonemic sequence is unclear. Once the student of child phonology rejects the idea that certain sounds are easier to produce than others, the way is paved to construct an alternate explanation of phonemic development.

MAPPING

Jakobson's search for an alternate explanation of the sequential order of acquisition is embedded in the scientific techniques of the late 19th century. Durkheim (1858–1917) and other researchers had championed the idea that problems such as suicide could be studied by the use of physical maps. Durkheim's technique, as explained in *Le Suicide,* involved plotting on a map the number of suicides found in specific geographical areas. To explain the given suicides, one merely develops a series of overlays that indicate the distribution of race, religion, creed, or social class on the same map. Theoretically, then, the map shows which variables are most closely related to suicide.

This co-relation or correlation has, of course, many serious logical flaws (see Hirst's *Durkheim, Bernard, and Epistomology,* 1975, p. 170). From the fields of psychology and statistics we know that it is wrong to infer that if A is found in the presence of B, A causes B. Even if A increases as B increases, one is not justified in inferring a causal relationship. All that can be done at this stage is describe the degree and order of the relationship.

Trubetzkoy, as related by Jakobson (1969, p. 323), used a similar technique of laying one pattern on top of another to determine the basic or universal patterns of language. In the period circa 1935, Trubetzkoy began developing an index card system in which he collected a description of the specific phonological characteristics of the numerous languages of the world. By comparing each of the languages, he felt he could "map" the most common phonological properties inherent in the systems. This desire to see the latent principles that underlie the phonological systems of the world typifies the structural approach. In all, Trubetzkoy's purpose was to seek that which unites amongst diversity. Three years after the formulation of the catalogue system, Trubetzkoy was dead. Jakobson preserved the importance of the work of Trubetzkoy by applying this work to child phonology in 1939 and 1941. In addition to this, he developed and refined the arguments behind the correlation/causality problem. These two contributions—the discussion of the historical developments of the universal pattern underlying phonological systems (stratificational patterns) and their initial logical relationship (laws of implication))—establish the first level of the theory.

chapter 8

Jakobsonian
Theory:

PHASE I

Jakobson began developing his theory of phonological acquisition by looking for the commonality of the language of the child and the languages of the world. As he said, "If we continue comparing the linguistic acquisitions of the child with the typology of the languages of the world, one glimpses the fact that the grouping of phonemes and the system of the grammatical meanings are equally subject to the rule of superposition of function" (Jakobson, 1939c/1971, p. 81). These typologies and their function were discussed extensively from a phonetic perspective in both the article in French in 1939 and the monograph in German in 1941.

THE LAWS OF IMPLICATION

Consonants

Pattern #1 In the comparison of the languages of the world, Jakobson noted an interesting latent pattern. All the languages of the world that have *back* consonants (velars and palatals) also have *front* consonants (labials and dentals). However, some languages have front consonants but do not have back consonants. But no language with back consonants is lacking front consonants! From this fact Jakobson concludes that one class of sounds implies the existence of the other:

The existence of back consonants in the languages of the world presupposes accordingly the existence of front consonants.... The solidarity is not reversible; the presence of front consonants (or individual classes of them) in no way requires the presence of back consonants (or individual classes of them). In other words, no language has back consonants without containing front consonants. On the other hand, there are some languages with labials and dentals, but without back consonants, as, e.g., the language of Tahiti in which both velars—k and ŋ—have changed to ' [*sic*], and Kasimov-Tatar, in which all velars—both stops (voiceless and voiced, oral and nasal) and fricatives—were also replaced by the glottal stop. In some languages the lack of palatovelar sounds is limited to oral consonants (e.g., in the languages of Samoa, where k became the glottal stop, but where ŋ was preserved), and in many languages the system of nasal consonants is represented solely by m and n, whereas we know of no language which possesses back but not front nasal consonants. (Jakobson, 1941/1968, pp. 53–54; cf. 1939c/1971, p. 77)

This law, which governs the *place* of articulation and its evolutionary sequencing, is not the only implicational rule.

Pattern #2   A second pattern that Jakobson discovered related to the *manner* rather than place of articulation. All the languages apparently have stops, but many languages may not have fricatives. All languages that have fricatives have stops. The converse relationship is not true. As Jakobson notes:

The acquisition of fricatives presupposes the acquisition of stops in child language; and in the linguistic systems of the world the former cannot exist unless the latter exists as well. Hence, there are no languages without stops, whereas P. Schmidt cites a number of Australian, Tasmanian, Melonesian, Polynesian, African and South American languages in which fricatives are completely unknown. In Kara-Kalpak and in Tamil, to cite additional examples from another continent, there is no autonomous category of fricatives; stops and fricatives appear as combinatory variants of the same phoneme—the first as basic variants, the others as variants conditioned by the environment. In Tamil, e.g., stops become fricatives after a vowel. (Jakobson, 1941/1968, pp. 51–52; cf. 1939c/1971, p. 77)

Thus, not only is the inherent implicational relationship important in the languages of the world, the child is constantly ruled by the same laws. "The child first changes fricatives to the corresponding stops—f to p, s to t, and insofar as the palatovelar series is established before the appearance of fricatives, x and ʃ to k" (Jakobson, 1941/1968, p. 52). In a subsequent discussion the full import of this fact will be expanded upon.

Pattern #3   It is commonly accepted that fricatives are complex elements made up of stop-like and fricative-like properties. Apparently for this reason, Jakobson simply states that the affricate class requires the formation of both classes, stops and fricatives. No specific languages are cited to validate this implicational rule. He does, however, note in a general way that no language has more affricates than fricatives (Jakobson, 1941/1968, p. 56). Formally stated, Jakobson's third law is as follows:

> The acquisition of affricates in child languages in opposition to the corresponding stops presupposes the acquisition of fricatives of the same series [place of articulation]; likewise in the languages of the world the opposition of the dental, labial and palatovelar affricate to the corresponding stop implies the presence of a dental, labial or palatal fricative. (Jakobson, 1939c/1971, p. 77; c.f. 1941/1968, p. 55)

These three laws of implication, relating the consonants to one another, far outnumber the number of laws that govern the vowels.

Vowels

Pattern #4   The discussion of vowels has been a weak element of distinctive feature theory. Few laws of implication were derived. In general, it might be said that a basic principle that implies a horizontal expansion of the vowel system must be preceded by a vertical expansion (from common logic), and subsequently the existence of the back vowels implies the existence of the front vowels of corresponding height:

> An opposition of two vowels of the same degree of aperture is not acquired by the child as long as a corresponding vocalic opposition of a narrower degree of aperature is lacking. . . . The phoneme æ, to which a as the palatal opposition of the same degree of aperature and e as the narrow opposition of the same series are opposed, appears relatively later in children and is explained by the laws of solidarity already mentioned. . . . The pair u ~ o cannot, therefore, precede the pair i ~ e, and there are no children who have an o-phoneme without having acquired an e-phoneme. On the contrary o is very often acquired considerably later than e. Accordingly, a number of languages have an e-phoneme without any o-phoneme (cf. Trubetzkoy op. cit., 98 on the Lezghian vowel system), but there is hardly any language with o and not e. (Jakobson, 1941/1968, p. 56; cf. 1939c/1971, pp. 77–78)

Summary

These four laws of implication/solidarity constitute an initial formulation of the actual steps in the evolutionary sequence of the phonemic system as it has developed diachronically. In 1939, Jakobson had indicated that an alternative set of laws, the laws of incompatibility, could be developed. This one aspect of the theory needs clarification and expansion. Each law of implication is based upon a threefold foundation. Given two sound classes, A and B, three conditions are necessary for an implicational relationship;

1. The presence of A
2. The presence of A + B
3. The absence of B without A

If sound class A exists alone (condition 1), and sound classes A and B coexist (condition 2), and if no language has B alone without A (condition 3), the existence of B implies the existence of A. In essence at this level, this simply states that A is a necessary precondition to B. All this is stated by Jakobson in abbreviated form as follows:

> All this goes to prove that the choice of differential elements within a language is by no means arbitrary and fortuitous, but is on the contrary ruled by laws (or tendencies) of universal and consistent validity. We have rapidly surveyed some laws of implication: the existence of unit Y implies the existence of unit X in the same phonemic system. It would be possible to examine another series of laws which are no less important for the typology of languages. They are the laws of incompatibility: the existence of unit Y excludes the existence of unit X in the same phonemic system. (Jakobson, 1939c/1971, p. 81)

A careful examination of this argument, however, reveals that the laws of incompatibility are the same as the laws of implication but are stated negatively. A fourth condition is a part of the law of implication. Following the impetus of the argument, in the confines of phonemic dissolution, it can be seen that incompatibility is the active destruction of factor A which produces a subsequent destruction of B:

4. $-A \rightarrow -B$ (cause + effect relationship)

This logical relationship can be recognized as a first order causal relationship. If an intervening variable occurs it must be discovered in subsequent orders. Once the four elemental relationships:

$$A$$
$$A + B$$
$$-B$$
$$-A \rightarrow -B$$

are demonstrated to exist, an inherent order is a certainty. It is for this reason that Jakobson entitled his book *Child Language, Aphasia and Phonological Universals.* What is universal in child language and the languages of the world is inherent, only, if incompatible relationships of the same order can be shown to exist in aphasia. Development and dissolution must be regulated by the same laws (Jakobson, 1941/1968, p. 90).

IRREVERSIBLE SOLIDARITY

The idea that certain sound classes imply the existence of other sound classes in the foregoing context is generally referred to as "irreversible solidarity," an important concept in Jakobsonian thought (see 1939c/ 1971, pp. 77, 78; 1941/1968, pp. 51, 58, 59(2), 90.). An inherently ir-reversible relationship is important to the theory for its implications for the various layers of the phonemic domain. Furthermore, these layers of development and their sequential order are the laws that govern linguistic evolution and child development (Jakobson, 1939c/1971, p. 77; 1941/1968, p. 59):

> Every phonemic system is a stratified structure, that is, consists of superimposed layers. The hierarchy of these layers is nearly universal and constant. It appears in the synchrony as well as the diachrony of language; we are therefore dealing with a *panchronic order* [emphasis mine]. When there is a relation of irreversible solidarity between two phonemic units, the secondary unit cannot be eliminated without the primary unit. This order prevails in the existing phonemic system and governs all its changes. The same order determines the language-learning, as we have just seen, a nascent system, and—let us add—it continues to prevail in language disorders, a system in dissolution. (Jakobson, 1939c/1971, p. 78)

THE SYNCHRONIC/DIACHRONIC RELATIONSHIP

What Jakobson is arguing in essence is that a nascent phonological class, "forward stops," was first used by primitive man. As man evolved, the back stops [k, g, ŋ] emerged. As the vocabulary increases the number of phonemes must increase. The preference for the back stops rather than the front fricatives, as the second step, can only be inferred from later writings (see Jakobson & Halle, 1956a, pp. 41–42). No comparative linguistic proof is offered to validate the sequence. The evolution of the front fricatives, following the back stops, permits the use of the back fricatives in the fourth stage. The development of the affricates can therefore be inferred to be a subsequent historic development:

Although this is a mere sketch of phonemic evolution, these four laws of implication, and the subsequent contention of irreversible solidarity (which was not always validated), are used to establish a working historical hypothesis.

THE BIOLOGICAL ORIENTATION

The idea that phonemic development may be directed by a person's genetic background has received renewed interest in recent years (Abbs & Sussman, 1971; Brosnahan, 1961; Chase, 1965a, 1965b; Menyuk, 1968). Brosnahan, in an extensive discussion of Darlington's hypothesis and its implications for phonemic development, has contended that speech sounds have a strong hereditary background:

> The role of the genetic component in the acquisition of speech is now becoming clear.... Each child passes through a sequence of distinct stages, both with regard to maturation of his vocal apparatus and with regard to the process of sound development, and in every aspect of this growth process it is the child's idiotypic abilities and the maturational potentialities which determined the nature, rate and course of his development. The actual norm of the community's sound complement acts as a goal toward which the development is directed, the norm to which the child adapts himself as a result of his own inherited patterns of growth and of drives and urges to communicate and interact with other members of the community.... As a result of the interaction of his heredity and this environment, the developing individual acquires a complement of sounds which, though approximating acoustically and articulatorily to the actual norm of the group, is yet as a whole individual to and characteristic of him alone. By the approximation he communicates with the other members of his language community, and by the individuality in his sound compliment he expresses the uniqueness of his genetic inheritance. (Brosnahan, 1961, p. 148)

This position, postulated by Franke in 1899, has been met with subsequent criticism (Leopold, 1948/1971, p. 3), but reappears periodically in current literature. The unfolding potential of the child, often referred to as "plasticity" in British and American literature, has been directly associated with the phonological component of language. As Chase noted in 1965:

> Two of the most remarkable features of verbal behavior are the early age during which the human infant acquires competent use of the phonological system of his adult culture, and the sensitivity with which the phonological system reflects adult vocalization patterns. These observations call attention to the plasticity of the developing nervous system, and the ability of the developing nervous system to replicate, in its own functional organization, features of the sensory environment. By the age of two years, young children have pretty good command of the phonemic ele-

ments of the adult language system. (Chase, 1965b, pp. 22–23; cf. Chase, 1965a, p. 2)

In 1968, Menyuk, working from the hypothesis that sound attributes are universally related to the physiological capacities of man irrespective of gene group (pp. 138, 142), tested the order of acquisition of the specific sound properties in two different language populations, English and Japanese. This study, which has been extensively criticized by Winitz (1969, pp. 61–62), does tend to imply that certain aspects of phonological growth are "innate" aspects of the child. But a careful reading of the article shows that Menyuk only claims that certain aspects are "inherent" to the acquisition process. Winitz had stated, "I do not mean to imply that distinctive feature principles have no use in the formal analysis of natural languages. My concern is their validity in the analysis of phonemic development when biological interpretations are made" (p. 62). In fact, what Menyuk (1968) had said was as follows:

> One can observe the same order in acquisition and relative degree of mastery or correct usage of sounds containing the various features by groups of children from two differing linguistic environments, indicating that a hierarchy of feature distinction may be a linguistic universal, probably dependent on the developing perceptive and productive capacities of the child. (Menyuk, 1968, p. 142; cf. p. 138)

The nature of the developing capacity of the child is a sensitive topic. One need only consider how many people died when one madman told an entire nation that their innate capacity was far superior to that of other nations.

ONTOGENY RECAPITULATES PHYLOGENY?

The idea that diachronic development of languages is used to explain the synchronic development of the child would seem to reinforce the position that Jakobson and his followers subscribe to the principle that "ontogeny," the growth pattern of the individual, recapitulates "phylogeny," the evolution of the species. However, this is not the case. Biological determinism has been discussed by Jakobson in passing on three different occasions (1939c/1971, p. 78; 1941/1968, pp. 65–66; 1949/1962, p. 424). The idea that a child is "preprogrammed to learn" according to evolutionary patterns is carefully avoided. Sigmund Freud, who came to the United States in 1909 (West, 1966, pp. 25–26), had repeatedly held that ontogeny recapitulated phylogeny. A. A. Brill (1960), in his book on Freudian analysis, states:

Psychoanalysis recognizes the direct path from ontogeny to phylogeny. The individual begins with the lawless Id psyche, which, as a result of struggle with the outer world, gradually becomes molded into a conscious ego and later into a super-ego. The race which constitutes an aggregate of individual beings is subjected to the same trials and vicissitudes and reacts to stimuli in the same manner, and with the same results as the individual. (p. 307; cf. Allers, 1955, p. ix; Strachey, 1965, pp. xvi–xvii)

In 1938, Barend Faddegan published *Phonetics and Phonology,* a structurally oriented text which reflected many of Jakobson's basic ideas. The review of this monograph by Farnsworth (1940) indicates the close perception of Freudian theory and structural phonology:

Several decades ago psychology was loath to admit the existence of her stepsister psychoanalysis. The latter, it may be recalled, did not wait for sisterly recognition; she introduced herself to a somewhat unfriendly world. Phonetics, too, has a so far but poorly introduced stepsister, phonology, a teleologically inclined discipline which holds to a "relational subconsciousness," as something or other which is composed of "perceptional and motoric" parts.... The theory is so similar to that of psychoanalysis one might guess that its future advocates will employ the now quite familiar Freudian arguments. (p. 169)

In fact, structuralism shares little in common with Freudianism or biological determinism. To Jakobson, diachronic evolution and synchronic development, as well as the biological evolution of the individual species, are all governed by higher laws:

On the other hand, the *universal* and *panchronic* validity, as well as inner logic, of the observed hierarchical sequence of phonological oppositions permits us to assume the same sequence for glottogony. Many earlier assumptions about the origin of language are, in this way, refuted, while others, on the contrary, are confirmed: e.g., Trombetti's view that stop sounds are more original than fricative sounds, or van Ginneken's brilliant hypothesis, which attributes an original priority to the first consonantal oppositions in contrast to the vocalic oppositions. *Both* ontogeny and, probably, the phylogeny of language are based on the same underlying principle, which governs the whole realm of language. [emphasis mine] (Jakobson, 1941/1968, p. 93; cf. 1939c/1971, p. 78; 1941/1968, p. 59)

In order to understand the concepts of the "panchronic law" and "universality," biogenetic determinism must be abandoned. Jakobson's theory is founded in a teleological perspective.

THE TELEOLOGICAL PERSPECTIVE

In 1928, Jakobson published a brief abstract of a paper delivered to the Prague Linguistic Circle the year before. This article, entitled "The concept of the sound law and the teleological criterion," sketches Jakobson's philosophical perspective. This orientation later came to be known as functionalism. Basically, a teleological perspective indicates a form of evolution that is directed with a particular end in sight. This purpose, of course, is often unknown. The process in and of itself is "natural," biogenetic as well as environmental. Furthermore, the process has a "supernatural" component, sometimes called Divine Providence, to quote Webster. In its entirety this concept is referred to as the "sound law" (Jakobson, 1928a/1962, p. 1). The sound law has two driving forces. One force tends to unite reality (unifying force), the other force tends to produce individual differences (particularist spirit). These two factors, which are mutually opposing, are always present and affect (perhaps effect) every linguistic event and generate historical growth (Jakobson, 1941/1968, p. 16). This concept, derived from Saussure, in essence merely states that phonemes, words, languages, individuals, the entire world, are evolving. Universal trends will be noted. Nonuniversal trends will be noted. The key concept for phonology is its final end. The purpose of the phonemic system is to make words different. If words, in their general sense, cannot be differentiated, communication cannot occur:

> Under the spell of the antiteleological (*antifialiste*) spirit of the end of the century, F. de Saussure—in spite of his pioneering courage—expresses the following conviction: "In contrast to the false idea which we often have of it, language is not a mechanism created and arranged for the sake of the concepts to be expressed." Now, however, we are often in a position to make this rejoinder: in contrast to the destructive, hypercritical attitude of the period, it is common sense, it is precisely the idea which we, the speaking subjects, often have of language which is perfectly valid: *language is actually an instrument governed and arranged for the sake of the concepts to be expressed.* It takes the sounds effectively and transforms this natural material into contrasting qualities suitable for carrying the meaning. The laws of phonemic structure just broached prove it. [emphasis mine] (Jakobson, 1939c/1971, pp. 81–82)

The child trying to learn this language is seen as a "separatist" constantly approximating the cultural norm like, interestingly enough, a small model builder (Jakobson, 1941/1968, p. 15). The unifying force of the language is constantly at odds with the continual hypotheses of the child that are being tested. The fact that a child is a model builder is implicit in the fact that children exhibit a constant type of deviation (Jakobson, 1939c/1971, pp. 75–76; 1941/1968, p. 18). Why the child builds models is inherent in the environment, the child, and the language—in other words, everywhere.

> The question inevitably arises: Why is one component of the linguistic system uncompromisingly and irrevocably rejected by the new generation, and why is it the same component for all its members? The answer obviously lies outside the specific problem of child language. Such a change is predetermined by the internal, inherent development of the

linguistic system; it is not an alien modification forced upon the linguistic system by children. Rather they anticipate those changes which are internally predetermined—in the air, so to speak. (Jakobson, 1941/1968, p. 18; cf. 1939c/1971, pp. 75–76, 1941/1968, p. 14)

When the question is asked, "Is the phonological acquisition process innate or environmental in character?", the only correct response is yes, as confusing as this might be. Biological determinism has little import for the Jakobsonian philosophical position. This is mainly because the perspective is too narrow and is only partially true as an explanation.

THE ABBS AND SUSSMAN POSITION

In 1971, two theoreticians from the University of Wisconsin, James Abbs and Harvey Sussman, put forth the concept that humans had sensory receptor fields, "feature detectors," which "were innately structured to detect, and respond to various distinguishing parameters of the acoustic sound system" (p. 23). Abbs and Sussman, working from their interpretation of Menyuk, drew direct analogies between these feature detectors and certain reflex patterns in lower animals: frogs, monkeys, pigeons, and rabbits. These innate trigger reflexes are seen as decoding mechanisms inherent in the entire animal world, including man. The classical position of distinctive feature theory has, however, never included this concept. The child's ability to differentiate is the only biologically inherent process in the theory (Jakobson, 1949, p. 424). Children learn to differentiate in their productive skills, in their discrimination skills, and in their auditory memory skills. Jakobson notes that these operations are first conscious endeavors that subsequently tend to be metalallic (1941/1968, p. 24). From the full perspective, distinctive feature theory requires a balanced position between the concepts of biological determinism and environmental determinism:

> Certainly, several striking points of contact have been observed between the linguistic development of the child on the one hand, and the languages of the world on the other. In particular, the interrelation between these two areas has been discussed. Romanticism stressed the *creativity of the child*, while the approach of scholars like Wundt or Meringer, considered realistic by its proponents, sought to explain the intellectual, and especially the linguistic, activity of the child as *mere imitation*. There is some truth in both points of view. On the one hand, the creativity of the child is obviously not pure creativity, or invention out of nothingness; on the other hand, however, neither is his imitation a mechanical and involuntary adoption. The child creates as he borrows. [all emphasis mine] (Jakobson, 1941/1968, pp. 13–14)

chapter 9

Prelinguistic
Behavior

A distinctive feature approach is strongly dependent upon the active intellectual process and a desire to communicate by expressing words. Furthermore, the desire to communicate must also be supported by the ability to communicate (Jakobson, 1941/1968, p. 424). These two prerequisites, adequate cognitive development and adequate motoric control of the articulators, have precluded emphasis on the prelexical or prelinguistic period from birth to 16 months. However, certain comments must be made concerning this period, quite apart from Jakobsonian writings. The brief comment that a period of silence may separate babbling from true linguistic behavior (Jakobson, 1941/1968, p. 29) is insufficient in terms of modern commentary and research.

THE PREPARATORY CYCLES

Whereas certain authors have contended that early phonetic and phonemic growth may be reflexive in nature, the data would seem to indicate that the converse is true. Basic reflexes, during the first year of life, are for the most part inhibited rather than enhanced or increased (Taft & Cohen, 1967, p. 92). This general process seems to be followed by increased sociovocal behavior that in turn leads to increased motor skills. These two processes, successive reflex inhibition and increased sociovocal behavior, constitute the preparatory stages of true linguistic behavior. The ability to control primitive biogenetic tendencies and the desire to assimilate into the adult linguistic culture set a foundation for phonetic/phonemic learning.

Nonlinguistic Reflexes

Many authors have concentrated on the significance of the birth cry as a beginning of verbal behavior (Berry & Eisenson, 1956, pp. 18–19; Carmichael, 1969, pp. 1–22; McCarthy, 1954, pp. 505–506; Tracy, 1909/1971, pp. 32–33). Kant opined that the birth cry represented an emotional expression of wrath, indignation, and lamentation (Carmichael, 1969, p. 11; Tracy, 1909/1971, p. 32). Blanton felt that it represented a feeling of inferiority (Carmichael, 1969). From a less pessimistic perspective, Semmig is noted as considering the birth cry as a triumphant song of life (Tracy, 1909/1971, p. 32). These early interpretations of the birth cry as expressions of intellectual or emotional significance have disappeared from the literature (McCarthy, 1954, p. 505). It is generally accepted today that the birth cry represents a physiological reflex triggered by the cold air passing into the lungs—the establishment of normal respiration for the oxygenation of the blood essential for the species.

Discussions that concentrated on the philosophical import of the cry detracted attention from the fact that the child's early life is innately preprogrammed for survival. In utero, 6 months postinsemination, the respiration reflex can be noted.

> The birth cry, for all its dramatic place in the history of thought about the infant, is not even the first sound of which the human individual is capable. There are reports in the medical literature, in cases of difficult birth, of *vagitus uterinus* or fetal crying. This phenomena is observed when the sac is ruptured before birth and the baby begins to breathe air prior to delivery (Graham, 1919). Minkowski (1922) and others have noted crying in operatively removed fetuses of approximately 6 months postinsemination age. Some components of the mechanism that makes crying possible are functional at even earlier fetal age. In operatively removed fetuses between 4 and 5 months of age the opening and closing of the mouth and rhythmic chest actions of the sort often named Ahfelds breathing movements have been observed. Air breathing, which is all-important in the first production of true human sound itself, has been reported in human fetuses in "fits and starts" before the sixth month. (Carmichael, 1969, pp. 12–13)

This onset of the reflexive phonatory power correlates with the onset of other basic reflex patterns of the third trimester of pregnancy: palmar (4–6 fetal months), plantar (4–6 fetal months), crossed extension (5–6 fetal months), pupillary (6–7 fetal months), doll's eye (6–7 fetal months), tonic neck (6–7 fetal months), Moro (7 fetal months), McCarthy's (7–8 fetal months), tibial adductor (7–8 fetal months), neck righting (7–8.5 fetal months), traction (8–9 fetal months), positive supporting (8–9 fetal months), stepping (8–9 fetal months), placing (8–9 fetal months), Galant (8–9 fetal months), and Perez (8–9 fetal months). With the exception of the persistent pupillary, sucking, and plantar reflexes, all reflexes are under control by the onset of lexical speech of the first year. Six of the major reflexes (McCarthy, rooting, doll's eye, positive supporting, stepping, and Galant) are under active inhibition by the second to the fourth month of the postgestational period. The palmar, tibial adductor, tonic neck, Moro, traction, and Perez are inhibited by the sixth postgestational month (Taft & Cohen, 1967, p. 92). These two periods of inhibition—the second to the fourth month, and the sixth to the eighth month—have been directly related to significant vocal behavior.

> There are in fact two discontinuities in the first year of life.... The two discontinuities mark off three periods. The first period, from birth through the third month, consists of a very rapid rate of change in the frequency and variety of vowel sounds and a somewhat lower though still rapid rate of change in the frequency and variety of consonant like sounds. At 4 months, the rate of change drops abruptly, thus ending the first period and starting the second.... A peak in the rate of change in the variety of vowel-like sounds occurs between the 5 and 6 months; then a peak in the rate of change in the variety of consonant like sounds at 7 months. (McNeill, 1970, p. 1132)

These stages or discontinuities emphasized by McNeill may be attributable to specific factors innate to man. As the infant is transformed from its embryonic environment, a semi-ichthyic condition, to a neonatal status, an air-breathing condition, extensive changes occur. Postembryonic differentiation, which is species specific, of course, is genetically coded. The neurological sophistication is not instantaneous and must take time, before and after the birth cry. Bever (1961) succinctly states the stages of the entire process:

> The cycles observed in vocal development are produced by phases of neurological maturation. a) The first cycle is concurrent with and presumably a manifestation of a primary level of neurological organization of vocal behavior. b) The end of the first cycle is a result of the end of the reflex stage of behavior due to cortical inhibition. c) The second vocal developmental cycle occurs as the cortex gradually reorganizes the activity it has inhibited. (p. 47)

The reflexive nature of postgestational vocalizations has long been noted by speech pathologists (Berry & Eisenson, 1956, p. 18; Van Riper, 1963, p. 83 [re: the deaf child see Ferguson & Garnica, 1975, p. 160]). Traditionally this stage has been considered a type of verbal beginning, as for instance the behavioral position (Staats, 1968, pp. 68–70; Winitz, 1969, pp. 32–48); but it may indeed be a neurological end point. In either case, whether or not one is willing to accept the broad maturational position of McNeill and Bever, the cessation of common nonverbal reflexes in the same time period is highly unusual.

THE STAGES OF DEVELOPMENT

Traditionally, the first year of vocal life has been viewed as a series of developmental stages (Berry & Eisenson, 1956, pp. 18–22) or basic building blocks (Van Riper, 1963, p. 79). A general pattern of these steps follows.

General Patterns of Prelinguistic Vocalization

Stage 1: Reflex Vocalizations   This period of language development is characterized by reflex sounds caused by discomfort. The crying is

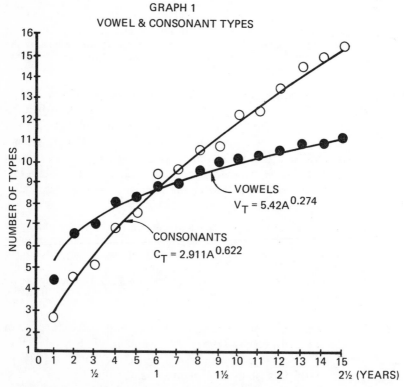

GRAPH 1
VOWEL & CONSONANT TYPES

$V_T = 5.42A^{0.274}$

$C_T = 2.911A^{0.622}$

Figure 1. Curves, with equations, showing the increase in the mean number of different vowels and consonants, respectively, in relation to increase in age for different subjects. (Adapted from Chen & Irwin, 1946, p. 28.)

an expression of hunger, cold, thirst, pain, etc. The vocalization is a total bodily reflex comparable to a startle reflex.

Stage 2: Babbling Stage (May Occur Between the Ages of 2 to 6 Months) Comfort sounds predominate. The child coos and gurgles. Sounds such as [ɪ, ɛ, ə, ʌ, k, g, ʔ, h] may predominate as single-unit gestures. This period is regarded as a play or experimentation period.

Stage 3a: Lalling Stage (May Occur Between the Ages of 6 to 12 Months) This stage is characterized by the repetition of consonant and vowel patterns, [pəpə - tətə - nənə] etc. With this behavior there is no conscious effort to socially communicate.

Stage 3b: Inflected Vocal Play (May Occur Between the Ages of 6 to 12 Months) We now find the child exercising the pitch, loudness, and duration of his or her voice. The speech is now inflected. It sounds like the child is asking questions, giving commands, acting surprised, or

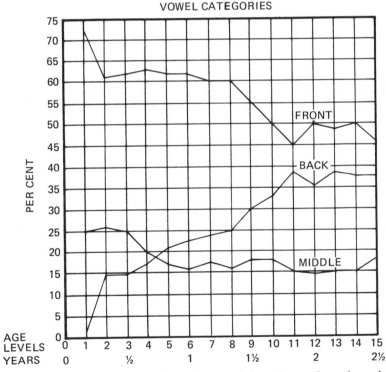

Figure 2.   Curves of progress with increasing age of three classes of vowel sounds (front, middle, back). (Adapted from Irwin, 1948, p. 32.)

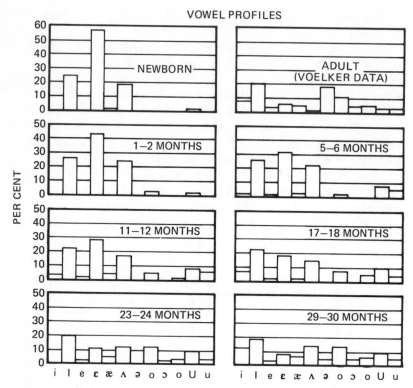

Figure 3.   Proportional values of vowels at selected age levels of the infant period. (Adapted from Irwin, 1948, p. 33.)

stating ponderous facts. However, the child still does not know any words and cannot be understood. This is the first stage when the child seems to indicate an awareness of the social importance of speech.

Stage 3c: Echolalia (May Occur Between the Ages of 6 to 12 Months)   At this stage the child is beginning to develop an acoustic awareness of the words that have been said. The child does not use words to communicate, but repeats them over and over again. This is comparable to lalling at the word level.

Stage 4: True Speech (May Occur Between the Ages of 12 to 16 Months)   This is the stage when the child begins to communicate. By talking we mean that the child intentionally uses conventional speech patterns (words), and his or her observable behavior indicates that he or she anticipates a response appropriate to the situation at hand.

VOLITIONAL VOCALIZATION

Nonreflexive, volitional vocalizations have been repeatedly reported in the studies of the 1930–1942 period (McCarthy, 1966, pp. 489–501). This nonsocial vocal behavior, commonly labeled "babbling," is associated with play and pleasure (Nakazima, 1975, p. 183; Winitz, 1969, p. 6). The child, once reflexive patterns are inhibited, is viewed as capable of producing several types of vocal output. "Cooing" (Bühler, 1930 [2 mos.]; Bühler & Hetzer, 1935 [3 mos.]; Cattell, 1940 [2 mos.]; Gesell, 1925 [4 mos.]; Gesell, Thompson, & Armatruda, 1938 [3 mos.]) and the vocalizations of pleasure (Bayley, 1933 [5.9 mos.]; Gesell & Thompson, 1934 [3 mos.]) predominate in the second to the fourth months. This self-motivated vocal activity seems to evolve concur-

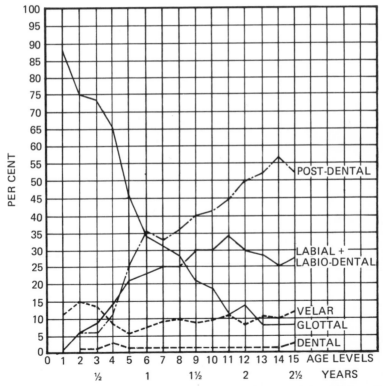

Figure 4.   Curves showing progress of developments of consonantal sounds in each of five major categories according to place of articulation. (Adapted from Irwin, 1947b, p. 399.)

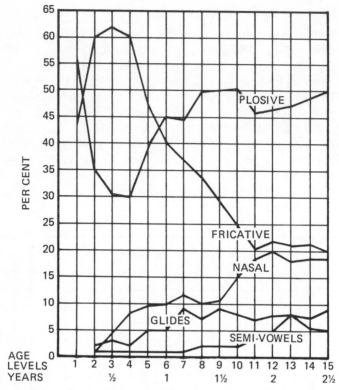

Figure 5. Curves showing the relative proportions of consonant categories according to manner of articulation. (Adapted from Irwin, 1947a, p. 404.)

rently with an increase in social awareness. Several authors have noted a consistent pattern of the child attending to the human voice (Bayley, 1933 [1.3 mos.]; Bühler & Hetzer, 1935 [2 mos.]; Cattell, 1940 [2–4 mos.]; Gesell & Thompson, 1934 [2 mos.]; Gesell, Thompson, & Armatruda, 1938 [4 mos.]). Furthermore, the child vocalizes to social stimulation (Bayley, 1933 [3.1 mos.]; Gesell & Thompson, 1934 [4 mos.]) in the same developmental period.

The type of phonetic output associated with the onset of babbling is of the most elemental forms: isolated vowels, isolated consonants, and simple consonant-vowel patterns. At birth vowel sounds predominate (see Figure 1). This pattern is maintained until approximately 1 year of age. The vowel types tend to be short in duration, and front and central in position. The [ɪ] sound (Irwin, 1948, p. 32; Van Riper, 1963, p. 78), the [ɛ] sound (Gesell, Thompson, & Armatruda, 1938; Irwin,

1948), and [ə] (Nakazima, 1975, pp. 82–83), the unstressed vowels, have a high degree of incidence. The central vowels, [ʌ] (Gesell, Thompson, & Armatruda, 1938; Irwin, 1948; Nakazima, 1975; Van Riper, 1933) and [a] (Berry & Eisenson, 1956, p. 20; Gesell, Thompson, & Armatruda, 1938), are often mentioned as early vowel-like items for babbling (see Figures 2 and 3).

In terms of consonants, "throaty" sounds (Shirley, 1933a, b) [1.3 mos.] are often mentioned. Considering the place of articulation, the glottal and velar sounds have a high degree of incidence in the second to the fourth month (Irwin, 1947a, p. 403; 1947b, p. 400). The [k] and [g] sounds (Nakazima, 1975, p. 182; Van Riper, 1963, p. 76) and the glottal stop, [ʔ], and aspirate [h] (Irwin, 1947a, p. 403) all indicate a high reliance on the posterior portion of the vocal tract in babbling activity (see Figure 4).

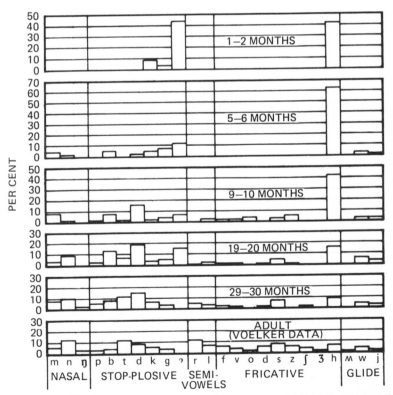

Figure 6.   Profiles for consonant usage according to manner of articulation. (Adapted from Irwin, 1947a, p. 403.)

From the point of view of manner of articulation, stop-plosives and fricatives are frequently observed. In the first 6 months, the stops appear less frequently, with a concomitant increase in the fricatives (Irwin, 1947a, p. 404). A converse trend can be noted in the post–8-month period (see Figures 5 and 6). In all, during the babbling period it may be said that the child's speech is characterized by the use of short, relaxed, front vowels; backward stop consonants; and fricatives. Furthermore, this period is highlighted by the beginning of social vocalizations (Winitz, 1969, p. 15).

APPROXIMATING THE ADULT MODEL

After the sixth month, several new aspects of prelinguistic behavior can be noted. The child, freed from nutritionally oriented behavior of the reflex period, begins to indicate a differentiated emotional system vocally. The emotional overtones of speech—the suprasegmental properties of pitch, stress, and duration—are the new object of play. The syllable patterns of the earlier babbling stage are lengthened to approximate the adult model of the social speaking pattern. These replications, or CV repetitions, permit the child to appear to speak in a strongly imitative pattern. As a culmination to this pattern, the child may produce entire words with little understanding of their real purpose. The progressively differentiated ego undergoes the social reinforcement to talk, much like any form of organic growth.

Inflected Vocal Play

The emotions of eagerness (Bayley, 1933 [5.6 mos.]; Gesell & Thompson, 1934 [5 mos.]), displeasure (Bayley, 1933 [5.9 mos.]; Gesell & Thompson, 1934 [5 mos.]), anger (Bühler, 1930 [6 mos.]), satisfaction (Bayley, 1933 [6.5 mos.]; Gesell & Thompson, 1934 [7 mos.]; q.v. Tracy, 1909/1971, p. 33), signs of recognition (Bayley, 1933 [7.4 mos.]; Gesell & Thompson, 1934 [8 mos.]), ventures into singing (Shirley, 1933 [7.3 mos.]), and interjectional sounds (Bayley, 1933 [8.1 mos.]; Gesell & Thompson, 1934 [8 mos.]) are commonly observed in the postbabbling period. It is easy to lose the forest for the trees in this stage when reviewing the basic studies. Inflected vocal play in essence is a variety of speaking states:

> Although some squeals and changes in pitch and loudness have previously occurred in babbling, it is not until about the eighth month that inflections become prominent. It is then that vocal play takes on the tonal characteristics of adult speech. We now find the baby using inflections which

sound like questions, commands, surprise, ponderous statements of facts, all in a delightful gibberish that has no meaning. We not only hear inflection and sounds of English but those of Oriental languages as well. No baby can be sure he will end up speaking English. So he practices a bit of Hottentot now and then. We have tried hard to imitate some of these sounds and inflections and have failed. (Van Riper, 1963, p. 81)

These little speaking states are best understood in terms of Mowrer's autism theory of acquisition (see Ferguson & Garnica, 1975, pp. 159–160; Winitz, 1969, p. 35). The basic theory postulates that a close bond is developed between people who bring pleasure (bird trainers, mothers, etc.) and vocal output on the part of a specific organism (bird, child, etc.). In subsequent states of isolation, the organism vocalizes in order to repeat or re-create the original state in a reminiscent pattern. This pleasurable play-acting is not a prerequisite of speech; it is merely an indication of the underlying growth in social awareness of normative suprasegmental patterns.

Echolalia

Staats (1968), as an extension of Mowrer's position, has postulated that acquisition, in its interpersonal context, is explained most readily as a form of instrumental conditioning. Whereas Mowrer's approach may be used to explain motivation, Staats's position has been formulated to explain the refinement in the production of the vocal signal. The successive growth in phonetic approximation is seen as directly under environmental control:

> The reason this [the reinforcing quality] is so important in the early development of speech is that the child's voice is so similar to the speech sounds of the parents. The more similar the child's speech sound is, the more reinforcing it will be. Following this analysis it would be expected that when the child made a vocal response that produced a sound like that in the speech of the parents, the vocal response would be more heavily reinforced than when the child produced a sound very unlike the speech sounds of the parents. (Staats, 1968, p. 68)

The ability to imitate or echo complicated words has long been observed by researchers in the 6- to 12-month period. The ability to imitate sounds (Bühler, 1930 [6 mos.]; Cattell, 1940 [9 mos.]; Gesell & Thompson, 1934 [10 mos.]; Nakazima, 1975 [10 mos.]) and words (Bayley, 1933 [11 mos.]; Bühler, 1930 [11 mos.]), the tendency to receptively attend to meaningful words (Bayley, 1933 [8.5 mos.]; Gesell & Thompson, 1934 [9 mos.]), and the ability to respond to them in a meaningful fashion (Bayley, 1933 [9.8 mos.]; Gesell & Thompson, 1934 [10 mos.], all indicate a growing sensitivity to lexemes and their components. This sensitivity no doubt results from the effects of instrumental conditioning. However, the ability to parrot or produce words does not indicate a knowledge of the importance or purpose of these elements.

> Echolalia appears markedly in some children during this period and it probably occurs in all children occasionally. By this we mean the parrot-like echoing of words he hears. Occasionally whole phrases and sentences will be repeated so faithfully that the parent fairly jumps. In one instance a year-and-a-half old girl almost wrecked a church service by saying "and ever and ever amen!" fourteen times in the middle of the preacher's sermon. She had only spoken a few words prior to this event and she never uttered the phrase again for years. (Van Riper, 1963, p. 91)

This form of vocal play, at the word level, like that of the suprasegmental or intonational level, illustrates the truth in the structural position that before true speech the child is capable of using the sounds of speech. This parrot-like behavior, however, is not communication or information exchange. The child does not need to know what a vocal cry means in order to utter it (Winitz, 1969, pp. 5–6). It is only when the child associates the vocal sign to the idea it represents, that true linguistic growth begins.

Lalling

Concurrently with the growth in intonational and phonetic skills, the child begins to appreciate basic patterns of syllable structure. Although Shirley (1933b) has noted two syllable patterns in children as young as 3 months, most authors note delineated syllabification in the post–6-month period. Bühler (1930), Gesell (1925), and Gesell and Thompson (1934) indicate 6 months of age; Bayley (1933), 6.3 months of age; Gesell, Thompson, and Armatruda (1938), 7 months. This use of repetitive syllables in the postbabbling period will set the foundation for the diminutive modifications of baby talk (see Ingram, 1974b, pp. 54–57).

$$[mama] \rightarrow [mami] \rightarrow [m\Lambda\eth\vartheta]$$
$$[dada] \rightarrow [dadi] \rightarrow [dædi]$$
$$[baba] \rightarrow [badi] \rightarrow [bad\mathbf{!}]$$

The behavior begun in play and crude imitation probably prepares phonotactic patterns for the morphophonemic rules of English. With the tremendous time requirements of the chain of speech—the need to process some 15 phonemes per *second*! (Liberman et al., 1967, p. 432; cf. House & Fairbanks, 1953, pp. 112–113; Peterson & Lehiste, 1960, p. 702)—the human productive and decoding system must have a certain degree of automaticity.

"Bob's"   [bɑbz]   Possessive

"lids"   [lɪdz]   Plural

"hides"   [haɪdz]   3rd person singular

This automaticity, that some would contend is genetic in nature, is probably a progressive motoric skill comparable to playing a musical instrument. What begins as a slow muscular motion in the early years, becomes an object of marvel in the accomplished adult.

SUMMARY

In the prelinguistic years, the successive suppression of reflexive behavior leads to the development of basic phonetic prerequisites in the acoustic and physiological domain. This behavior, nurtured and rewarded by the environment, sets the stage for cognitive-phonemic growth. The early recognition of the human voice in the babbling period leads to the demonstration of this awareness in inflected vocal play. This vocal play with its social awareness indicates a lack of phonetic skills. From the self-motivated sounds of babbling, to the syllables of lalling and the demonstrated imitative abilities of echolalia, it may be concluded that by the end of the first year of age the child, in addition to having the motivation to speak, also has the skills to speak (Berry & Eisenson, 1956, p. 21; Brown, 1968, pp. 198–199). This growth in the motivation and speech production skills is paralleled by a concurrent development in intellectual skills (Ames, 1967, passim; Ingram, 1975, pp. 7–9; 1976b, p. 16; Kessen, Haith, & Salapatek, 1970, pp. 326–328). At the age of 1½ years, the child will increase his or her vocabulary size at the rate of approximately 263% at each 3-month interval. From the third to the sixth year, the average child will add three new words to his or her vocabulary every other day (Smith, 1926). This tremendous growth rate points toward the significance of the first year. This explosive development would seem to be a result of a proper mixture of social motivation, basic motoric skills, and adequate cognitive growth. The catalyst, in turn, could be the realization of the power of the spoken word as a method of manipulating reality. As Brown (1968) points out, the ability to use a word is the essence of language (pp. 7–16). Once the sign is associated with the idea to be conveyed, the phonological process can begin. As Jakobson (1960/1971) notes, "At first child's language is devoid of any hierarchy of linguistic units and obeys the equation: one utterance–one sentence–one word–one morpheme–one phoneme–one distinctive feature" (p. 215). Distinctive feature theory is a word-oriented theory:

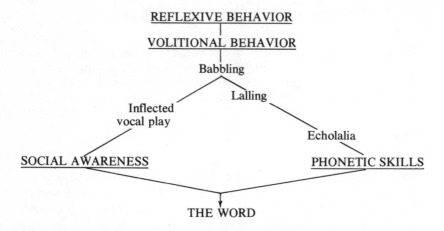

chapter 10

Jakobsonian Theory:

PHASE II

THE COGNITIVE LEVEL
  Infantemic Expansion Model
  Free Variation Model
THE PHONETIC LEVEL
  Physiological Model
  Acoustic Model
STAGES OF DEVELOPMENT
THE NONPHONEMIC STATUS OF PRELINGUISTIC VOCALIZATIONS
THE PERIOD OF SILENCE
MAXIMUM CONTRAST

In Chapter 8 it was noted that, historically, certain sound classes (velars, fricatives, back vowels, etc.) were assumed to evolve from a basic class of sounds called forward stops. In the growth of the theory this formative information is essential, for it establishes in part the validity of the theory. However, in the post–1940 period, emphasis is not placed on these evolving sound classes. With the publication of *Fundamentals of Language* (Jakobson & Halle, 1956a), the focus shifts to the properties inherent in these classes (velarization, continuation, palatalization, etc.). This emphasis was not new but served to stress the importance of the property over the phoneme. In earlier writings, circa 1929, Jakobson had tended to emphasize the collective aspects of the sound classes and referred to their emergent properties as "distinctive correlations" (Jakobson, 1962, p. 634). It was not until 1933 that he used the term "distinctive feature." This term, which emphasized the oppositional aspects of the system, he adopted from two American structuralists, Bloomfield and Sapir (Jakobson, 1962, p. 636).

In the 1956 monograph no discussion was devoted to the diachronic aspects of the theory. The broad and rich philosophical frame was missing. The emphasis was placed totally on the distinctive features, their motoric and acoustic definitions. To date, no one has integrated these definitions of the later phase with the philosophy of the earlier phase. In the following discussion the distinctive features as described in *Preliminaries to Speech Analysis* and *Fundamentals of*

Language are explained in their phonetic aspects from an acoustic and physiological point of view. These components, as will be remembered, were prerequisites from the linguistic sign level of the Genevan and Leningrad Schools. In addition to this, the type of conceptual development stressed by Baudouin de Courtenay and Saussure is used in the discussion to describe the thinking process involved in the ordering of these features into a sequence of acquisition. These two levels, *langue* and *parole,* are used in a sequenced discussion as found in the initial Jakobsonian format. In order to do this, four types of explanatory models are used: 1) an infantemic model, 2) a free variation model, 3) a physiological model, and 4) an acoustic model.

THE COGNITIVE LEVEL

The Infantemic Model

As noted earlier, no sound property or distinctive feature has a phonemic status until it is used to differentiate words (Jakobson, 1932/ 1962, pp. 231–232). It must be noted that the base of reference is the child's language and not the adult's (Jakobson, 1941/1968, p. 29). If a child interchanges the expressions [pɪn] and [bɪn], as well as [tɪn] and [dɪn], it is assumed that the voicing contrast is not relevant for the speaker. Until the child uses a distinctive feature to separate words, it is classified as allophonic in status, that is, only important to the adult system. As the child makes his or her initial phonemic distinctions, they are integrated with the previous distinctions.

This form of inhibition or refinement, from when everything (such as babbling) is possible to when no tolerance for interchange is permitted in the adult model (phonemic maturity), is seen as the basic acquisition process. These intervening cognitive categories, so confusing to the adult, are referred to as infantemes. An infanteme is a set of concurrent sound properties that serve to differentiate words of unlike meaning *in the language of the child.* These infantemes, initially broadly defined (macrophonemes in Twaddel's [1935] terminology), become narrower and narrower with successive learning. When the inclusion rules of the child equal that of the adult, the infantemes become phonemes; macrophonemes become microphonemes. The infantemic expansion model (Figure 1) illustrates these changing phonemic categories. Each category and its prerequisite criteria, which are found at higher nodes, represent the number of cognitive categories relevant to an infanteme at each step of development. From the end of the prelinguistic utterances to maturity, the child is constantly expand-

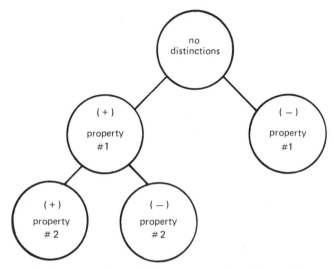

Figure 1.   Explanatory model 1: Infantemic expansion. This model represents a series of categorical refinements in the specifications of the sound system until the adult phonemic definitions are reached.

ing his infantemic definitions to meet adult phonemic rules. Ten major stages of development pertinent to the American English system are discussed in Chapters 11–18. At the end of the last stage, each end node will be labeled with the appropriate phonemic marker (/p/, /b/, /t/, etc.).

The Free Variation Model

To compare the adult model to the child's, an additional explanatory model is used. This model, the free variation model (Figure 2), represents an array of adult phonemes to which the child is being exposed. As the child uses a distinctive feature certain "substitutions" or "transformations" are observed from the adult's point of view.

In the classical linguistic sense certain sounds are in free variation. For example: ([p] = [t] = [k]) and ([b] = [d] = [g] = [m] = [n] = [ŋ]). Those sounds within a class are interchangeable, whereas those transformations across a class are not permitted. The former relationships are allophonic, the latter are phonemic. By using a larger array of sounds, it is possible to continually compare the adult system to that of the child. However, one must be cautious in making inferences from the adult model to that of the child (Winitz, 1969, p. 8). The child is not perceiving adult sounds as such; he or she is responding to the features or properties that are known. It is only those properties that have been learned that are significant. D. B. Fry (1967), from

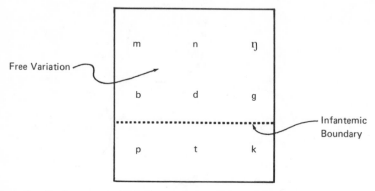

Figure 2.   Explanatory model 2: Free variation. This model represents a comparison of the child's phonemic rules as compared to the adult system.

University College London, has described the entire process with precision:

> The child's changes of articulation under the pressure of adult responses to his utterances are the first steps toward establishing the phonemic system. The goal of being understood by everyone is not reached until the system is complete. Naturally, the forty-odd units of the English phonemic system, for example, do not crystallize simultaneously in the child's speech. In the earliest utterances that are used consistently, that is to say, in specific situations and with specific referents, only two or three phonemes may be involved. The boy who uses /mama/ and /dada/ and no other words in this meaningful way has a system of just three units, for *the system must be thought of as being at each stage complete in itself* [emphasis mine]. The English child does not start with a set of forty pigeonholes of which the majority remain to be occupied during the development of speech; he is actively constructing the framework, and, as each pigeonhole is added, the shape of the whole structure and particularly the interrelationships are changing. (p. 194)

The free variation model illustrates the pigeonholes as they are being constructed. As each new property is added to the system, it is illustrated by a dotted line. This line represents a restriction in free variation; it serves as a boundary that no longer can be crossed. Sounds within an unrestricted space are in free variation, meaning they are used interchangeably from the adult point of view. From the child's perspective, there are no differences. In reference to the boundary, the sounds are not interchangeable because they make words different in the language of the child.

The infantemic model represents the same information as that found in the free variation model. However, certain aspects of phonemic development are emphasized by each. In the infantemic model, the sequence of the development of the child is of paramount importance. Furthermore, the adult phonemic system is ignored. The free variation model constantly compares the child's system to the adult's but ignores for the most part the sequence of development. The commonality of the two models is the infanteme. The number of end nodes of the generating phonemic system is equal to the number of "pigeonholes" in the free variation model. A combined model, of course, could be created, but it would be at the expense of the highlights, the infantemic sequence and the adult/child comparisons.

THE PHONETIC LEVEL

Two additional explanatory models can be used to monitor the phonetic substance of the two infantemes. One model illustrates significant *acoustic* information, the other model illustrates significant *physiological* information. Each aspect of the infanteme, the acoustic and physiological parameters, is essential to the distinctive feature models previously discussed.

The manner in which the child learns to discriminate between two sound classes, using auditory information, is an important prerequisite to the production of the linguistic utterance. This process establishes the language-specific goals. The subsequent comprehension of the physiological requirements that will produce the target sound completes the acquisition process. The comprehension and internalization of the goal utterance is linked, so to speak, with the specific postures needed to produce the goal utterance. These two aspects of the phonetic level, once they are internalized, form the basic feedback loop. While the child is producing, he/she is constantly monitoring his/her own acoustic product in comparison to the perceived cultural norm.

The Physiological Model

The physiological model is simply a series of anatomical drawings that incorporates basic knowledge of articulatory phonetics into the larger theory. It is presumed that all students of the theory are familiar with midsaggital displays of the human articulatory apparatus. This information, contained in basic texts in phonetics, is essential for a full appreciation of the eclectic power of the theory. Distinctive feature theory organizes contemporary information in articulatory phonetics and speech science into its larger linguistic/cognitive domain. These midsaggital displays, unlike contemporary information, illustrate the cognitive emphasis placed on certain articulatory structures by the evolving infantemic system. These illustrations represent one aspect of

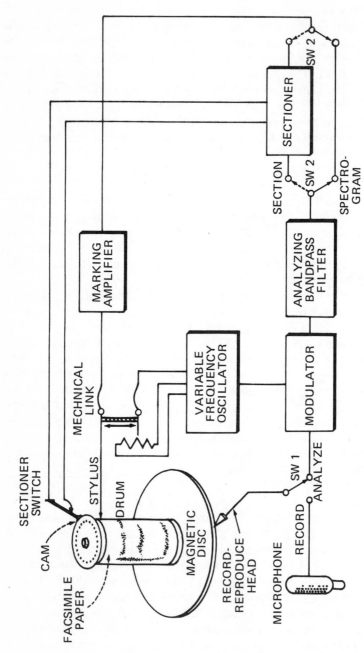

Figure 3.   Functional diagram of the sound spectrograph. (Based on Flanagan, 1965, p. 127.)

the phonetic substance incorporated into the basic differential unit. In other words, the illustrations picture the physiological posture and motions that are perceived as important. It is the perception of the articulation that is of essence, not the posture in and of itself.

The Acoustic Model

Whereas the physiological model emphasizes information derived from articulatory phonetics, the acoustic model is based upon illustrations of the speech signals and their concomitant properties in the domains of frequency, intensity, and time. Most typically, the acoustic manifestation of the infantemes are illustrated by means of sonographic displays (spectral displays) sometimes referred to as sonograms. A basic understanding of the typical phonemic representations presented by the sonogram can enhance the same information portrayed by the physiological model.

The sonogram is a 12.5 × 4 inch piece of heat-sensitive paper printed by means of a complicated acoustic analyzer (see Figure 3). This paper, in a very real sense, represents a three-dimensional display of the speech sounds. The picture displays the frequency of the sound, the intensity of the sound, and the time of the sound (Figure 4). The frequency of the sound is displayed vertically from the baseline to the top of the print. The range usually encompasses a span from a low component of 0 Hz (approximately) to 8000 Hz, the upper limit. This does not represent the range of human hearing, roughly 20–20,000 Hz, but it does represent the range of human hearing considered most significant for human speech. From the point of view of the sonogram, the lower the frequency component the lower the indication on the vertical dimension.

The time production of the sound is represented horizontally from left to right on the display. In terms of each sonogram, the duration is 2.4 seconds long. As previously mentioned, this is a long period when

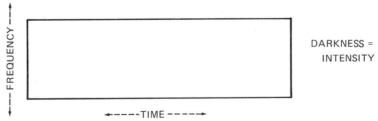

Figure 4.   Representation of sonogram illustrating the coordinates of frequency, intensity, and time.

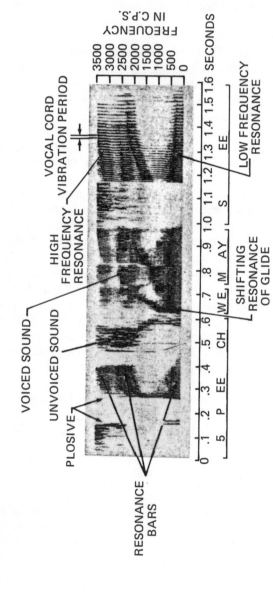

Figure 5. Sound spectrogram of the words, "Speech we may see," using a wide-band analyzing filter (300 Hz) to emphasize vocal resonances. (Adapted from Potter, Kopp, & Kopp, 1966, p. 12.)

one considers the average time needed in the production of each speech segment. Common expressions for initial study—"Joe took father's shoe-bench out!" (approximately 23 segments), or "Wee Willie ate many apples" (21 segments)—fit fairly easily into the 2.4-second time span. Longer sonograms are possible, but this length is most typical. In all, short sounds, such as consonants, occupy little horizontal distance, whereas longer sounds, such as vowels, occupy more space. As noted in Figure 5, the visual perspective of the consonants appears to "go up and down" whereas the vowels appear to "go across" in terms of the display.

The intensity of the sound is indicated by the darkness of the print. Areas with darker print are more intense than gray or white areas. Where the sonogram is white no significant sound was detected by the filters. It sometimes helps to think of the darker areas as being comparable to the peaks of a mountain rising upward from the paper; the lighter areas are comparable to valleys hidden beneath the clouds.

As might be guessed, the inexact nature of the intensity component of the sonogram causes problems. Because of this, a second type of display is available. This type of display, a "section," illustrates one moment in time, with the frequency and intensity being the objective coordinates (Figure 6). In Figure 6, intensity, measured in decibels, is displayed vertically. The more intense the sound at any given frequency, the higher the "peaks of the mountain"; the less intense, the lower the "valleys." By relating the sections to the sonogram it is possible to create a three-dimensional display of any sound. Although this three-dimensional display (Figure 7) represents the complexity of the acoustic substance the child is being exposed to, all discussions are oriented to one or the other displays for the sake of clarity. It is easier to see the acoustic portrayals of the distinctive features by using either the section or the sonogram, but not both.

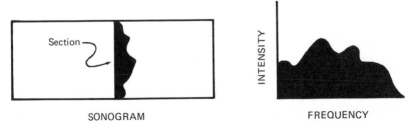

Figure 6.   Representation of sonogram illustrating the coordinates of frequency and intensity as portrayed on a sonographic display of a section.

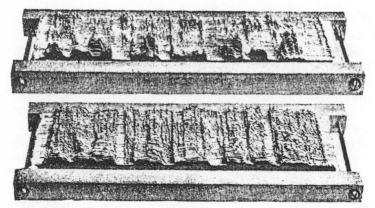

Figure 7.   A solid model built up of oscillograms similar to those of Figure 5, for 222 overlapping frequency bands. The words are, "visual telephone for the deaf." The two models differ in the amount of amplitude compression. (From Koenig, Dunn, & Lacy, 1946, p. 23.)

STAGES OF DEVELOPMENT

By a total integration of the cognitive and phonetic components of the infantemes, a comprehensive linguistic description of the developmental sequence is possible. The stages of infantemic development, and their implications for the adult model, take on more meaning in their acoustic and physiological contexts. There are 10 basic stages of development discussed in this format, and each stage is presented by means of each of the explanatory models: infantemic, free variation, acoustical, physiological.

1. Consonantal/ vocalic
2. Nasal/ non-nasal
3. Labial/ dental (I. Consonants)
4. Compact/ diffuse (I. Vowels)
5. Grave/ acute (II. Vowels)
6. Compact/ diffuse (II. Consonants)
7. Flat/ plain
8. Continued/ interrupted
9. Tense/ lax (Voiced-voiceless)
10. Strident/ mellow

Each of these stages represents significant cognitive milestones in the child's paradigmatic development. The evolutionary process, which begins with no phonemic distinctions in the prelinguistic stage, is developed through to the adult model at stage 10 (Chapters 11–18).

THE NONPHONEMIC STATUS OF PRELINGUISTIC VOCALIZATIONS

Although, by the end of the first year the child has acquired the basic skills for phonemic differentiation and is highly motivated to communicate, no culturally specific consistency is maintained in day-to-day output. To test this idea Olney and Scholnick (1976) asked 59 college students, ages 18–20, to determine whether speech samples of young children's babbling could be identified when the children were selected from two different linguistic communities, English and Toisanese (a Chinese dialect). The students were asked to identify the cultural background of the children from three age groups: 6 months, 12 months, and 18 months. In this and a subsequent design, the authors concluded that adult speakers could not identify the linguistic community of the children, but they could identify the age levels. As the authors note:

> It is possible that before the use of language in a meaningful way the child's vocalization is also characterized by cues which distinguish it clearly as prelinguistic. The child may use different prosodic features or draw from a different phoneme pool than when he uses language meaningfully. This distinctly prelinguistic vocalization may be universal. If so, then the samples used should not differ despite their linguistic origins. This interpretation is, of course, similar to Jakobson's (1968) and is one of the contrasting views which inspired this research. (Olney & Scholnick, 1976, p. 154)

This ability to produce the sounds most common to the languages of the world, the universals, marks the diminution of prelinguistic behavior and the onset of true speech.

THE PERIOD OF SILENCE

Just before the child's acquisition of the first word, Jakobson (1941/1968) reports that the child undergoes a period of silence. "As all observers acknowledge with great surprise, the child then loses nearly all his ability to produce sounds in passing over from the prelanguage stage to the first acquisition of words, i.e., to the first genuine stage of language" (p. 21). This phenomenon, it may be concluded, is a result of confusion and disorganization. The child, who can speak so many languages in general, must learn to speak one in particular. Each particular language has a set pattern of phonemic acquisition that is optimal. These sound properties have an optimal learning sequence.

MAXIMUM CONTRAST

Although Jakobson rejects Buffon's and Schultze's contention that sounds which are easiest to produce are learned first, he does have a similar approach. The order of acquisition of the sound properties, as opposed to phonemes, is governed by a principle referred to as maximal contrast:

> Only in light of an inherently linguistic and comprehensive procedure does the sequence of stages of phonemic systems turn out to be meaningful and rigorously consistent. This sequence obeys the principle of maximal contrast and procedes from the simple and undifferentiated to the stratified and differentiated. (Jakobson, 1941/1968, p. 68; cf. 1939c/1971, p. 79)

Also:

> This system is by its very nature closely related to those stratified phenomena which modern psychology uncovered in the different areas of the realm of the mind. Development proceeds "from an undifferentiated original condition to a greater and greater differentiation and separation [citing Jaensch (1928)]." (Jakobson, 1941/1968, p. 65)

What Jakobson is saying is that the grossest phonemic contrasts are learned before the more refined, more difficult contrasts. In comparison to Schultze they seem to agree! For example:

> In which sequence do the vowels gradually emerge in the child language ... in the series A-U-O, the extremes are A and U because the lips and tongue are least removed from their position of rest in the case of A, most in the case of U. In this regard O occupies a midway position.... The latter apparently requires a more practiced and experienced feeling of accomodation and innervation, as in general coarser contrasts are perceived more easily than the intermediate, more delicate transitions. (Schultze, 1880/1971, pp. 28–29)

Whereas both authors may be compared on the general agreement that gross motor contrasts are learned before fine motor contrasts, Jakobson goes several steps further. Schultze's position was restricted to the motoric manifestation of the contrast, whereas Jakobson retained the position that gross and fine distinctions need not necessarily be restricted to the motoric aspect of the phonemic decision. Phonemic decisions are based upon acoustic contrasts. They are also based on semantic contrasts. At each stage the semantic, acoustic, and motoric contrasts are simultaneously bound and maximal in character. The reception, retention, and production of these infantemes are centered around this psychological Gestalt. At each end of the 10 developmental stages, the maximal character of the semantic, acoustic, and motoric contrasts (Figure 8) are used as discussion points for the following chapters.

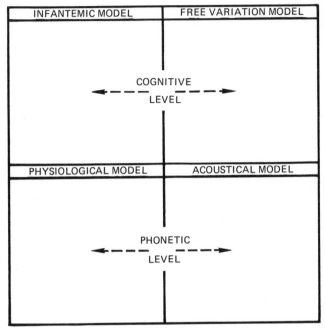

Figure 8.   Basic diagram for illustrating each of the 10 stages of development. The elements being maximally contrasted will be found in each of four quadrants.

chapter 11

Stages of
Development:

STAGE 1—
Consonantal/Vocalic

THE COGNITIVE LEVEL
THE PHYSIOLOGICAL MODEL
THE ACOUSTIC MODEL

With the learning of the first meaningful word, the child begins the construction of the phonological system (Jakobson, 1941/1968, p. 85). This period generally appears between 12 and 18 months (Cattell, 1940 [11 months]; Johnson, Darley & Spriestersbach, 1963 [before 18 months]; Shirley, 1933b [14 months]; q.v. Darley & Winitz, 1961; McCarthy, 1966, pp. 523–526). This first sound contrast, the consonantal versus vocalic feature, establishes two major infantemic classes, the consonants and the vowels.

THE COGNITIVE LEVEL

In terms of sound categories, this dichotomy is the most primitive or nascent. Sounds that generally represent the consonantal class are the forward stops (Jakobson, 1941/1968, p. 47). As noted in phase I of the theory (Chapter 8), these include [p], [b], [t], [d], etc. Although any consonant is *possible* to meet the requirements of the class, [p] is understood to be more highly *probable* (Jakobson & Halle, 1956a, p. 37). The vowel class, it is generally posited, is represented by the "wide, neutral vowel" (Jakobson, 1941/1968, pp. 47, 71, 85; Jakobson & Halle, 1956a, p. 37). A word such as "papa" is typical and representative (Jakobson, 1960/1971, p. 213).

Not only does the consonantal/vocalic property indicate the first restriction in the free variation model (see Figure 1), it has implications for the syntagmatic axis. The labial stop in conjunction with the /a/ vowel forms the basic pattern of the syllable (Jakobson, 1941/1968, p. 71). The CV pattern, as Jakobson notes (1941/1968, p. 85), is repeated in the child's speech in a CV-CV format. This pattern indicates the

PHONEMIC STAGE #1

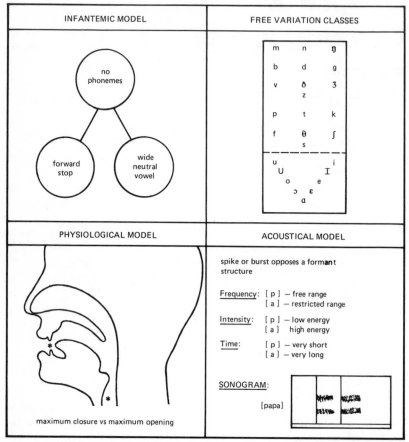

Figure 1.   Four different representations of consonantal/vocalic as viewed from cognitive and phonetic perspectives.

freedom of the syllable and its true independence. These two significant developments—the first distinctive feature and the basic syllable—are cognitive milestones; they are predetermined because of maximal contrast.

THE PHYSIOLOGICAL MODEL

From a physiological point of view, the consonant represents maximal closure (Jakobson, 1941/1968, p. 69; Jakobson & Halle, 1956a, p. 37) or restriction (Jakobson, 1939c/1971, p. 79), whereas the vowel represents maximum opening or dilation. This vertical contrast, open versus closed tract, is maximal because no closure is greater than [p] and no opening is greater than [a]:

> From the articulatory point of view, the two constituents of this utterance represent polar configurations of the vocal tract: in /p/ the tract is closed at its very end while in /a/ it is opened as widely as possible at the front and narrowed toward the back, thus assuming the horn shape of a megaphone. (Jakobson & Halle, 1956a, p. 37)

Although the point of emphasis is the vertical axis, it should be noted that the horizontal axis is hinted as being significant.

Unlike the current-day American phonetician's orientation, Jakobson's theory is European in derivation. This causes problems in certain areas. During the formulation of the theory, Lepsius's conception of the cardinal vowel system was the working vocalic model (see Albright, 1958, p. 28; cf. Jakobson, 1941/1968, pp. 79, 82/84; Jakobson & Halle, 1956a, pp. 38–40). In this array five vowels are used as optimal reference points in the system:

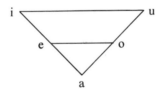

This system, which is basic to Japanese (Ishiki, 1957, p. 392), is a true triangle. Many authors (Albright, 1958, p. 7; Kantner & West, 1960, pp. 103–166; Ladefoged, 1975, pp. 194–198; Leutennegger, 1963, pp. 36–37; Pike, 1964, pp. 15, 18) following the lead of Jones have opted for an eight-point quadrilateral labeled a "triangle." (See abovementioned authors, as well as Carrell & Tiffany, 1960, p. 32; Faircloth & Faircloth, 1973, pp. 11–12.) It can be seen that European authors such as Karlgren (1968, p. 131) and Malmberg (1963, pp. 14–15) and the early editions of the International Phonetic Association alphabet (Albright, 1958, p. 55 [1900]; p. 56 [1914]) rely or relied on this model. Without going into the merits of the two configurations as physiological predictors, it can simply be observed that the triangle should be accepted for pedantic convenience. The quadrilateral format is not incompatible with the theory, and the triangle simplifies the discussion.

Now, in reference to the feature consonantal/vocalic, it should be noted that /a/ is the one vowel which represents maximal opening. Furthermore, the /a/ is implied to be "passive" in production, whereas

the consonant is implied to require muscular energy in the supralaryngeal articulatory areas (Jakobson, 1941/1968, p. 85). Not only is
the presence or absence of articulatory energy maximal in its own
domain, the horizontal distance is maximal. The forward stop, such as
[p], occupies one end point of the vocal tract; the infralaryngeal closure
necessary for the voicing of the vowel occupies the other end point of
the vocal tract. All sounds that are produced in subsequent stages will
occupy positions within these limits.

The maximal contrasts possible in the vertical domain, the horizontal domain, and the energy component each serve as natural factors
that begin and shape the organization process. What is universal to
man are the human vocal tract and articulatory structures (Lieberman
et al., 1971, pp. 725–726; Stampe, 1973, pp. 1–2). The natural structures
and the limitations of these functions serve as a cognitive frame for the
onset of phonemic growth.

THE ACOUSTIC MODEL

Maximal contrast is also demonstrable in the acoustic domain. The end
points of the frequency, intensity, and time scales of the world of
physics are used as references to the sound system.

> The labial stop presents a momentary burst of sound without any great
> concentration of energy in a particular frequency band, whereas in the
> vowel /a/ there is no strict limitation of time, and the energy is concen-
> trated in a relatively narrow region of maximum aural sensitivity. In the
> first constituent there is an extreme limitation in the time domain but no
> ostensible limitation in the frequency domain, whereas the second con-
> stituent shows no ostensible limitation in the time domain but a maximum
> limitation in the frequency domain. (Jakobson & Halle, 1956a, p. 37)

Referring to the acoustic model, it may be seen that the consonant /p/
makes use of the entire frequency range; it is restricted maximally in
terms of time, and it tends to be very weak in terms of energy output
(Flanagan, 1965, pp. 50–51). The vowel, on the other hand, especially
/a/, is restricted in terms of the frequency range to a central domain
(Peterson & Barney, 1952, p. 183) with two relatively close formants.
The time of production, in contrast to the stop, is optimal. The vowel is
maximally long. The energy of the vowel /a/ is unimpeded. Each of
these parameters—frequency, intensity, and time—establish, again,
natural parameters to guide the acquisition process. It would seem that
these features are inherent to the acoustic domain and predetermined.
As Lafon (1968) notes, "Phonetic mistakes in identification increase
with the subtlety of the discrimination involved: the distinction be-

tween vocoids and contoids is certainly the easiest, and is the one in which the deaf subject with identification troubles makes the least mistakes'' (p. 96). The developmental predominance of the consonant in the initial position, although it is not essential to the theory, is found in American English (Irwin, 1951, p. 161). (Refer to Figure 1, Chapter 9).

Finally, the primary cycle of the syllable, from a physiological viewpoint, aids in the integration of the paradigmatic theory of Jakobson with the coarticulatory theory of McDonald (1964, pp. 5–9). Although the latter theory is more restricted in nature, because of its physiological base (McDonald has an abiding interest in cerebral palsy), it carefully avoids direct contradiction with the more abstract theory (McDonald, 1964, pp. 14–16).

chapter 12

Stages of
Development:
STAGE 2—Nasal/Non-Nasal

THE INFANTEMIC MODEL
THE FREE VARIATION MODEL
THE SEMANTIC CONTRAST
A POSSIBLE EXPLANATION
THE PHYSIOLOGICAL MODEL
THE ACOUSTIC MODEL
  A Personal Observation
FORMAL DEFINITIONS

Once the child begins to establish an understanding of the properties that signal consonantal versus vocalic characteristics, the focus of attention shifts to the consonantal class (Jakobson, 1939c/1971, p. 81). Considering the passive aspects of the vowel, this is not unusual.

THE INFANTEMIC MODEL

The forward stop infantemic class is subdivided into two subclasses, a nasal class and a non-nasal class (Jakobson, 1941/1968, pp. 47–48). (See Figure 1.) The resultant number of infantemes is three. At this stage it is possible to split the vowels into two groups, a nasal class and a non-nasal class. However, this contrast is not pertinent to American English. Nasal vowels are not used in our language. It is interesting to note that the denasal node is culturally bound in English, whereas its counterpart is bound for languages such as French. Transposition of either property in either culture creates qualitative or dialectical differences rather than phonemic problems.

THE FREE VARIATION MODEL

From the adult perspective /m/, /n/, and /ŋ/ may vary freely in the nasal, forward stop class; the remaining consonants vary freely in the non-nasal class. Of course, the vowels themselves are free-varying, with /a/ being the most probable. Whereas /p/ was the most probable forward stop for all the consonants in stage 1, it is retained as a representative

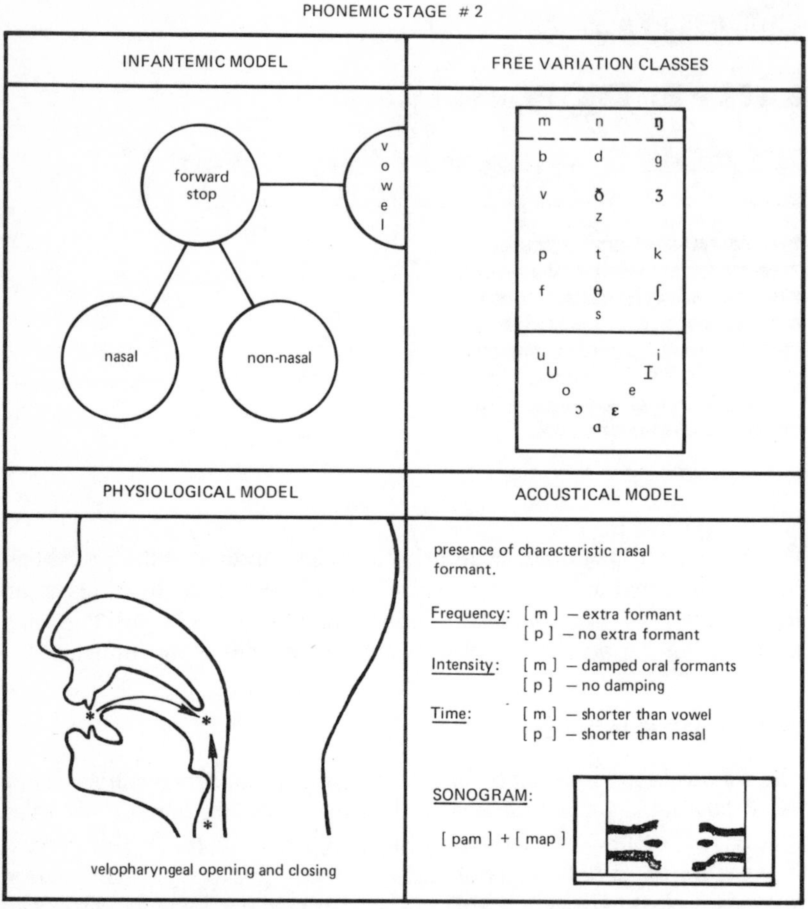

PHONEMIC STAGE # 2

Figure 1.   Four different representations of nasal/non-nasal as viewed from cognitive and phonetic perspectives.

for the non-nasal subclass. The most probable nasal stop is /m/. This infanteme produces the significant minimal pairs' contrast *mama* versus *papa* (see Jakobson, 1960/1971).

THE SEMANTIC CONTRAST

At the semantic level several observations can be made. Jakobson has long maintained that nasality is a universal property contained in all languages (1941/1968, pp. 47–48; cf. 1966, p. 265). He has held this contention because of an unusual aspect of the phonemic properties of the kinship terms for the father and mother as found in various societies (Jakobson, 1960/1971, p. 538). Almost all the utterances used to designate the mother, for instance, begin with the bilabial nasal /m/ (see Figure 2). This characteristic has been corroborated by Murdock (1959) and Ferguson (1964). Jakobson, although not inclined to Freudian explanations (q.v. 1939c/1971, pp. 78–79), does connect this sound property to emotion (1941/1968, pp. 72–73) and the maternal cultural role (1960/1971, p. 543).

Unlike other Indo-European languages, English is syntactically and morphologically sex free. However, the older languages have constantly maintained sex-specific articles, prefixes, suffixes, and declensions. This tendency has created an intensive classification of the world into male and female objects. Trying to break friends of the habit of referring to my bitch as "he" and my Tom cat as "she" sensitized me to this phenomenon. The early recognition of the face by infants, as

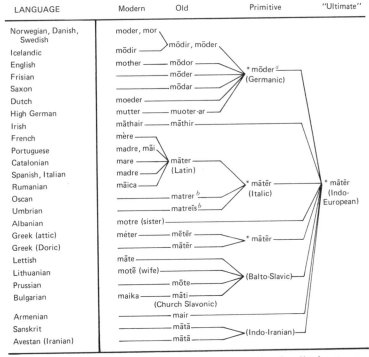

Figure 2.   Evolution and distribution of the kinship term "mother." [a] denotes reconstructed forms by asterisks. [b] genetive forms of the word, corresponding to Latin *māter*. Extant inscriptions contain no nominative form. (Adapted from Gray & Wise, 1969, p. 341.)

demonstrated by Kagan (1967, pp. 336–348), would lead to the conclusion that the nurturing object is of major importance to the young child. It is hard to forget, even now, the olfactory and visual cues that separated my father and my mother. The occupational cues (in this case the white paper pulp on pants legs—he was a paper maker), six o'clock chin whiskers (which I thought could saw wood), and perspiration contrasted sharply with adipose tissue, long hair, and perfume. This male/female dichotomy is a general way of classifying the world, from rough to smooth, so to speak.

> Since the mother is, in Gregoire's parlance *le grande dispensatrice,* most of the infant's longings are addressed to her, and children being prompted and instigated by the extant nursery words, gradually turn the nasal interjection into a parental term, and adapts its expressive makeup to their regular phonemic pattern. (Jakobson, 1960/1971, p. 216)

Although some may find the semantic dichotomy difficult to accept at face value, additional support is available in the physiological realm.

A POSSIBLE EXPLANATION

During nursing behavior, the child is often reported to emit a "nasal murmur" (Jakobson, 1960/1971, p. 542). As the child ingests liquid, from breast or bottle, the velopharyngeal port is closed, allowing a negative pressure buildup for "sucking." Once the liquid passes into the esophagus, the velopharyngeal port opens, permitting life-sustaining respiration. The lips are generally not removed from the food source. This opening and closing of the velum, triggered by cycles of ingestion and respiration, is naturally associated with the mother. This property in a period of months apparently is associated with the child's favorite object, "le grande dispensatrice." It should be noted in passing from the maximal contrast at the semantic level to the physiological level that the velar activity is the one articulatory movement not under ready conscious control. To elicit nasalization or velar activity diagnostically, it is common to ask the child to imitate a nasal sound, [a - ã - a - ã], rather than instruct the child to move the articulators.

THE PHYSIOLOGICAL MODEL

The physiological model shows that the velopharyngeal port is located at an intermediate point horizontally between the forward stop and the laryngeal activity of the passive vowel. Once the end points of the bipolar scale have been used, the midpoint then becomes the next optimal contrast. This aspect of the nasal/non-nasal contrast was not emphasized by Jakobson. Instead, he stressed the idea that the obstructed tract of the consonant and the open tract of the vowel could be contrasted by a tract that is *both* open at the port and closed at the lips (Jakobson, 1941/1968, p. 71). The presence and absence of a closed tract (Jakobson & Halle, 1956a, p. 38) seems to violate the logical properties of the theory. The (+) versus (−) signs have a phonemic meaning until one presents the (±) as an alternative. This choice, in symbols, may shift the frame from a phonemic to a phonetic concept in the minds of many people. In any case, the theory was brought forward with the former, phonemic, strategy in mind.

THE ACOUSTIC MODEL

No authors challenge the early onset of the acoustic property. This supports the feature's hierarchical validity. In the acoustic domain, the property is less clearly maximal. The idea that the significant cues are a result of subsidiary resonance (Jakobson & Halle, 1956a, p. 37) was simplified from the work with Fant in *Preliminaries to Speech Analysis*. An additional formant (citing Joos—Jakobson, Fant, & Halle, 1952–1967, p. 39) and a higher formant density or additional spectral poles and zeros were used as the working acoustic definition (Fant, 1968, p. 237). In Fant's strategy (1973, p. 13), he has ranked the formant restrictions as being the most important aspect. From the child's primitive viewpoint, however, the extra formant, or the damping characteristics of the spectrum, may be of secondary importance. The nasal sounds are longer than consonants and shorter than vowels (see Potter, Kopp, & Kopp; 1947/1966, pp. 166–201). This again is an intermediate contrast.

There is general agreement that nasality is a valid phonemic property. It appears in all the major distinctive feature systems proposed since the first one in 1952 (Blache, 1970, p. 3; Singh, 1976, pp. 90–91). Jakobson, Fant, and Halle (1952–1967), Miller and Nicely (1955), Halle (1961), Wickelgren (1966), Singh and Black (1966), Voiers (1967), Chomsky and Halle (1968), Ahmed and Agrawal (1969), and Singh, Woods, and Becker (1972) have all proposed nasality as a significant sound property. The separation of [m + n + ŋ] from all other consonants, as a class, seem to be one logical operation that all theoreticians would support as crucial to the adult model.

A Personal Observation

At the time of this writing my 10-month-old son, Nathan, is just beginning to communicate socially. His first expression, used with consistency, was learned at the changing table. Our cat is in the habit of lying on the table with the child as his diapers are being changed by my wife. She in turn tried to teach him to say the word "kitty." He began to use his approximation [θʌθʌ - θɛθɛ - θ̬ʌθ̬ʌ], which represents little more than a bisyllabic, consonant/vowel contrast, at the beginning of the ninth month. This production was apparently an approximation of the place characteristics of the medial consonant [t], plus an approximation of the continuous, dragging characteristics sometimes found with velars (see Potter, Kopp, & Kopp, 1947/1966, pp. 94–104). This durational cue (manner) specific to the velar, and the lingua-alveolar/dental cue (place), apparently are the significant properties perceived. For the consonant, neither /t/ or /k/ is realized; what is produced is an unclear approximation of both sounds. This phenomenon, a form of progressive/regressive/reciprocal assimilation, was observed by Schleicher as early as 1861 (see Bar-Adon & Leopold, 1971, p. 19 [condition 3]).

Incidentally, Nathan consistently uses his approximation of "kitty" in the presence of small, furry, four-legged animals. He also calls our bitch, a white sheltie, [θʌθʌ - θɛθɛ - θ̬ʌθ̬ʌ]. Because he has labeled both objects in the same way, and has never used this expression in any situation without either animal, this expression constitutes his first word.

The adult expression "No! No!" was Nathan's second target approximation. [nʌnʌ - nɛnɛ - n̬ʌn̬ʌ] are used interchangeably for forbidden behavior: attempts to destroy books, eating dirt, removing pens and pencils from his father's pockets. Little conscience is apparent, for the "words" are chanted as the acts are going on! It is interesting to note that my wife does not believe in negative verbal reinforcers but prefers to distract the child with more suitable toys. "No! No!" is my expression. Somewhere between the world of mother's dressing table and father's plants, pens, and books the child has learned a significant minimal pair. The [nʌnʌ, etc.] versus [θʌθʌ, etc.] contrast, although atypical from the realm of probability of representative sounds, does meet the requirements of stage 2 behavior, a nasal/non-nasal contrast. Furthermore, the labels seem to be associated with sociosexual roles.

FORMAL DEFINITIONS

Nasal (versus Non-Nasal or Oral)

Acoustic Definition

1) a. Spreading of energy over wider (versus narrower) regions by
    b. A reduction in the intensity of certain (primarily the first) formants and

    c. Introduction of additional (nasal) formants. (From Jakobson & Halle, 1956a, p. 30; 1956b/1962, p. 485)

2) a. A higher formant density

    b. A nasal murmur that produces two constant and clear formants (one at about 200 Hz and another at about 2500 Hz)

    c. The additional poles and zeros, caused by nasalization, are a local distortion in the spectrum without any influence on the other resonance features. (From Jakobson, Fant, & Halle, 1952/1967, pp. 39–40)

Physiological Definition

1) a. Mouth resonator supplemented by the nasal cavity versus the exclusion of the nasal resonator. (Jakobson & Halle, 1956a, p. 30; 1956b/1962, p. 485)

2) a. Formed by the air stream that escapes from the larynx through the mouth cavity only.... Produced with a lowering of the soft palate, so that air is bifurcated and the mouth resonator is supplemented by the nasal cavity. (Jakobson, Fant, & Halle, 1952/1967, p. 40; Halle, 1964, p. 327)

chapter 13

Stages of
Development:

STAGE 3—Labial/Dental
(Grave/Acute I)

THE INFANTEMIC MODEL
THE FREE VARIATION MODEL
  A Semantic Aside
THE PHYSIOLOGICAL MODEL
THE ACOUSTIC MODEL
PROBLEMS WITH TERMINOLOGY
RESEARCH SUPPORT
ANOTHER PERSPECTIVE
THE NOISE COMPONENT

The third stage of infantemic development centers around further development of the consonantal system. As noted by Faircloth and Faircloth (1973, pp. 78–79) some 75% of all syllables are released by consonants. In addition to this, 57% of all syllables are arrested by consonants. This reliance upon consonants in adult language, a phenomenon that can be corroborated by the works of Dewey and others (Flanagan, 1965, p. 5), would seem to mirror infantemic development in the child.

THE INFANTEMIC MODEL

In Jakobson's third stage (1941/1968, pp. 67–68, 84; Jakobson & Halle, 1956a, p. 41) the nasal consonantal class and the non-nasal consonantal class are both subdivided into more refined infantemes. This cognitive decision, in gross detail, separates "lip sounds" from "tongue sounds." This operation yields five infantemes: four consonantal and one vocalic (see Figure 1):

1. A *labial,* non-nasal consonant
2. A *dental,* non-nasal consonant
3. A *labial,* nasal consonant

PHONEMIC STAGE # 3

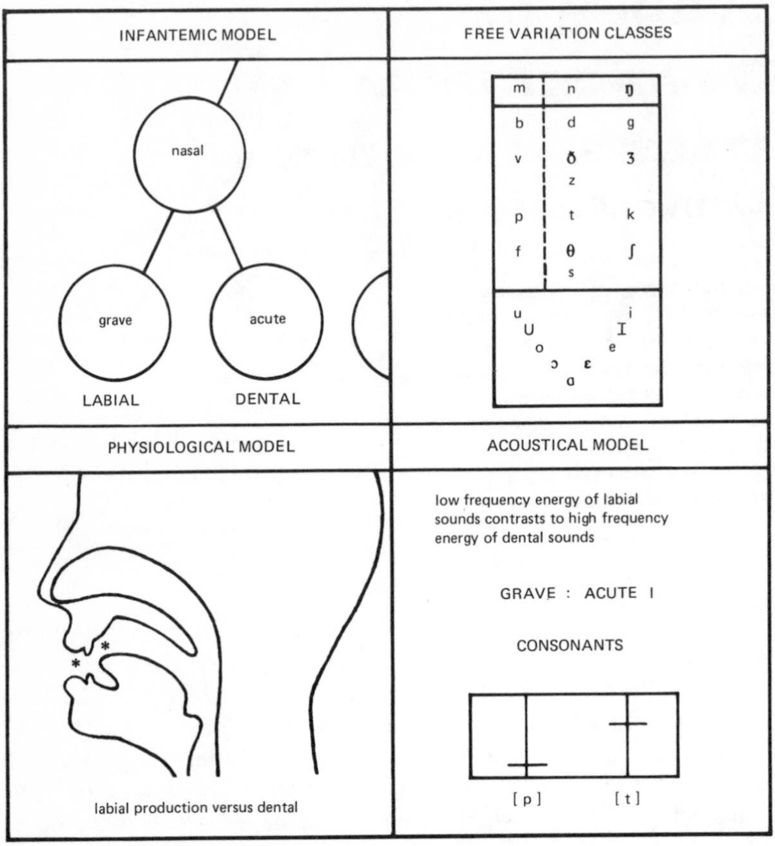

| INFANTEMIC MODEL | FREE VARIATION CLASSES |

Figure 1.   Four different representations of labial/dental (grave/acute I) as viewed from cognitive and phonetic perspectives.

4.   A *dental*, nasal consonant
5.   A passive vowel
These five classes contain a different number of allophones from the point of view of the adult model.

THE FREE VARIATION MODEL

In the labial, non-nasal class /p/, /b/, /f/, and /v/ vary freely to form the /p = b = f = v/ infanteme. In the dental, nasal class /n = ŋ/ is phonemic. The adult phoneme /m/ is realized in the generative sense at this stage such that the infanteme equals the adult phoneme. All the remaining adult phonemes will appear to vary freely in the non-nasal, dental class. Finally, all vowels are in free variation.

A Semantic Aside

From a lexical point of view certain possible phonetic variants are of interest. [nana] is a childhood term often heard in Italian communities and is the term used for the maternal grandparent. [n]-like bisyllabics are often used to denote "baby," as in the talk of Commanche, Gilyak, and Spanish. Another common childhood concept, "sleep," has the same phonetic/phonemic property in Arabic and Marathi (Ferguson, 1964, pp. 107–108). One of my nieces chose the expression [nini] as the term to represent her grandmother. This incidence in the use of post-dental nasals for common kin and object terms of baby talk, contrasted to the bilabial forms, seems in the least unusual. Paternal referents seem to be drawn from the non-nasal class irrespective of the place of articulation (Ferguson, 1964).

THE PHYSIOLOGICAL MODEL

Physiologically the labial versus dental contrast is a further restriction in the velar to forward-stop scale. This intermediation represents a successively finer distinction. The contrast of the lips versus the tongue at first glance appears minute in terms of horizontal distance. However a casual review of the well known sensory "homunculi" (Gray, 1948, p. 8) shows the tongue and lips as disproportionately larger than originally supposed. The perceptual independence of the fleshy pre- and postdental structures, as a cognitive operation, would seem quite apparent.

THE ACOUSTIC MODEL

From the acoustic perspective, all labial sounds are low in pitch. All dental sounds are high in pitch (Jakobson, Fant, & Halle, 1952/1976, p. 29; Jakobson & Halle, 1956a, p. 31). The formal term for low pitched is *grave*. This term with its musical characterization in tonal parameters is easily remembered for its morbid solemnity. *Acute,* a term used to denote the rising intonations of ancient Greek, is used for all high pitched sounds. The feature grave versus acute is the acoustic equivalent of the physiological contrast labial versus dental.

Table 1.   Terminology

Physiological term	Acoustic term
Consonants: 1. Labial/dental = labial/lingual	1. Grave/acute = high pitch/low pitch
Vowels: 2. Narrow/wide = high/low	2. Diffuse/compact = non-central/central energy
3. Palatal/velar = front/back	3. Grave/acute = high pitch/low pitch
Consonants: 4. Backward/forward flanged	4. Diffuse/compact = non-central/central energy
Vowels: 5. Rounded/spread	5. Flat/plain
Consonants: 6. Tense/lax (voiceless/voiced)	6. Same
7. Rough/smooth edged	7. Strident/mellow = sibilant/fricative

Note: All terms are presented in the order of discussion. The Jakobsonian terminology is presented first followed by the more common terminology.

PROBLEMS WITH TERMINOLOGY

It should be noted at this juncture that the number of terms used in distinctive feature theory is large. Oftentimes, two different terms mean the same thing but differ in the emphasis (acoustic or physiological). Furthermore, the terms are complicated in that European terminology, such as "dental," "wide," "pharyngeal," etc., do not mean the same thing to American phoneticians. Europeans such as Jakobson often refer to the vocal tract rather than the articulators as a basis of reference, and this is a common American practice. From the physiological perspective, [i] is a "narrow" vowel in reference to the vocal tract (European) or a "high" vowel from the perspective of the tongue position (American). Table 1 simplifies the multiple orientations of the theory. It arranges the various terms into their basic relationships from the multiple perspectives. One final note: certain features in certain subclasses such as consonantal or vocalic are defined different physiologically, but when the same subclasses are compared in the acoustic domain they result in equivalent terms: grave/acute and compact/diffuse in particular.

RESEARCH SUPPORT

All the distinctive feature systems consider the bilabials, [p], [b], [m], versus the front lingual stops, [t], [d], [n], as minimal, or one distinctive feature in difference. However, for Jakobson the voiced and voiceless fricative couplets (f/θ - v/ð - f/s - v/z) remain minimal into the adult model (Jakobson, Fant, & Halle, 1952/1967, p. 43). (See Appendix A.) Miller and Nicely (1955, p. 351), Wickelgren (1966, p. 390), Singh and Black, (1966, p. 384), Voiers (1967, p. 11), and Singh (1968, p. 3) each consider the (f/θ) and (v/ð) contrasts minimal (1 feature difference) and the (f/s) and (v/z) contrasts larger in terms of the number of differential properties. (See Appendices D, E, F, G, respectively.) Halle, working alone (1961, p. 90) and in collaboration with Chomsky (1968, pp. 176–177), has posited a converse relationship: (f/θ) and (v/ð) are greater (2 feature differences) than (f/s) and (v/z), which he considered minimal. (See Appendices B and C.)

	Pairs	
System	(f/θ + v/ð)	(f/s + v/z)
1. Jakobson, Fant, & Halle	1	1
2. Voiers	1	2
3. Miller & Nicely	1	2
4. Singh; Singh & Black	1	2
5. Wickelgren	1	2
6. Halle	2	1
7. Chomsky & Halle	2	1

A casual review of the Olmsted data (1971, p. 71) reveals only a slight trend indicating (f/θ + θ/f) and (v/ð + ð/v) substitutions being more likely than (f/s + s/f) and (v/z + z/v): 55% versus 45%, the position taken by most authors. (Notice that the fewer the feature differences the greater the similarity. The greater the similarity the higher the probability of articulatory error.) Black (1969, p. 22) has ranked (f/θ), (θ/f), (v/ð), and (ð/v) as much more similar perceptually in adults than (f/s), (s/f), (v/z), and (z/v). They were ranked (5, 2, 2, 2) versus (15, 14, 6, 12), respectively.

Abbs and Minifie (1969) attempted to test young children's ability to discriminate between [f, v, θ, ð, s, z]. Seventeen preschool children, ages 3:0–5:1 years, were asked to identify all the 15 possible diadic combinations of those sounds in three vowel contexts in both a CV and VC order. Using a Modern Teaching Association (MTA) "Scholar," a back-lit visual display board, the researchers presented two pictures serially. The children heard one of the pictures "say" one-half of the diadic combination. Subsequently a second picture was identified with the other half of the phonetic item. The child's task was to recall which picture "said" the target phoneme. To begin, there was no difference in the recall in the various vowel contexts, [i, aɪ, a]. The results of the consonantal contrasts are interesting. The (f/s) and (v/z) contrasts were more easily perceived (implying more dissimilarity) than the (f/θ) and

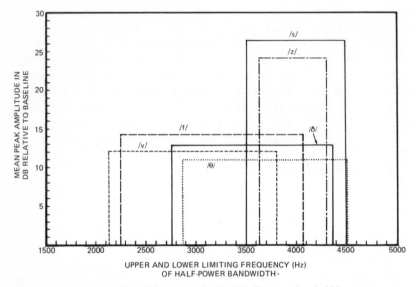

Figure 2.   Representation of frequency limits of half-power bandwidth versus mean peak amplitude for each fricative (90 representations for each sound). (Adapted from Abbs and Minifie, 1969, p. 1540.)

(v/d) contrasts. This indicates greater proximity or fewer feature differences separating the latter two classes. This information matches the Black (1969) and Olmsted (1971) data. Subsequently, Abbs and Minifie analyzed their presentation tapes for frequency, intensity, and time differences. This post hoc analysis indicated that [s] and [z] are set apart significantly from [f, v, θ, ð] by a higher frequency of resonance [4000 Hz], a shorter spectrum, and a 10- to 15-dB difference in intensity (Abbs & Minifie, 1969, p. 1542). Among the fricatives, [f, v, θ, ð] no significant sonographic differences could be found in the spectrum (see Figure 2).

     Similar findings concerning the difficult identification of the sonographic properties separating (f/θ) and (v/ð) were noted by Bush (1964, pp. 140–141). In general, it can be concluded that Jakobson's contention that (f/s) and (v/z) are minimal (grave/acute) through to adulthood must be questioned. Systematic predictions, such as those presented by Miller and Nicely (1955, p. 351), Wickelgren (1966, p. 390), Singh and Black (1966, p. 384), Voiers (1967, p. 11), and Singh (1968, p. 3), have been supported on this one issue. Halle's contention that (f/θ) and (v/ð) are greater in terms of difference than (f/s) and (v/z) can be rejected barring further evidence to the contrary.

ANOTHER PERSPECTIVE

Concerning the stops, the (p/t), (b/d), and (m/n) contrasts have been very extensively studied. (Alvin Liberman once quipped that he would go down in history as an individual who knew only six sounds: p, t, k, b, d, and g.) Before reviewing the work of the Haskin's Laboratory, it should be noted that Jakobson many times relied on the works of Potter, Kopp, and Green (Jakobson, 1962, p. 649), today known as Potter, Kopp, and Kopp. *Visible Speech,* one of the first comprehensive texts to present the visual configurations of the sonograms as they represented the speech sounds, can be used to illustrate the grave/acute dichotomy. /p/ and /b/ are both noted for having a concentration of energy in the *lower* frequency domain; /t/ and /d/, on the other hand, have a *higher* or more acute concentration of energy in the upper frequency domain (see Figure 3). Symbolically, this hub is indicated by a perpendicular line drawn through the spike or rapid noise onset of the stop (see Figure 4).

In 1951, Franklin Cooper, Pierre Delattre, Alvin Liberman, John Borst, and Louis Gerstman published a study of the stop consonants in which they used the Pattern-Playback machine. This machine, which "reads" painted sonograms and converts them into acoustic signals, was extensively used to determine the significant sound properties of American English (see Figures 5 and 6). In one of their initial articles

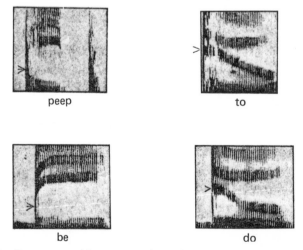

peep

to

be

do

Figure 3.   Four sonographic representations of grave/acute. The lower frequency hubs of [p] and [b] contrast with the higher frequency hubs of [t] and [d]. (Adapted from Potter, Kopp, & Kopp, 1947/1966, pp. 83, 90.)

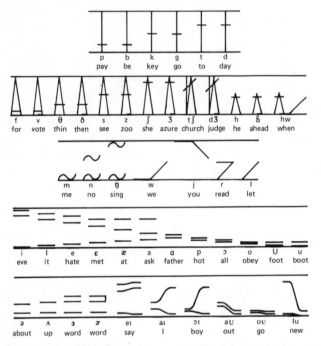

Figure 4. Manual symbols for visible speech adapted for use in the experimental Visible Speech Training Program. (Adapted from Potter, Kopp, & Kopp, 1947/1966, p. 60.)

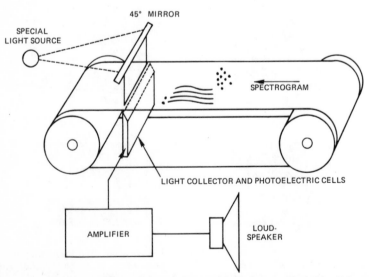

Figure 5. Highly simplified schematic diagram of the Pattern-Playback. (Adapted from Denes & Pinson, 1963, p. 128.)

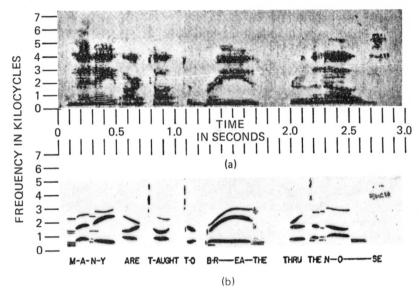

(a)

(b)

Figure 6.   The (a) portion of the figure is the sound spectrogram of a naturally produced sentence; (b) is a painted pattern that can be played on the Pattern-Playback to hear the same sentence. (Adapted from Denes & Pinson, 1963, p. 129.)

(Cooper et al., 1952), the authors reported that the center frequency of small noise bursts (see Figure 7) could trigger phonemically significant behavior in college students.

> In general, it appears that this one variable—the frequency position of the burst—provides the listener with a basis for distinguishing among *p*, *t*, and *k*. We see that high frequency bursts were heard as *t* for all vowels, bursts at lower frequencies were heard as *k* when they were on the level with, or slightly above, the second formant of the vowel; otherwise they were heard as *p*. (Cooper et al., 1952, p. 597)

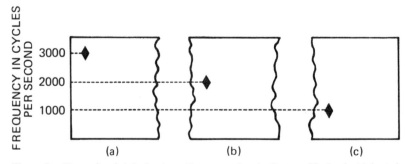

Figure 7.   Example of "plosive burst" patterns for the Pattern-Playback. (Adapted from Denes & Pinson, 1963, p. 131.)

(For those without a speech science background, see Denes & Pinson's *The Speech Chain,* Chapter 8, pp. 125–147.)

If one compares the relative position of these bursts, it can be noted that they match the "hub" positions of Potter, Kopp, and Kopp. However, the Haskins Laboratory group continued:

> It is clear that for *p* and *k* the identification of the consonant depended, not solely on the frequency position of the burst of noise, but rather this position in relation to the vowel. (Cooper et al., 1952, pp. 597–598)

This study and subsequent studies went on to question the "hub" concept, and eventually replaced it with the "locus" concept (Delattre, Liberman, & Cooper, 1955). (For a succinct listing of the subsequent theory, see Liberman et al., 1967.) The locus is different from the hub. As sounds are joined together in connected speech, in a coarticulatory fashion, especially in a CV or VC context, the second formant or vowel tone can be seen to shift rapidly depending upon the place of articulation of the adjoining consonant (see Figure 8). The labial sounds have a "downward" shift or point of origin (grave locus). The lingua-alveolars have an "upward" shift or point of origin (acute locus). This use of the transition and the noise burst has remained an essential part of distinctive feature theory (Jakobson, 1972, pp. 74–75).

The maximal contrast involved in the (p/t), (b/d), and (m/n) is obvious within the stop category itself (cf. Potter, Kopp, & Kopp,

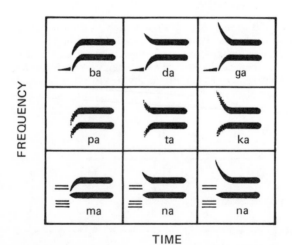

TIME

Figure 8.   Hand-painted spectrograms of nine consonant-vowel syllables, showing some of the principle acoustic cues for the perception of the stop and nasal consonants. (Adapted from Liberman et al., 1956, p. 159; q.v. Liberman et al., 1959, p. 336.)

1947/1966, p. 60). The hubs of /t/, /d/, and /n/ are higher (more acute). The hubs of /p/, /b/, and /m/ are lower (more grave) than their counterparts. From the relative perspective of the fricative class, /f/ and /v/ have lower hubs than the remaining fricatives /θ/, /ð/, /s/, and /z/. The hubs of the latter class, tongue tip sounds, do not remain in a frequency region that may be labeled grave (see Figure 4). This apparent contradiction between "graveness" residing in the frequency range (therefore, in man himself) or the sequential decision process (relative to previous decisions) is hard to reconcile. A review of the original cycle of the theory (phase I) indicates a sequential class form of evolution, rather than a pure binary form. The stop class may be organized at a different stage of development than the fricative class. This aspect of the theory is never fully expanded upon or detailed. In any case, it may be assumed that the feature grave/acute may be of a varying nature in various subclasses. (For similar schemes see Crocker, 1969, passim; Edwards, 1974, passim; and Stampe, 1969, p. 443. For a full presentation of current issues see Kornfeld, 1971.)

THE NOISE COMPONENT

The question subsequently is why the stop class is more likely than the fricatives to be organized at an earlier time. A partial answer may be inferred from Olmsted's theory of acquisition. In his theory speech sounds are the objects of learning. Phones that are more discriminable are learned first (Olmsted's postulate 10). Furthermore, sounds that are learned first are learned in a background of noise:

> Postulate 17: The conditions under which talk is directed at the child vary constantly, there being sometimes steady partially masking noise, and sometimes loud interruptions at various frequencies.
> Postulate 18: While such interference never, for the physiologically normal, results in the failure of the language-learning, it gives an advantage (higher probability of being learned earlier) to those phones whose components are more easily discriminable. (Olmsted, 1966/1971, p. 3; q.v. Olmsted, 1971, pp. 39–40)

Turning from the sound to the sound property, it may be assumed that certain sound classes, in their natural setting of noise, present more difficult or more unlikely tasks for the learner (Miller & Nicely, 1955; Singh & Black, 1966; Voiers, 1967; Singh, 1968). This may be why man has evolved the forward stops rather than the fricatives. Either feature, fricative versus stop, is apparently possible as an early phonemic goal (Velten, 1943/1971, p. 283). All the possibilities, as in the free variation model, are not possible in a natural context. Jakobsonian principles require an ideal state, *ceteris paribus,* as he would say, all things being equal. Blesser (1972) has shown that man in a short time can learn to decode speech that is presented spectrally "upside down," low frequencies being transposed into high frequency components, and the converse. This result apparently implies that the acoustic characteristics of speech are not paramount, as sometimes implied (Jakobson & Halle, 1956a, p. 8). Although the grave/acute feature has a formal definition (Jakobson, Fant, & Halle, 1952/1967, pp. 29–30), it may be that this feature is relative to each subclass, that is, *lower* frequency components rather than *low* frequency components.

chapter 14

Stages of Development:

STAGE 4—
Narrow/Wide Vowels
(Compact/Diffuse I)

THE INFANTEMIC MODEL
THE PHYSIOLOGICAL MODEL
THE ACOUSTIC MODEL
  Lepsius's Triangle
  Sound Color
  Stumpf's Triangle
RESEARCH SUPPORT

Once the child separates the nasal and non-nasal sounds into those made by the lips versus those made by the tongue tip (grave/acute I), the child then turns his/her attention to the passive or neutral vowel. In the subsequent two-step process, which begins before the third year, the neutral vowel will be transformed into a cardinal point vowel system (Jakobson, 1941/1968, p. 49). The triangular phonemic framework, so to speak, will subsequently be refined into the vowel quadrilateral commonly seen in textbooks on phonetics.

THE INFANTEMIC MODEL

In the first step of the process, the vocalic infanteme is split into two subclasses, the wide versus narrow vowels. This produces a full infantemic sound system containing six macrophonemes. The high vowels /i = ɪ = u = U/, perhaps /o = e/, are contrasted to the low vowels /ɔ = ɛ = a/ (see Figure 1). This results in an infantemic system with four consonants and two vowels. Expression such as [pipi - bibi - mimi - titi - didi - nini] and/or [pupu - bubu - mumu - tutu - dudu - nunu] would tend to be generated. It is interesting to note that three of the latent expressions are euphemisms for toilet training functions, [pipi - pupu - dudu]. Several other expressions are common baby talk items, [bibi - titi]. Two expressions are for exotic dress patterns, [mumu - tutu].

PHONEMIC STAGE   # 4

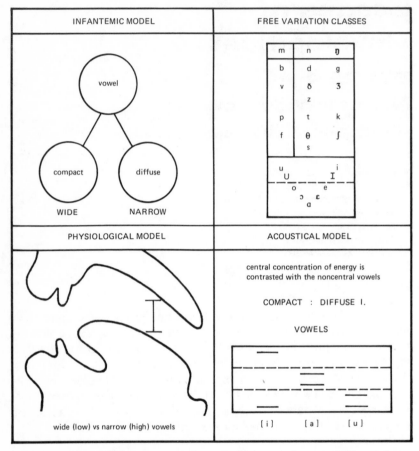

Figure 1.   Four different representations of wide/narrow (compact/diffuse I) from cognitive and phonetic perspectives.

These unusual phonetic patterns, which tend to disappear from adult vocabularies, until the children in question have their own children, tend to bridge the gap between the child's restricted lexical world and the immense vocabulary pool of the adult world (60,000 words in some individuals).

Jakobson apparently has based his timing of this stage, before the third year, on the work of Pavlović (Jakobson, 1941/1968, p. 49). Templin (1957) noted that almost all vowels are learned before the third year:

In the present study, approximately the same level of accuracy is reached in the production of vowels and diphthongs by the 3-year-olds as in con-◦ sonant elements by 7-year-olds and in the consonant blends by 8-year-olds. (p. 32)

If one is willing to concede an early date of onset of the vocalic expansion, one can note that bladder and bowel control is concomitant with onset of the high vowels. As fantastic as this appears, the same phonemonon, the association of high vowels with expressions, euphemisms, or baby talk forms for urination and defecation, appear in languages other than American English. [kaku] is the Spanish baby talk form for defecation; [ʔasí], Commanche; [(i)ši], Marathi. [mumu] and [šu] are used in Arabic for urination; [hisa], Gilyak; [wiwi], an alternative English form; [pipi - pichi - chichi], Spanish (Ferguson, 1964, p. 107). Whereas the child's constitutional and natural setting aided in the development of nasality (velar movement) and labiality (bilabial closure), concentration on toilet functions in the second year by the society may sensitize the child to the muscular masses necessary for the raising of the tongue, or at least present a social situation in which high vowels are more probable through baby talk items. In either case, the observation merits, at least, a smile in passing.

THE PHYSIOLOGICAL MODEL

Physiologically, narrow versus wide constitutes the bipolar end points of the vertical axis of the vowel system. Narrow vowels are termed diffuse; wide vowels are termed compact. Because these terms are essentially acoustic terms, they are explained in the section below. The maximal contrast, a high versus a low vowel, establishes a foundation for the horizontal axis that will be learned in the following stage. This two-dimensional orthogonal system, in its full form a vertical versus horizontal place of articulation grid, has been used to analyze both the consonants and the vowels (Peterson & Shoup, 1966a, pp. 45, 54–56; 1966c, pp. 108, 119). Jakobsonian theory, as opposed to Peterson and Shoup, tends to treat the consonants and vowels as separate developmental forms, initially. In subsequent stages Jakobson's concepts combine both the consonants and vowels onto the same perceptual grid.

THE ACOUSTIC MODEL

In the acoustic domain, the terms "compact" and "diffuse" have caused several problems (Chomsky & Halle, 1968, pp. 303–309). These problems, however, are only apparent in the physiologically based phonological theories (re: Halle, see Blache, 1970, pp. 31–32). To begin, the terms "compact" and "diffuse" were developed in the years following the beginning of acoustic phonetics, the 1940's. For instance, Chiba and Kajiyama's, *The Vowel: Its Nature and Structure,* the first extensive instrumental discussion of the acoustics of the vowel system, appeared in 1941. Koenig, Dunn, and Lacy's, "The sound spectrograph," the first formal discussion of the instrument, appeared in 1946. Potter, Kopp, and Kopp published *Visible Speech* for the first time in 1947. Luchsinger and Arnold published their encyclopedic report on speech science in the same period (West, 1966, pp. 29–30).

In 1949, Jakobson proposed a phonetic/phonemic property he labeled "saturation." This term was worked out in joint efforts with John Lotz, an early collaborator (Jakobson, 1949/1962, p. 42). It was defined as follows:

> Saturated/Diluted. The saturated vowels are characterized by a *compactness* [emphasis mine] of their formant spectrum (especially by the rise of the lower formant), and they exhibit a higher energy than the diluted vowels; the latter presents a lower energy and are characterized by some loosely composed, widely separated formants in the spectrum (particularly by the depth of the lower formant)[7] [citing Delattre (1948), Stumpf (1926) and Hála (1941)] *ceteris paribus,* saturation involves a longer duration, a higher perceptibility, and a greater resistance to distortion. The data so far published on the formant spectrums of the consonants are still incomplete[8] [citing supportive data re: consonants from Bell Telephone Laboratories]; but the difference between saturated and the corresponding diluted consonants in energy, audibility, resistibility and natural duration justifies the proposed identifications. (Jakobson & Lotz, 1949/1962, pp. 427–428)

This feature was subsequently relabeled and termed "compact" versus "diffuse" (Jakobson, Fant, & Halle, 1952/1967, pp. 27–29). In later works, Chomsky and Halle (1968, pp. 303–309) would abandon this terminology altogether. They revised the terminology by dividing the terms into more than one feature.

Lepsius's Triangle

To really understand these terms, it is necessary to return to the controversial work of Lepsius. Lepsius, as noted previously, established a triangular vowel system that closely resembled the models in Jakobsonian writings. More important is another fact:

> One of the most controversial contributions made by Lepsius was his vowel triangle. G. Oscar Russell [1928] believed that, of all vowel triangles, "... one of the most clearly conceived, ingenious, and applicable

right at the present time, was that of Lepsius." Russell considered Lepsius's use of the analogy between vowels and colors in the construction of his triangle to be supported by modern vowel research in its assumption that there were three primary vowels and that intermediate vowels were "... formed between the three as all the colors between red, yellow, and blue." Following is the pyramid which Lepsius used to diagram the vowels with their analogous colors:

```
                      a
                    (red)
          e          ö          o
      (orange)    (brown)   (violet)
          i          ü          u
      (yellow)    (green)     (blue)
```

(Albright, 1958, p. 28)

Now to begin, the five-point outer triangle is commonly found in Jakobsonian writings (1929/1962, pp. 59, 61, 62, 80, 87). The inverted and/or reversed triangle, sometimes called a pyramid, is frequently also found (Jakobson, 1931a/1962, p. 224; 1931b/1962, p. 204; 1939c/1971, p. 80; 1941/1968, p. 74). This correlation is attributable, no doubt, to intervening sources, which a review of the sources will show. However, the essential aspect of the correlation is not the triangle itself, but the concept of vowel color.

Sound Color

Sound color, which is extensively discussed by Jakobson (1941/1968, pp. 73/84), is not a new concept to the American phonetician. Many authors in the United States have held to a phonetic system which separates /l/ into two allophones: a light and a dark form. (For this coloration dichotomy, see Faircloth & Faircloth, 1973, pp. 52–54; Kantner & West, 1960, pp. 91–92; Leutenneger, 1963, p. 34.) For those unfamiliar with the concept, an /l/ that occurs in the postvocalic position—such as in the words "ball," "all," "tall"—does not need lingua-alveolar contact in its production. A dark [l]-like quality will be created by merely raising the *back* portion of the tongue toward the supralaryngeal region. This "dark" quality results from the unusual shape of the oral cavity, the high back tongue position. A different quality is detected in the lingua-alveolar or tongue-tip production of /l/. This is the "lighter" counterpart. This color dimension and its discussion in American texts is, I believe, a remnant of the same concept found in European literature.

Compact/diffuse (or saturated/diluted) is this same perceptual dimension, a light/dark dimension. This dimension, which Jakobson labels achromatism (1941/1968, pp. 78–79), is derived from two cases of sound-color perception. K. Langenbeck and an additional unidentified 32-year-old female Czech painter had been reported to exhibit an unusual color-phoneme association pattern:

a
(red)

e   o
(yellow)   (blue)
i   u
(silver white)   (dark brown)
CASE 1

a
(red)

e   o
(light green)   (blue red)
i   u
(canary yellow)   (dark blue)
CASE 2

(Adapted from Jakobson, 1941/1968, p. 83)

In each case, it was noted that certain physiological productions were associated with specific light/dark, and chromatic/achromatic properties. Without trying to adjust the directions of the orthogonal axes for the two perceptual fields (sound and color), it can be noted that certain light colors—white, yellow, etc.—are associated with the high front vowels. Dark colors—brown, blue, etc.—are associated with high back vowels. The low central vowels are "red," understood to mean intense and vibrant (see Torgerson, 1958, pp. 280–292; Wicker, 1968, pp. 178–188). Incidentally, the same color relationship can be found in Lepsius's example! Now, the color system is oriented to two color dimensions: hue (color) and saturation (intensity). Jakobson conjectured that a two-dimensional perceptual system separated the vowels, compact/diffuse and grave/acute. Compact/diffuse is comparable to a saturation concept (note the original term). Grave/acute, the pitch dimension, is comparable to the graduated color spectrum.

Stumpf's Triangle

The acoustic data that reinforce this idea had been discovered during Jakobson's formative years, 1912–1926:

> We might survey briefly and concisely the fundamental discoveries of Kohler [1919/1925] and Stumpf [1926], which unfortunately still is insufficiently made use of in linguistics. These two great scholars of modern

acoustics deserve the credit for having uncovered and made precise two kinds of indissoluble quantities of speech sounds.

Like visual sensations, speech sounds are, on the one hand, light or dark, and on the other hand, chromatic and achromatic in different degrees. As the chromatism (abundance of sound) decreases the opposition of lightness and darkness becomes more marked. (Jakobson, 1941/1968, p. 73)

Stumpf (1926) had posited that two orthogonal dimensions were used to decode speech. One dimension, a /i/-/u/ dimension, was comparable to a light-dark contrast; the /a/ versus /i/ and /u/ dimension was comparable to the chromatic-achromatic concept:

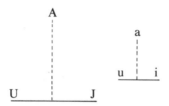

(Adapted from Jakobson, 1941/1968, p. 74)

The /a/, the "red" vowel, was seen as more colorful, more pigmented, or more intense—therefore, compact. The /i/ and /u/ were less colorful—therefore, diffuse. In 1952 this same feature was defined formally as follows:

> 2.411 Stimulus. Compact phonemes are characterized by the relative predominance of one centrally located formant region (or formant). They are opposed to diffuse phonemes in which one or more non-central formants or formant regions predominate. (Jakobson, Fant, & Halle, 1952/1967, p. 27)

This shift in terminology from "saturation" to "compactness" to "centrality" merits further attention.

RESEARCH SUPPORT

In the 1950's two research teams working at Bell Telephone Laboratories, Potter and Steinberg (1950) and Peterson and Barney (1952), discovered some unusual properties of the vowel system. The acoustic formants or resonating frequency regions of the vocal tract could be transformed into the physiological vowel triangle. Peterson and Barney analyzed the acoustic properties of 10 different vowel sounds uttered twice by males (N = 33), females (N = 28), and children (N = 15). This total list (2 × 76 × 10) of 1520 words was analyzed by

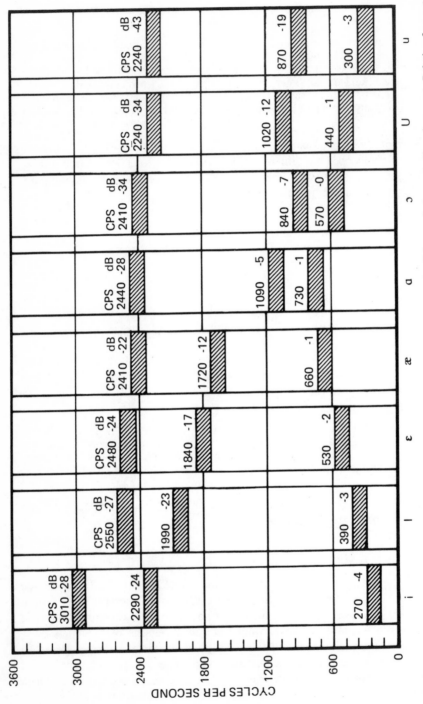

Figure 2. Mean formant frequencies and relative amplitudes for 33 men uttering the English vowels in an /h-d/ environment. Relative formant amplitudes are given in decibels re the first formant of /ɔ/. (Diagram adapted from Flanagan, 1965, p. 131, after the works of Peterson & Barney.)

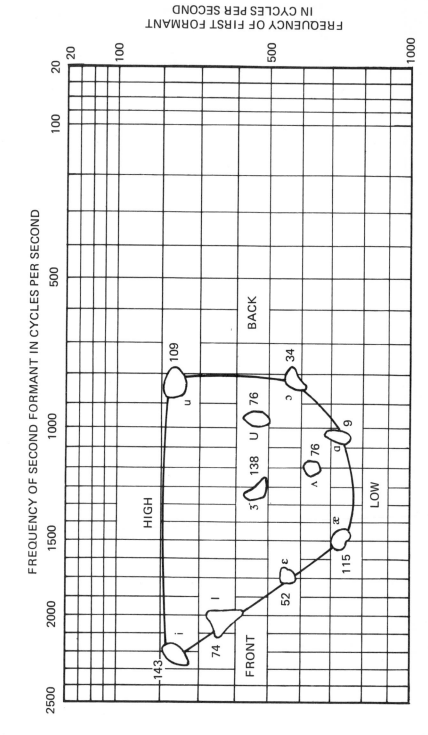

Figure 3. Vowel loop with numbers of sounds unanimously classified by listeners; each sound was presented 152 times. (Adapted from Peterson & Barney, 1952, p. 177.)

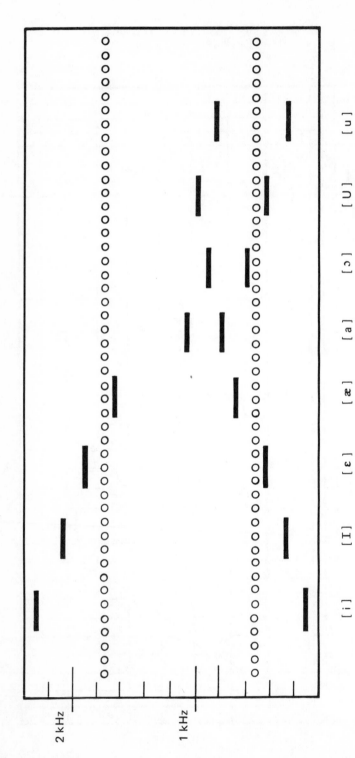

Figure 4.   Schematic representation of centrality. (Norms from Peterson & Barney, 1952).

[i]   [I]   [ε]   [æ]   [a]   [ɔ]   [U]   [u]

2 kHz

1 kHz

means of the sound spectrograph. The average results revealed a uniform pattern of change as one procedes from the high front vowel, to the low central vowel, to the high back vowel, (/i/ to /a/ to /u/) (see Figure 2). The first, or lowest frequency formant, begins in the lower frequency regions and rises until the central vowel /a/ is reached. At that point the formant lowers in pitch as the tongue is raised to the high back position of /u/. In essence the configuration forms a "hill." The second formant, on the other hand, begins very high in frequency (circa 2290 Hz) and lowers in frequency as one travels around the vowel triangle. Now when the frequencies of the first and second formants are plotted on a Cartesian coordinate system, the physiological vowel triangle is reproduced (see Figure 3).

As will be seen the second formant is uncomplicated. It distributes itself in one direction on the graph, from 2200 Hz to 800 Hz, displayed from left to right. Because the first formant rises then lowers, a triangle can be formed. Incidentally, if the coordinates were not reversed the triangle would closely approximate the original Lepsius pyramid. The central redirection point of the first formant is a key factor in compactness. If an artificial line is drawn across the spectrum from 500 Hz to 1750 Hz, it will be noted that centrality, having *both* formants in the central region, separates the low vowels /æ/, /ɔ/, /a/ from the narrow vowels /i/, /ɪ/, /ɛ/, /ʊ/, /u/ (see Figure 4). The /u/ and /ʊ/ vowels, although they have their formants close together, do not fall in the central region. The centrality is more important than the saturation or compactness.

The central frequency regions have long been known to be more sensitive to speech sounds. When humans are asked to judge the difference between sounds of two different intensities, they tend to overestimate the differences in the central domain. (For a simplified discussion of this phenomenon read Bergeijk, Pierce, and David's *Waves and the Ear,* 1960, pp. 75–83.) This sensitivity or increased awareness is a unique characteristic universal to all men. The psychophysical ability would indicate that, perhaps, compactness may not be totally embedded in the phonetic signal.

Returning to the child and his/her natural abilities, the vocal expansion begins initially with a consonant versus vowel comparison. The consonants such as /p/ or /t/ are characterized by a "spike," meaning a diffusion of noise throughout the frequency spectrum. This is the initial example of diffuse. The wide neutral vowel /a/ has two centrally located formants, that is, compact. This dichotomy, consonant versus vowel, represents the maximal compact/diffuse dichotomy. This comparison is seen as a catalyst for the vocalic expansion (Jakobson, 1941/1968, pp. 75–78).

chapter 15

Stages of Development:

STAGE 5—Palatal/Velar Vowels (Grave/Acute II)

THE INFANTEMIC MODEL

Once the child has actively learned to raise the tongue, that is, produce diffuse vowels, he or she begins to work on the development of the front versus back vowel contrast. Characteristically in Jakobsonian writings, front vowels are referred to as "palatal" and back vowels are referred to as "velar." This splitting of the high front vowel into the front and back classes creates the triadic vowel system. It may be inferred that the subsequent application of this feature to the low vowels (Jakobson & Halle, 1956a, p. 4) creates a vowel quadrilateral. However, this idea is never expanded upon by the authors. Returning to the high vowels, it may be noted that the horizontal expansion, although a necessity in American English, is not universal in character. The vowel triangle or quadrilateral is not developed in many languages. These systems have a simple *linear* [i-e-a] vowel system (Jakobson, 1941/1968, p. 49).

Lieberman et al. (1971) have studied the human vocal tract in neonatal crying and compared the infant's potential with that of nonhuman primates. In their conclusions, they point out an essential characteristic of the human digestive/respiratory tract:

> The upper pharynx also differs markedly in the neonate and as a result is much less mobile than in the adult. In the newborn, the upper pharynx is a narrow tube, the longest diameter of which runs anteroposteriorly rather

155

PHONEMIC STAGE #5

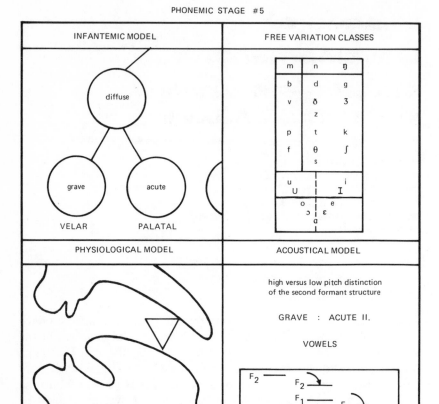

Figure 1.   Four different representations of palatal/velar (grave/acute II) from cognitive and phonetic perspectives.

than superoinferiorly as it does in the adult (Braislin, 1919). The roof of the infant's pharynx slopes gently downward from the chonae to the dorsal wall of the mesopharynx and, therefore, the epipharynx of the infant does not have a dorsal or posterior wall (Bosma and Fletcher, 1961). The newborn infant, like a nonhuman primate, thus lacks a pharyngeal region that can vary its cross sectional area. In fully developed human speech, pharyngeal volume changes over a ten-to-one range as the root of the tongue, which forms the anterior pharyngeal wall, moves. (Lieberman et al., 1971, p. 725)

THE FREE VARIATION MODEL

In terms of the free variation model, the initial palatal/velar distinction separates the /i = ɪ/ class from the /u = u/ class (see Figure 1). The gross contrast between the two infantemes is distinguished, but the class elements are still free varying. It is unclear at what stage the front/back contrast is applied to the low vowels. (The pattern of Jakobson and Halle [1956a, p. 40] contradicts the order of #0.1111 preceding #0.112 [p. 41]). For the sake of the presentation of the original theory, it should be presumed that grave/acute vowels are marked by the diffuse vowel. I believe that this contradiction is inherent in the training and background of the co-authors. Jakobson, I believe, formulated the theory on the assumption of a triangular system, whereas Halle, who did not formulate the acquisition theory, corrects the theory for the American audience. It is the contention of this book that a theory must first be understood in detail before revisions that alter basic assumptions of the viewpoint are examined.

THE ACOUSTIC MODEL

Acoustically, palatal vowels have a higher frequency second formant component than low vowels. In other words, they are high pitched or "acute." This is the same term that is applied to the consonantal system. Velar vowels are low in pitch because the frequency of their second formant is low. The compact/diffuse distinctive feature, with its central/noncentral energy orientation, and the grave/acute feature, with its high pitched versus low pitched dimension, serve as the basic acoustic dimensions or axes for the entire sound system. From this perspective Jakobson's ideas share much in common with Peterson and Shoup. Both theoretical frames attempt to place the consonants and vowels onto an analysis grid. Whereas Peterson and Shoup begin with the physiological component and evolve an acoustic facet, Jakobson evolves an acoustic grid to integrate physiological differences.

In terms of the acquisition sequence, the vowels are organized first. In the following stage the consonants will be placed on the same perceptual grid. The concept of sound color, as expressed by Lepsius, in subsequent years turned out to be the inspiration for connecting data from experimental phonetics and the hue and saturation of color perception. Although somewhat unclear in orientation, as seen in the number of changes in terminology, this feature (compact/diffuse) in conjunction with normal pitch perception establishes what is called Stumpf's triangle, the coordinates of the sound system.

COMPACT
↑
A
┆
U ┆ J
GRAVE ←   K   → ACUTE
┆
P ┆ T
↓
DIFFUSE

(Adapted from Jakobson, 1941/1968, p. 74)

These coordinates, the grave/acute and compact/diffuse axes, are basic to Jakobsonian theory. Two subsequent distinctive feature systems (Halle, 1961, p. 90; Voiers, 1967, p. 11) retain the triangular similarity relationship in their design.

PSYCHOPHYSICAL SUPPORT

The psychophysical properties of the vowel system have been studied rather extensively in recent years (Singh, 1976, pp. 75–87, 147–152). Once the relevant acoustic specifications of the vowels had been published by Potter and Steinberg (1950), Peterson and Barney (1952), Fairbanks, House, and Stevens (1950), and House and Fairbanks (1953), the way had been paved for the theoretical discussions of how the vowels were actually produced by the vocal tract (Fant, 1956; Stevens & House, 1961) and their implications for the speech of the deaf (Tiffany, 1953a, 1953b). The significant work of Chiba and Kajiyama (1941), which predates this work by some 10–12 years, suffered the same fate as *Kindersprache* in terms of wartime discrimination. From our modern perspective it is hard to imagine the sound spectrograph as having a "top secret" classification.

The first major psychophysical study of the vowels—"An experimental study of the acoustic determinants of vowel color: Observations of one- and two-formant vowels synthesized from spectrographic patterns" (Delattre et al., 1952)—in essence reversed the Potter and Steinberg (1950) and Peterson and Barney (1952) studies. Whereas the former studies analyzed the acoustic properties of the vowels by means of the sonograph, Delattre et al. used a Pattern-Playback machine. Painting sonograms of the ideal parameters of the vowels, the authors attempted to trigger, in the listener, the specific phonemic identifications of 16 cardinal vowels. By varying the amplitude of the formants relative to one another they were able to produce the proper vowel-like qualities.

In 1955 Moser and Dreher examined the information alphabets used by police and other communication systems [ALPHA - BRAVO - COCOA - DELTA - etc.). In their experiment they presented the code of the ICAO, the International Civil Aviation Organization, to subjects from 28 different countries. To test the adequacy of the alphabet they presented the words in the presence of noise. The authors concluded, after 1½ years of testing, that more than the alphabet was affecting the results:

> Since the confusions noted throughout the testing period were so remarkably consistent and recurrent, it was evident that some law seemed to be operating. It was further observed that the first syllable, which incidentally, was in most cases the accented one, seemed to be the most important in determining the identity of a word with succeeding (or unaccented) syllables apparently having but little effect on recognition. (Moser & Dreher, 1955, p. 876)

These underlying laws were the perceptual dimensions of the vowel system.

The full scope of these mental or cognitive dimensions was not discovered until later experimentation was done. By 1955, the method of formant construction as described by Delattre et al. (1952), and the values derived sonographically by Potter and Steinberg (1950), Peterson and Barney (1952), and others were thought of as a theory of vowel perception (q.v. Pickett, 1957, p. 613, note #1, and p. 620, conclusion #2). By the early 1960's the formant relationships were being used to program computers to recognize vowel sounds (Cohen, Slis, & Hart, 1967; Foulkes, 1961, p. 8; Plomp, Pols, & van de Geer, 1967, p. 711; Welch & Wimpress, 1961, p. 426). Just one step remained to be taken in order to link the acoustic properties to the perceptual system. If one could program a computer to recognize the vowel sounds, human recognition could be compared and contrasted.

COMPUTER IDENTIFICATION OF VOWELS

In 1969 Pols, van de Kamp, and Plomp published a succinct summary of the current research concerning the vowel system (pp. 458–460). At that time it was known that 87% of the time computers could identify vowels of the basis on the F_1 versus F_2 relationship. If only one speaker was used to produce the stimuli, the rate was shown to be as high as 97.5% (Gerstman, 1968). However no one had shown that humans perceptually analyzed the vowel sounds of speech in the same manner as the computer. In their experiment 15 subjects (11 male, and 4 female) were asked to judge 11 vowel-like sounds as to their similarity and dissimilarity, [i, y, e, ø, œ, ɛ, a, ɔ, o, ɑ, u]. Three vowel items were presented to the subjects at one time. Each subject was asked to determine which combination (XZ, XY, or YZ) was the most similar. These estimates were in turn analyzed by a computer program (Kruskal, 1964b) to derive the number of perceptual dimensions needed to cognitively separate each vowel-like item. Once the perceptual dimensions were derived, the speech signals were acoustically analyzed. This second set of data was then matched to the perceptual estimates. The results were encouraging though not ideal:

> Projections on the points of the superimposed planes given in [see Figure 2]. It is apparent that there is a large correspondence between both configurations, which brings us to the conclusion that the F_1 and F_2 information is almost completely present in our multidimensional physical representation, despite the fact that one is derived from a broad-band (⅓-octave) analysis. The correspondence with the two-dimensional physical space (68.0% variance) appears to be less good, thus indicating that if one wants to describe the spectral information of vowel sounds as positions of points in a plane, the F_1-F_2 plane is not the most proper one. (Pols, van de Kamp, & Plomp, 1969, pp. 464–465)

This experiment suffered from the fact that only balanced segments of the vowels, that is, *vowel-like* stimuli, were presented to the subjects. The signals were so brief that some subjects did not know they were hearing sounds derived from speech. However, this study did set the pattern for the extensive psychological studies of later years. These latter studies (Singh & Woods, 1971; Singh, Woods, & Becker, 1972) derived the dimensions of both the consonants and the vowels.

SUMMARY

In review, at this stage of development (stage 5) a previously learned distinctive feature is generalized to previous vowel classes, the compact and diffuse classes. The grave (low pitch) category is contrasted to the acute (high pitch) category on the basis of the second formant of the vowel sounds (see Figure 2). From the maximal viewpoint, the second formant of /i/ is the highest in the vowel system and the second formant of /u/ is the lowest.

The grave (low frequency) vowels in physiological terms are the "back" or "velar" vowels. All back vowels have a low frequency second formant. The acute (high frequency) vowels in physiological terms are the "front" or "palatal" vowels. All front vowels have a high frequency second formant. The front versus back dichotomy establishes the cornerpoints of the vowel triangle. It should be noted that high versus low was acquired in the previous stage.

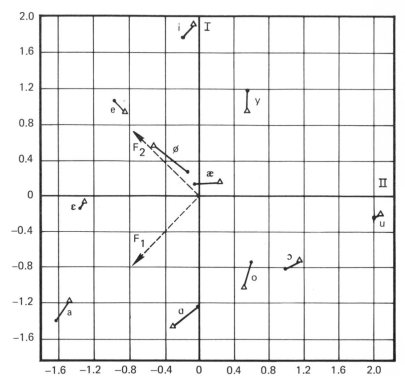

Figure 2. Position of the points when the F_1-F_2 configuration ($\cdot$) is matched maximally with the subdimensional physical configuration (Δ). The original orientations of the F_1 and F_2 axes are also given. (Adapted from Pols, van de Kamp, & Plomp, 1969, p. 465.)

In terms of free variation four vowel phonemes can be noted:

/u = ʊ/   A variable high back vowel
/o = ɔ/   A variable low back vowel (if grave/acute is applied to compact vowels)
/i = ɪ/   A variable high back vowel
/e = ɛ/   A variable low front vowel (see condition above)

The [a] vowel will have to be considered both front and back for this explanation. It should be noted that this ambiguous status should not be present in theory. However, this option serves to simplify the discussion and avoids certain confusions.

chapter 16

Stages of Development:

STAGE 6—Velar/Nonvelar Consonants (Compact/Diffuse II)

THE INFANTEMIC MODEL
THE FREE VARIATION MODEL
THE ACOUSTIC MODEL
FORMAL DEFINITIONS
   Compact (versus Diffuse)
   Grave (versus Acute)

THE INFANTEMIC MODEL

In stage six, the lingual sounds (acute) are subdivided into front tongue sounds versus back tongue sounds (Jakobson, 1941/1968, pp. 79–81). This process increases the number of infantemes from eight to ten (see Figure 1). This extension of the velar consonants equates to the diachronic evolution of language. Jakobson's law of implication, which stated that the existence of velars implied the existence of forward stops, constitutes the relevant theme here. From the child's perspective, and perhaps man in the historical sense, it is presumed that a delay in the velar consonants is attributable to the need to establish the vowel triangle beforehand. While the child is in the process of organizing the vowels, the velar consonants are precluded from the field of development, for they occupy the same physiological space, the back of the tongue.

THE FREE VARIATION MODEL

In terms of free variation, the sound classes /n/-/ŋ/ and /d, ð, z, t, θ, s/-/g, ʒ, k, ʃ/ are contrastive, the former two having a phonemic status (equal to the adult) and the latter having a macrophonemic or infantemic status (not yet adult). Common substitution patterns just prior to this stage are (t/k), (d/g) and (n/ŋ). This variety of error, attributable to

PHONEMIC STAGE # 6

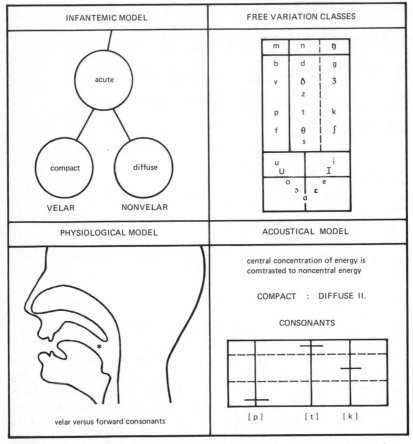

Figure 1.   Four different representations of velar/nonvelar (compact/diffuse II) from cognitive and phonetic perspectives.

a lack of understanding of compact/diffuse, has been reported in the literature as early as 1865:

Schleicher (re Ernst, almost 3 years old):
   The change of k and g into t and d in the pronunciation of children is familiar. Before my oldest boy, who had earlier an actual t for k learned to pronounce a pure k, he pronounced a palatal ç... (1861/ 1971, p. 19)
Schleicher (re Ethart, 3 years old):
   The same child transforms initial *s* and *sch* into a dark, faintly articulated d (t is not used in the region it occurs only exceptionally)... Since the same language artist also changes *g* and *k* and, of course, *t*

into *d*, she pronounces no fewer than six different sounds in the same way [i.e., [ɖ] = all six]. (1861/1971, p. 20)

Ament (re Irma, 3 years old):

A blending phenomena is contained, for example in Irma's *kalerne* (laterne, 'latern'), 1086th day. The child converted t into k and performed a metathesis with them [if t = k then k = t]. (1899/1971, p. 40)

As Franke (1912/1971, p. 41) concludes, "Apparently children in the first speaking period have no difficulty articulating at least m. b. or p., n. d. or t. The difficulty lies only in the change of place or manner of articulation of consonants in one word". This group of sounds, the forward stops, in this stage are opposed to the back place consonants. Whereas maximal contrast has operated until this stage, a new dynamic principle, a privilege of occurrence concept, may be in operation. However, no further interpretation of this concept is developed. Subsequent stages are described without details as to ontogeny. It may be that for the theory maximal contrast establishes a universal foundation. With the subsequent developments, the addition of continuants and velars, the diachronic pattern predicts the most probable pattern of subsequent evolution, which is simply not apparent to the observer.

The child possesses in the beginning only those sounds which are common to all the languages of the world, while those phonemes which distinguish the mother tongue from the other languages of the world appear only later. Thus Van Gunneken appropriately characterizes the manner of language development of the Dutch child: "From general human language to Dutch." (Jakobson, 1941/1968, pp. 50–51)

THE ACOUSTIC MODEL

Acoustically the velar stops are characterized by a central concentration of energy as opposed to the diffuse non-central hubs of the lingua-alveolars and the bilabials, [t], [d] and [p], [b], respectively (see Figure 2). This central region is presumably more sensitive for consonants as

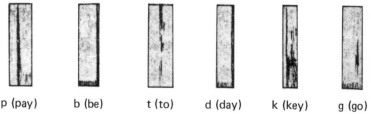

p (pay)   b (be)   t (to)   d (day)   k (key)   g (go)

Figure 2.   Voiceless and voiced stop sounds. (Adapted from Potter, Kopp, & Kopp, 1947/1966, p. 54.)

well as vowels. "But what is only a secondary phenomenon, or epiphenomenon of the vocalic chromatic oppositions, is an essential characteristic of palatovelar consonants. Stumpf carried out an acoustical decomposition of sounds *k, t, p* by means of acoustic filters, and the results showed that, when *t* and *p* are on the point of disappearing the velar stops still remain in the form of a 'dry knocking noise'" (Jakobson, 1941/1968, p. 81). This desire to place perception of consonants and vowels onto the same perceptual dimensions is an attractive aspect of the theory. If both the consonants and the vowels are decoded by the same features, acoustic and physiological, the solution will meet the goal of parismony.

FORMAL DEFINITIONS

Compact (versus Diffuse)

Acoustic Definition

1) a.   Compact phonemes are characterized by the relative predominance of one centrally located formant region (or formant). They are opposed to diffuse phonemes in which one or more

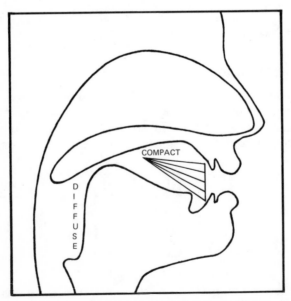

Figure 3.   Physiological model of compact/diffuse.

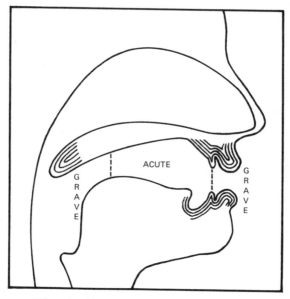

Figure 4.   Physiological model of grave/acute.

non-central formants or formant regions predominate. (Jakobson, Fant, & Halle, 1952/1967, p. 27)

2) a.   Higher (versus lower) concentration of energy in a relatively narrow region of the spectrum

   b.   Accompanied by an increase (versus decrease) of the total amount of energy. (Jakobson & Halle, 1956a, p. 29)

Physiological Definition (Figure 3)

1) a.   Forward flanged versus backward flanged... the resonator of the forward flanged phonemes (wide vowels, and velars and palatals, including postalveolar, consonants) has a shape of a horn, whereas the backward flanged phonemes (narrow vowels, and labial and dental, including alveolar consonants) have a cavity that approximates a Helmholtz resonator. (Jakobson & Halle, 1956b/1962, p. 485)

Grave (versus Acute)

Acoustic Definition

1) a.   Predominance of one side of the significant part of the spectrum over the other. When the lower side of the spectrum predomi-

nates, the phoneme is labeled grave. (Jakobson, Fant, & Halle, 1952/1967, p. 29) ["relative emphasis"]

2) a.   Concentration of energy in the lower (versus upper) frequencies of the spectrum. (Jakobson & Halle, 1956a, p. 31) ["absolute emphasis"]

Physiological Definition (Figure 4)

1) a.   The gravity of a consonant or vowel is generated by a larger and
   b.   Less compartmented mouth cavity, while acuteness originates in a smaller, more divided cavity. (Jakobson, Fant, & Halle, 1952/1967, p. 30)

2) a.   Peripheral versus medial: peripheral phonemes (velar and labial) have ampler and
   b.   Less compartmented resonators than corresponding medial phonemes (palatal and dental). (Jakobson & Halle, 1956a, p. 31)

chapter 17

Overview and Evaluation

SUMMARY OF EARLY STAGES
  The Binary Unfolding Model
STUMPF'S TRIANGLE (ANOTHER PERSPECTIVE)
EVALUATION OF STUMPF'S TRIANGLE
INFORMATION THEORY
  Orders of Approximation
  The Crocker Revision (Prime Features)
HALLE AND THE PHYSIOLOGICAL PERSPECTIVE

SUMMARY OF EARLY STAGES

The first six stages of phonological development are involved in the intricate interplay between consonantal and vocalic properties and Stumpf's triangle. The application of compact/diffuse and grave/acute to the vowels and consonants represents six major stages of development that ultimately could be resolved into four perceptual decisions in the final process. To review, these are the distinctive features learned up to this stage:

1. Consonantal–vocalic
2. Nasal–non-nasal
3. Grave–acute (consonants)
4. Compact–diffuse (vowels)
5. Grave–acute (vowels)
6. Compact–diffuse (consonants)

The Binary Unfolding Model

The binary unfolding model is one manner in which the acquisition of the first four distinctive features may be viewed in all their detail (see Figure 1). In review, the first step is the separation of speech sounds into a vowel or consonant category (level 1). This is followed by the separation of the consonants into a nasal or non-nasal category (level 2). Note that under the vowels this distinction is not relevant linguistically. In French all vowels tend to be nasal. In English the non-nasal property predominates. The third step in the binary unfolding process is the separation of consonants into the labial (grave) versus dental

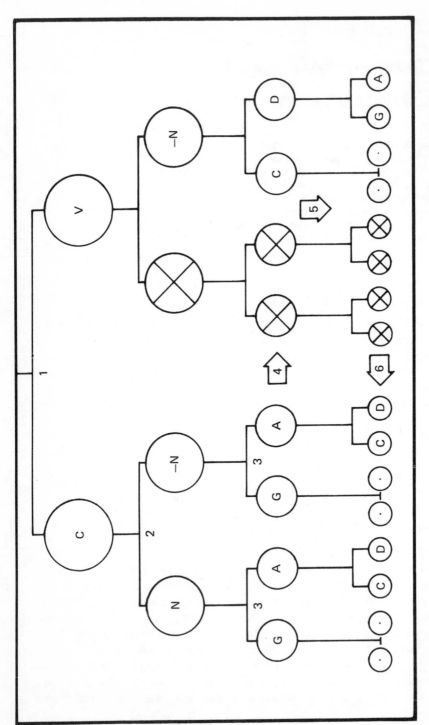

Figure 1.   A binary unfolding model of the acquisition of the first four distinctive features: 1) consonantal/vocalic; 2) nasal/non-nasal; 3, 5) grave/acute; 4, 6) compact/diffuse.

(acute) classes (level 3). In the fourth stage the child begins by comparing the diffuse consonants with the compact vowel. This intermediate step permits the analysis of the vowel system. In this stage the high (diffuse) vowels are opposed to the low (compact) vowels (level 4). The "diffuse-like" nature of the consonants and the "compact-like" nature of the vowels serve as a foundation for the application of this feature to the vowel system alone. In stage five, the high vowels are split into the front (acute) and back (grave) categories (level 5). Finally, the area of concentration of effort returns to the consonantal class. In this stage the lingual sounds are separated into front lingual (diffuse) and back lingual (compact) categories (level 6).

From a critical viewpoint this six-stage decision process is wasteful because the same questions are being asked twice in some cases. Grave and acute is applied to consonants and vowels (stages 3 and 5). Compact and diffuse is applied to vowels then consonants (stages 4 and 6). For this reason, the redundant decision process, it may be assumed that the child with repeated practice reduces the six perceptual steps to four:

1. Consonantal–vocalic
2. Nasal–non-nasal
3. Compact–diffuse (consonants and vowels)
4. Grave–acute (consonants and vowels)

The order of preference here for stages 3 and 4 is based upon the order of the matrix decisions (see Jakobson, Fant, & Halle, 1952/1967, p. 43). The compact/diffuse feature is now applied to both the consonants and the vowels at the same time. This is followed by the application of grave/acute to all sounds. It is reasoned, as previously discussed, that the compact/diffuse and grave/acute axes form the foundation of perceptual judgments (cf. Peterson & Shoup, 1966a, b). The use of Stumpf's triangle is the major mechanism for this type of decision process.

STUMPF'S TRIANGLE (ANOTHER PERSPECTIVE)

Another way in which to present the acquisition of the first four distinctive features is by means of Stumpf's triangle (Jakobson & Halle, 1956a; McNeil, 1970). This explanatory model emphasizes the compact/diffuse and grave/acute axes. In stage 1 (see Figure 2), the child separates the consonants (represented by /p/) from the vowels (represented by /a/). Note that the vertical consonantal/vocalic axis later is redefined as compact/diffuse in stages 4, 5, and 6. In stage 2 the nasal sounds (represented by /m/) are separated from the non-nasal

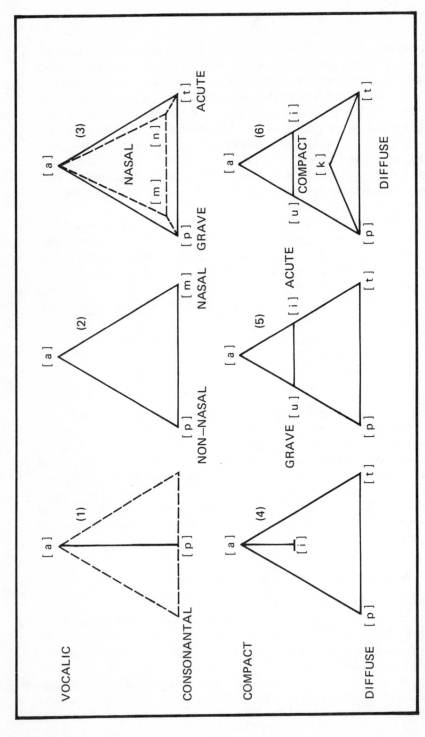

Figure 2. Stumpf's triangle through six stages of phonemic development: 1) consonantal/vocalic, 2) nasal/non-nasal, 3) grave/acute (consonants), 4) compact/diffuse (vowels), 5) grave/acute (vowels), and 6) compact/diffuse (consonants).

sounds (i.e., /p/). Throughout this process /p/ takes on more meaning because the child is learning what /p/ is by learning what /p/ is *not*. This is the relativity component. This stage is sometimes referred to as the "mama-papa" stage. Using the nasal/non-nasal contrast the child may begin to orient his perception of the environment into "maleness" and "femaleness" in the largest and most abstract sense. In stage 3 (the labial/dental split) the child uses the grave/acute axis to separate low frequency consonants [p, m] from the emerging high frequency consonants [t, d]. As can be seen in Figure 2, the nasalization axis lies in a rotated position, orthogonal to the grave/acute axis. This perpendicular relationship supplies the third dimension to the illustration. Stage 4 begins the development of the vowel triangle. Note the inversion of the high/low axis. The high vowels (represented by [i]) are separated from their low counterparts (i.e., [ɑ] etc.) on the basis of diffuse or noncentral energy. This diffuse quality, which has been mentioned before, is generalized from the "spike" component of the stops and is applied directly to the vowel system. In stage 5 the high vowels are categorized into front (high pitched or acute) vowels (represented by [i]) and back (low pitched or grave) vowels (represented by [u]). With the addition of this feature, the vowel triangle has been established, upside down and reversed. Note the relationship of grave/acute as it applies to *both* consonants and vowels. The final stage, 6, makes use of the compact/diffuse axis. The velar consonants with a central concentration of energy are added to the child's infantemic system.

In the final analysis it should be noted that this system, Stumpf's triangle, is a two-dimensional structure. The major axes are: 1) compact/diffuse (vertical dimension), and 2) grave/acute (horizontal dimension). Superimposed on this structure are two fields. The vocalic field is "north," so to speak; the consonantal field is "south." At stage 3 the nasalization feature can be seen, but then it is hidden behind the pyramid. With an active imagination, for that is the only way to see six-dimensional (!) objects, the reader can relate the four features through the six basic stages.

EVALUATION OF STUMPF'S TRIANGLE

Three distinctive feature systems (Halle, 1961, p. 90; Jakobson, Fant, & Halle, 1952/1967, p. 43; Voiers, 1967, p. 11) have utilized Stumpf's triangle as a working base. The configuration posits the following relationships:

p/k = t/k	b/g = d/g	m/ŋ = n/ŋ
∴k/p = k/t	∴g/b × g/d	∴ŋ/m = ŋ/n

because each contrast is equal to one distinctive feature difference, a compact/diffuse difference. (See Appendices A, B, and D.) The remaining systems (Chomsky & Halle, 1968, pp. 176–177; Miller & Nicely, 1955, p. 351; Singh, 1968, p. 3, or Singh & Black, 1966, p. 384; Wickelgren, 1966, p. 390) predict the following relationships:

$$
\begin{array}{lll}
\text{p/k} > \text{t/k} & \text{b/g} > \text{d/g} & \text{m/ŋ} > \text{n/ŋ} \\
\therefore \text{k/p} > \text{k/t} & \therefore \text{g/b} > \text{g/d} & \therefore \text{ŋ/m} > \text{ŋ/n}
\end{array}
$$

The latter distance estimates are because place of articulation (front-middle-back) is considered a linear relationship. Sounds that are made toward the front (labials) are considered more dissimilar than the middle sounds (lingua-alveolars) when they are compared to the back (velar) consonants:

Miller and Nicely linear model   *Jakobsonian triangular model*

```
   p----t----k                              k
     1   1                              1 /‾\ 1
                                       p <------> t
   p/k = 2                                   1

                                         p/k = 1
```

The linear presumption is apparent not only in Miller and Nicely (1955), which uses a front-middle-back orientation (three-point scale). It is apparent in Singh and Black (1966) and Singh (1968), which use a bilabial-labio/linguadental-linguapalatal-velar/glottal orientation (four-point scale); Wickelgren (1966), bilabial/labiodental-linguadental/lingua-alveolar-postdental (sibilant)-palatal (strident/semivowel)-velar/glottal (four-point). Chomsky and Halle (1968) have a hybrid system that attempts to bridge the linear and triangular system.

	Pairs		
System	p/t or t/p	t/k or k/t	p/k or k/p
1. Miller and Nicely	1 +	1 =	2
2. Singh; Singh and Black	1 +	2 =	3
3. Wickelgren	1 +	3 =	4
4. Chomsky and Halle	1 +	4 =	3 !

Whereas a relationship such as AB + BC = AC is shown to exist, a linear assumption is all that is needed to explain the relationship:

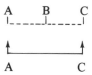

When AC < AB + BC, a two-dimensional explanation or relationship is needed:

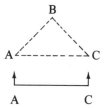

However, when AC + AB = BC, point B is again in a linear relationship, but B lies 180° outside of the original linear domain:

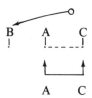

The simplicity of the Chomsky and Halle (1968) model may have been at the expense of common logic. This does not obviate the relationship, for it is a mathematical possibility, but it does call the hypothesis into question. From the Jakobsonian viewpoint the elegance of the theory must not override the predictive power, for the explanation must be grounded in the data at hand.

> The establishment of these general and necessary parallels presupposes the study of the structural laws of linguistic systems—a task much neglected until a short time ago. In addition, the uncovering of generally valid structural principles of child language requires *very careful and exact observations* concerning the linguistic development of the child [emphasis mine]. (Jakobson, 1941/1968, p. 19)

To test the adequacy of the three models—the American linear, the Jakobsonian equilateral, and the Chomsky and Halle reversed linear— three hypotheses were formulated:

H_0: There is no difference in the number of times labials and velars of the same phonetic nature are interchanged as opposed to the number of times lingua-alveolars and velars of the same phonetic nature are interchanged. (Jakobsonian "equilateral hypothesis")

H_{A1}: The number of times labials and velars of the same phonetic nature are interchanged is greater than the number of times the lingua-alveolars and velars of the same phonetic nature are interchanged. (Chomsky and Halle "reversed linear hypothesis")

H_{A2}: The number of times lingua-alveolars and velars of the same phonetic nature are interchanged is greater than the number of times labials and velars of the same phonetic nature are interchanged. ("Simple linear hypothesis")

A post hoc analysis of the Olmsted data (1971, p. 71) was then performed to test the three hypotheses. The results are unambiguous.

Olmsted data

Labials		Lingua-alveolars	
p/k = 9	→	t/k = 35
k/p = 7	→	k/t = 36
p/g = 0	→	t/g = 3
g/p = 1	→	g/t = 2
b/k = 4	→	d/k = 17
k/b = 0	→	k/d = 4
b/g = 2	→	d/g = 12
g/b = 3	→	g/d = 35
m/k = 0	→	n/k = 3
k/m = 0	=	k/n = 0
m/g = 0	→	n/g = 2
g/m = 0	=	g/n = 0

As can be seen, lingua-alveolar/velar interchange is much more common than labial interchange (85.14% versus 14.86%). The χ^2 value of 86.4 exceeded the .001 level of significance. Furthermore, the fact that all (10/12 to 12/12) of the pairs held the same relationship is significant in and of itself (exact probability .0002). For this reason the null hypothesis (Jakobsonian "equilateral hypothesis") may be rejected in favor of the second alternative ("simple linear hypothesis").

The immediate question to be asked is, "Is Stumpf's triangle a good predictor of children's phonemic patterns?". On the surface it would appear that natural data such as Olmsted's contradicts the triangular perceptual arrangement. However, it may be that Stumpf's triangle (an acoustic model) may be a mere step in the progression to the linear arrangement (a physiological model). The child may triangulate acoustically, evolve into an ideal linear system, and then shape the system considering the language at hand.

Jakobson's theory, then, from this frame of reference is transitory but essential. Although it appears that the theory indicates a triangular vowel system that results in a quadrilateral, the theory, as mathematically arranged in 1952, may be too static and mechanical. Whereas from phase II of the theory (the matrix predictions) the predictions are inaccurate, but from phase I (the sound class concept) one would expect a close relationship between the velars and the tongue tip sounds. The logical/mechanical nature of the second phase may override the organic power of the initial formulation.

INFORMATION THEORY

In 1953 Jakobson, Cherry, and Halle published an article entitled, "Toward the logical description of languages in their phonemic aspect." This article attempted to integrate the mathematical principles of information theory as developed by Claude Shannon with the works of Jakobson (see Shannon & Weaver, *The Mathematical Theory of Communication,* 1949/1963). In this work, the mathematical aspects of the either/or cognitive process were directly related to *bits* or binary digits.

Shannon had postulated that for any given set of communication symbols the most parsimonious method of transmission was to subdivide the entire set (and subsequent subsets) until each unit had a unique code.

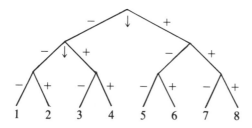

By asking a certain number of yes/no types of questions the unknown symbol may be determined. For instance, in the example above it can be shown with absolute certainty that any number chosen can be determined with three questions, that is, whether it lies above the midpoint of the subset. If the number chosen had been 1, the questions:

1. Is it 5 or above?   No.
2. Is it 3 or above?   No.
3. Is it 2 or above?   No.

tells you it is 1. This process of elimination so to speak is a method for determining the best trial and error method of guessing when no information is known about the frequency of occurrence of the elements in the array. All elements are presumed to be equiprobable (Shannon & Weaver, 1949/1963, pp. 3–5). This process of elimination, as a potential, establishes the fewest number of questions that will evaluate the basic array:

> Successive subdivisions eventually identify any object in a set. If there are N objects in the set, and if N happens to be a power of 2 [if not you will waste part of a question], the number of yes-or-no answers necessary to identify each of the objects in the set is $\log_2 N$. The complete identification of any object is then a chain of plus and minus signs; thus, the object G in Fig. 1 is identified by the chain $(++-)$

A	B	C	D	E	F	G	H
−	−	−	−	+	+	+	+
−	−	+	+	−	−	+	+
−	+	−	+	−	+	−	+

Jakobson, Cherry, & Halle, 1953, p. 36

In a natural situation all elements are not equiprobable. The answer to one question may be used to reevaluate the subsequent questions. In terms of the decision diagram, deviations may deflect on either side of the node from the probability figure of .5. This is the "unbiased coin" assumption. If the deviations are subtracted from the ideal transmission values the amount of information transmitted will be reached. In a sense, information theory is set up in such a way that redundant information is removed from the array. It is this ideal cognitive strategy that forms the Jakobsonian base (Hultzen, 1965). What is missing are the natural effects of the language setting. Triadic decisions do not permit a process of elimination for removing redundancy. In reality this type of decision is a "stacked binary decision" (see Shannon & Weaver, 1949/1963, pp. 18–21).

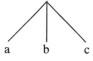

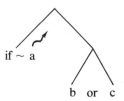

In a balanced array, if one tract of a three-node tier does not contain the element in question, a second question must be asked to determine with certainty the location of the item. In essence this means that the binary digit or bit (or the binary feature) is the *simplest* way of viewing an operation (Cherry, 1956, 1966). Tertiary, quaternary, etc., decisions may be made, but they all can be reduced to their simplest binary form. The former terms imply a process while the latter term involves the purest decision.

Orders of Approximation

Not only was a direct analogy shown to exist between the binary digits (+, −), (0, 1), etc., and the distinctive feature concept; Jakobson, Cherry, and Halle (1953) began to incorporate the concept of orders of approximation into the matrix process itself. The original matrix system is based upon a zero order approximation. Each phoneme in the matrix is considered equiprobable (Jakobson, 1949; Jakobson & Lotz, 1949/1962; cf. Shannon & Weaver, 1949/1963, p. 13). In the normal course of events the ideal binary system concept should have given way to a probability concept where the frequency of occurrence of the sounds of American English are used to weight the decision nodes (Martin, 1973). This would have been a first order approximation of the phonemic system. Instead, the authors opted to retain the pure binary code and presented a quasi-second order approximation. In this format the occurrence of two features is used to produce general sound categories recognizable on the basis of phonetic similarity. Because the original argument is worked out on Russian, an analogous situation will be presented for American English.

In 1941 Jakobson had used consonantal/vocalic as a bipolar feature in his theory of acquisition. However, in subsequent writings this feature was divided into two features: consonantal/nonconsonantal and vocalic/nonvocalic (cf. Jakobson, 1949/1962, p. 492; Jakobson, Fant, and Halle, 1952/1967, p. 43 to Jakobson & Lotz, 1949/1962, p. 434). This strategy, at first an apparent contradiction, permits the creation of four similarity classes: a sound class coded as a consonant and not a vowel (pure consonants), a sound class coded as not a consonant and plus vowel (pure vowel), a sound class coded as *both* a consonant and a vowel (semivowels), and finally a class coded as neither a consonant nor a vowel (null phoneme). This hypercode produces a semivowel class that can include /r/, /l/, etc., which were not included in the acquisition series; and this class still is not formally integrated into the model. The unusual hypercode of −consonant and −vowel fits an unusual situation. When one compares [ɪl] and [pɪl], it will be noted the absence of a phoneme in the initial position has a phonemic status.

$$[\# \; \text{ɪ l}]$$
$$\uparrow$$
$$[\text{p ɪ l}]$$

This phoneme, /#/, the null phoneme, is neither a consonant nor a vowel. Again, it has not been formally integrated into the acquisition theory, but it does have definite implications for syntagmatic development. In all, the splitting of consonantal/vocalic into two separate distinctive features, as a second order approximation, permits the establishment of four important sound classes: true consonants, true vowels, semivowels, and the null phoneme.

The Crocker Revision (Prime Features)

In 1969, John Crocker adapted this idea in his revision of the Jakobsonian model (p. 296). In his strategy there are three class features: primary, secondary, and cognate. Primary features are those which "establish a class" (p. 205). Crocker posited vocalic and consonantal (±), and +nasal, and +strident as basic for the establishment of five classes: vowels, consonants, liquids, nasals, and stridents. The secondary features—continuency, diffuseness, voicing, and graveness—were used to separate sounds within the major subclasses. The cognate features were defined as any feature that separates two sounds that are identical in all other perspectives. The general evolution of the child was seen as the establishment of prime feature sets that were successively refined until terminal definitions of each phoneme were reached.

The foregoing discussion in Chapter 6 of the function of the distinctive features shows that any feature may be used as prime feature (when combined with other features), secondary feature (when a previously learned feature is being generalized), and a cognate feature (when the situation is minimal). However, this formulation of Crocker's does have certain advantages. On the positive side the second order approximation cycle of the theory was integrated into an acquisition model. Furthermore, this work points out the importance of defin-

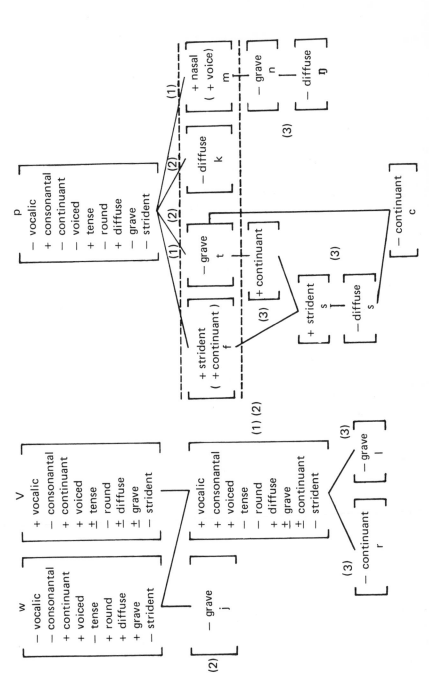

Figure 3. Diagram of the phonological model of children's articulation competence as it develops from prime feature sets, through the formation of base sets, to terminal feature sets. (Adapted from Crocker, 1969, p. 217.)

ing the various functions of the distinctive feature: to establish classes, to be generalized, and to separate words. On the negative side Crocker's article tended to violate the basic assumption of distinctive feature theory, that is, a distinctive feature is a binary decision. Rather than retain the concept that features were indissoluble bipolar attributes, it was posited that one-half of a feature could be learned irrespective of the other bipolar term. In a sense Crocker was trying to integrate the class evolution theory (phase I) with the implications of the matrix notation and bipolarity (phase II) (see Figure 3).

HALLE AND THE PHYSIOLOGICAL PERSPECTIVE

In 1961, Halle, in constant collaboration with Jakobson, evolved a concept of "natural class":

> We shall say that a set of speech sounds forms a *natural* class if fewer features are required to designate the class than to designate any individual sound in the class. (Halle, 1961, p. 90)

This tendency to categorize sounds into classes had long been a tradition in phonetics. The desire to see the phonemic system of a language as a series of simple sound categories could be traced to the IPA charts developed in Europe. In the United States, the tradition of using manner, place, and voicing (physiological dimensions) had begun as early as Sapir (Blache, 1970, pp. 40–41):

> Any such sound may be put into its proper place by the appropriate answer to four main questions: What is the position of the *glottal cords* during its articulation? Does the breath pass into the mouth alone or is it also allowed to stream into the nose? Does the breath pass freely through the mouth or is it impeded at some point and, if so, in what *manner*? What are the precise *points* of articulation in the mouth? This fourfold classification of sounds, worked out in all its detailed ramifications, is sufficient to account for all, or practically all, the sounds of language. [all emphasis mine] (Sapir, 1921/1949, p. 53)

In his writings, Halle tends to return to the physiological frame, in preference to the motoric/acoustic balance of the original theory. In 1964, he began to separate speech sounds along a continuous physiological axis. In his article he noted that sounds may be placed into four general categories depending upon the "degree of narrowing of the vocal tract" (Halle, 1964, p. 326). Considering sounds from the greatest degree of constriction to the least, stop consonants are termed "contacts"; fricatives and sibilants, "occlusives"; glides, "obstructives"; and high vowels, "constrictives." Although this strategy did not affect the binary code in the matrix, it presented a shift in emphasis from a motoric/acoustic feature to a physiological feature concept. Each feature, for the first time, was defined only from an articulatory viewpoint (Halle, 1964, pp. 326–327).

This radical reorientation of distinctive feature theory is best typified by a quote from an article Halle wrote in collaboration with Kenneth Stevens, "Speech recognition: A model and a program for research":

> In producing a utterance the speaker looks up, as it were, in the table the individual phonemes and there instructs his vocal tract to assume in succession the configuration or gestures corresponding to the phonemes. (1964, p. 605)

In 1968, with the publication of *Sound Patterns of English,* Chomsky and Halle broke with the Jakobsonian framework and tradition. The issue was Stumpf's triangle, the compact/diffuse and grave/acute axis:

> One of the many contributions of R. Jakobson is a phonetic framework in which many of these parallels are properly captured. As is well known, the salient characteristic of the Jakobsonian framework is that the same three features—"gravity," "compactness," and "diffuseness"— are used to describe the primary strictures in both vowels and consonants. This complete identification of vowel and consonant features seems in retrospect too radical a solution... (Chomsky & Halle, 1968, p. 303)

Although the differences between the systems of Chomsky and Halle (distinctive feature = physiological rule) versus Jakobson's (distinctive feature = binary decision) are great, these differences have only currently come to the light of discussion (Parker, 1976, pp. 23–31). It is beyond the scope of this book to develop the Hallian viewpoint. It may simply be observed that the orientation of *Sound Patterns of English* is too one-sided physiologically to explain paradigmatic development holistically. By analogy, Jakobsonian theory attempts to decide on the number of elements in the periodic table, whereas Chomsky and Halle are evolving a scheme for organic chemistry. The models are different because they serve different purposes. Chomsky and Halle are bound to a "transformational" orientation in order to develop a syntagmatic theory. Attempts to integrate both viewpoints may be fatal. Whereas Stumpf's triangle may be too drastic as a total solution for paradigmatic development—a statement that is still debatable—a transformation of the basic assumption of the feature (its differential property) may be too drastic as an explanation of syntagmatic phenomena. The paradigmatic theory will suffer at the expense of the syntagmatic theory. The paradigmatic theory, furthermore, needs revision to incorporate the "linear" phonemic model, for this model has more predictive power. The psychophysical researchers who have developed this model have not attempted to build an acquisition model. They have concentrated on the perceptual task in adults. It would appear that Crocker's (1969) work, which emphasizes feature function, may be the necessary catalyst for further efforts on paradigmatics in the midst of current emphasis in syntagmatic theory (Ingram, 1976b; Smith, 1973).

chapter 18

The Remaining Stages: STAGES 7-10

The remaining four stages of phonemic development, unlike the previous six stages, are easily understood because they entail phonetic properties easily discernible to the student of phonetics. Furthermore, each stage has readily understandable acoustic and physiological properties. Finally, these remaining stages, because they involve distinctive features of a less universal importance, received little, if any, discussion by the authors of the theory. These three factors—the simplicity of the features, the ease of explanation, and the lack of extensive treatment—point toward the need for brief rather than extensive discussion. It would be safe to say that the heart of Jakobsonian theory lies in its development (phase I) and the first six developmental stages. In fact, it is hard to find a source to justify the ordering (!) of the last four stages.

STAGE 7: FLAT/PLAIN VOWELS

With the establishment of the foundation of the vowel triangle, the child is free to pursue the intermediate vowels. At the level of the present discussion it may be presumed that a perceptual structure resembling a quadrilateral has been detailed with four free variation classes (see Figure 1 in Chapter 15). A high front class [i, ɪ], a low front class [e, ɛ], a low back class [o, ɔ], and a high back class [u, ʊ] serve as infantemes. The last remaining operation is to split each of the classes into their true phonemic, that is, adult, status. This restriction in free variation is accomplished by the flat/plain feature.

STAGE 7: FORMAL DEFINITIONS

Flat (versus Plain)

Acoustic Definition

2.4221 Stimulus. Flattening manifests itself by a downward shift of a set of formants or even of all the formants in the spectrum. (Jakobson, Fant, & Halle, 1952/1967, p. 31)

Physiological Definition

2.4222 Production. Flattening is chiefly generated by a reduction of the lip orifice (rounding) with a concomitant increase in the length of the lip constriction. (Jakobson, Fant, & Halle, ibid.)

Discussion

Although they are very similar acoustically, the composition of [ɪ] has a slightly lower (flatter second formant) than its counterpart [i] (see Figure 1). In the same manner [ɛ] is flatter than [e]; [ɑ] is flatter than [æ]; [o], [ɔ]; [u], [ʊ]. This acoustic or musical flattening is accomplished by an increase in rounding, that is, more lip protrusion. (See Figure 1.)

From a critical viewpoint several comments must be made. The three distinctive features—compact/diffuse, grave/acute, and flat/plain—used for the vowels, are insufficient to explain vocalic perception. To begin, three distinctive features can only be used to accommodate eight vowels ($2^3 = 8$). In addition to this, Jakobson's theory only discussed the evolution of six vowels (Jakobson, Fant, & Halle, 1952/1967, p. 43). Using the broadest estimates, 11 vowels [i, ɪ, e, ɛ, æ, a, ɔ, o, ʊ, u, ʌ], a minimum of three diphthongs [aɪ, ɔɪ, aʊ], and the unstressed [ə], a very restricted number of symbols, we can see that at least four features are needed ($2^{3.90689} = 15$). Furthermore, the specific problems of a changing phonetic configuration, such as found in the diphthongs, have not been discussed for their phonemic and perceptual implications. Further revisions of distinctive feature theory will have to take these deficiencies into account. Even the distinctive feature system of Chomsky and Halle (1968, pp. 176–177), which has the capacity to code 8192 phonemes (2^{13}), is not arranged to correct these deficiencies.

PHONEMIC STAGE   # 7

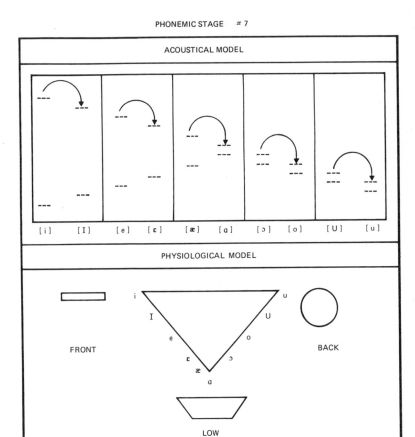

Figure 1.   Two phonetic representations of the flat/plain distinctive feature.

On the positive side, the Jakobsonian treatment of vocalic acquisition does seem to generate broad brush strokes of development. The idea that the child begins with a passive vowel, learns high versus low, triangulates with front versus back, and then begins an intermediating process or differentiation has been reported in the literature:

In the case I studied the speaking stage began in the last three months of the first year, overlapping with babbling, which continued for many months. The low vowels were carried over from babbling. The [æ] of crying and babbling, however, was now dropped. Standard [æ] was replaced by [a]. Standard central [ʌ] was also replaced by [a]... Thus phonemic contrasts became more clearcut. The highest front vowel [i] was acquired in the tenth month in an imitated word, with the allophones [ɪ] and [y], the latter being used after the bilabial phoneme [p b]. In the first month of the second year, the high [i] was contrasted with low [a] and experimentally with the high back [u], so that briefly the coarsest three-vowel system was realized. However, the [u] did not yet become established. Instead two months later (1;2) the mid front [e] was learned in the new word *baby*, which had long remained passive in spite of its great interest value for the child. In this word a clear contrast between mid front and high front vowels existed.

Thus three series of front vowels were learned before the contrast front-back was tackled in earnest. High back [u] and [ʊ] were added lastly to the vowel system in the middle of the second year, that is, four and five months later (1;6–7). Both functioned as representatives of all standard high and back vowels. Mid back vowels were either raised to [u], or

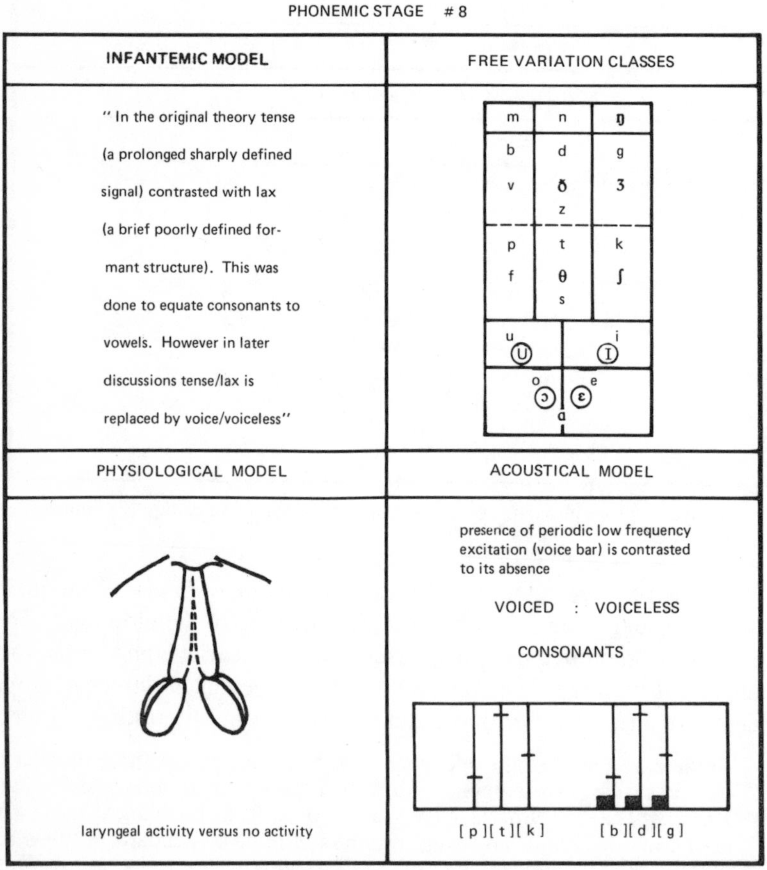

PHONEMIC STAGE   # 8

INFANTEMIC MODEL	FREE VARIATION CLASSES

" In the original theory tense

(a prolonged sharply defined

signal) contrasted with lax

(a brief poorly defined for-

mant structure). This was

done to equate consonants to

vowels. However in later

discussions tense/lax is

replaced by voice/voiceless"

m	n	ŋ
b	d	g
v	ð	ʒ
	z	

p	t	k
f	θ	ʃ
	s	

u ⓤ   i ⓘ

o ⓞ ⓔ e

a

PHYSIOLOGICAL MODEL	ACOUSTICAL MODEL

presence of periodic low frequency
excitation (voice bar) is contrasted
to its absence

VOICED : VOICELESS

CONSONANTS

laryngeal activity versus no activity

[p][t][k]   [b][d][g]

Figure 2. Four different representations of voiced/voiceless as viewed from phonemic and phonetic perspectives.

lowered to [a], and sometimes split into both contrasting vowels as [aʊ]—eloquent testimony to the fact that the mid back vowels did not yet exist as phonemes in the child's vowel system. (Leopold, 1953/1971, p. 137)

To date, there is little doubt that approximately four distinctive features are needed for vocalic acquisition (Singh, 1976, pp. 75-87). It remains for the theoreticians of acquisition to determine the full details of their interaction beyond the grossest configuration.

STAGE 8: VOICED/VOICELESS CONSONANTS

The eighth stage of development in the original theory is devoted to the acquisition of tense/lax. The use of this terminology, if it had been retained, would have permitted a further analysis of consonants and vowels as a simultaneous operation. The *tense* property implied an articulating vocal tract that is under intense muscular control, as in the production of whispered speech. This stage of production generates long sounds. The *lax* property indicated a vocal tract relaxed or at rest. This condition produces short sounds. However, these terms were changed in later revisions of the feature(see supplement to Jakobson, Fant, and Halle, 1967). For reasons beyond the scope of this work, *tense* translates into *voiceless*, and *lax* can be equated to *voiced* production. To simplify the discussion, it might be imagined that the presence of vocal band activity (voiced) is contrasted to the lack of vocal band activity (voiceless) (q.v. Eimas & Corbit, 1973; Lisker & Abramson, 1964). In acoustic terms, voice onset time (VOT) or the presence or absence of the voicing bar might trigger this distinctive feature. (See Figure 2.)

STAGE 8: FORMAL DEFINITIONS

Voiced (versus Voiceless)

Acoustic Definition
  2.331 Stimulus. The voiced or "buzz" phonemes as /d, b, z, v/ vs. the voiceless or "hiss" phonemes are characterized by the superposition of a harmonic source upon the noise source of the latter.... For the voiced consonants this means a joint presence of two sound sources. (Jakobson, Fant, & Halle, 1952/1967, p. 26)
  Physiological Definition
  2.332 Production. Voiced phonemes are emitted with concomitant periodic vibrations of the vocal bands and voiceless phonemes without such vibrations. (Jakobson, Fant, & Halle, ibid.)

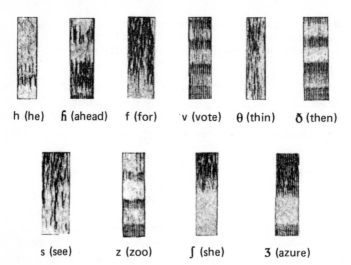

h (he)   ɦ (ahead)   f (for)   v (vote)   θ (thin)   ð (then)

s (see)   z (zoo)   ʃ (she)   ʒ (azure)

Figure 3.   Voiceless and voiced fricative sounds. (Adapted from Potter, Kopp, & Kopp, 1947/1966, p. 54)

Discussion

As noted in Figure 3, the "superposition of a harmonic source" is very apparent when the fricatives are under consideration. The stop class with their "spike" or brief duration, on the other hand, seem to be handled in a different fashion than the former sounds. The idea that a child can learn a series of decisions, as in the binary unfolding model, places great stress on the explanation, when the discussion is definitive. As in the previous classes it becomes apparent that voicing differs as an acoustic cue depending upon the sound class. This implies that a feature is not learned as one decision that is superimposed across the entire sound mass. It would appear that voicing is learned at different stages as a generalization process, perhaps; but a uniform type of acquisition explanation needs revision and refinement to fit the data at hand.

STAGE 9: CONTINUED/INTERRUPTED CONSONANTS

The ninth stage of development is devoted to the time dimension. As has been shown in many texts and experiments, the major use of time is to separate the stop-plosive sounds from the fricative class. The *continued* (fricative) sounds are produced through prolonged physiological contact at the place of articulation. Acoustically this is equated to the production of a "fill." (See Figures 3 and 4.) The *interrupted* sounds

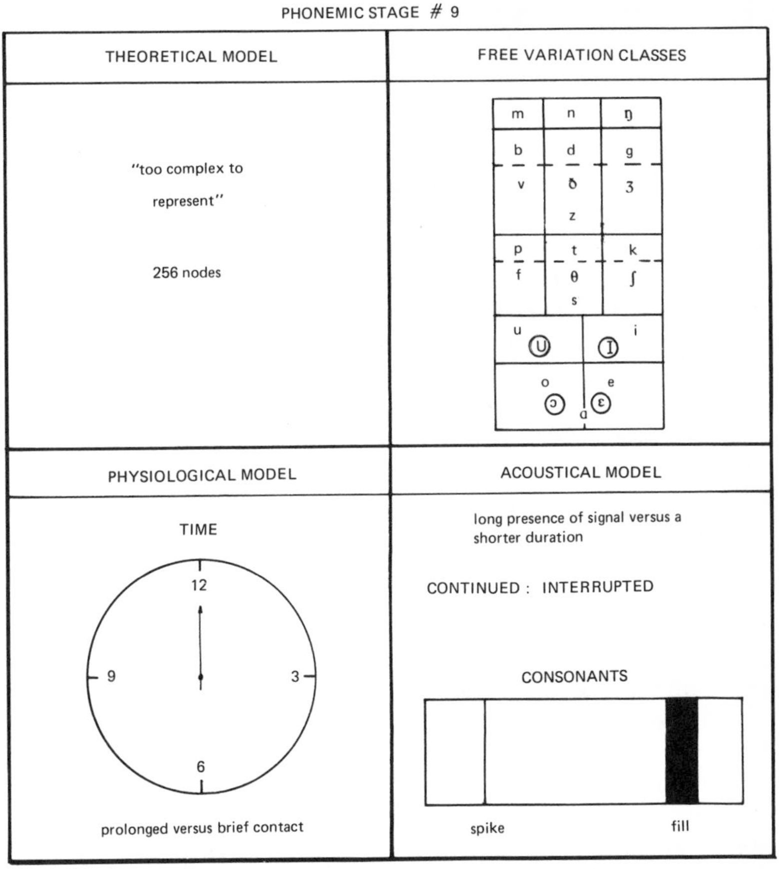

PHONEMIC STAGE # 9

THEORETICAL MODEL	FREE VARIATION CLASSES
"too complex to represent" 256 nodes	(phoneme grid)

m	n	ŋ
b	d	g
v	ð	ʒ
	z	
p	t	k
f	θ	ʃ
	s	

u (ᴜ) (ɪ) i
o (ɔ) (ɛ) e
a

PHYSIOLOGICAL MODEL	ACOUSTICAL MODEL
TIME	long presence of signal versus a shorter duration CONTINUED : INTERRUPTED CONSONANTS
(clock diagram 12, 3, 6, 9) prolonged versus brief contact	spike fill

Figure 4.   Four different representations of continued/interrupted as viewed from phonemic and phonetic perspectives.

(stop-plosives) can be characterized by a brief excitation of the vocal tract. This rapid production creates a "spike" of energy. This time property separates [p, t, k], as well as [b, d, g], from their prolonged counterparts (see free variation classes, Figure 4). As can be noted, the amount of free variation left within the child's phonemic system is very restricted. Only [ð] and [z] and the additional pair [θ] and [s] are used interchangeably. This condition is referred to formally as a "lisp" in the therapeutic fields. In retrospect, a [θ/s] substitution has a more mature quality than a [b/v] (stage 8) or a [t/k] (stage 5). This quality is perhaps inherent in our understanding of the developmental stages as we went through them.

STAGE 9: FORMAL DEFINITIONS

Interrupted (versus Continuant)

Acoustic Definition

2.3111 Stimulus. The abrupt onset distinguishes the interrupted consonants (stops) from the continuant consonants (constrictives). The onset of constrictives is gradual. The main characteristics of stops, on the contrary, is a sharp wave front preceded by a period of complete silence, for which, under certain conditions, a mere vibration of the vocal folds may be substituted. The spectrograms show here a sharp vertical line preceded either by a period of silence or a "voice bar. . . ." (Jakobson, Fant, & Halle, 1952/1967, p. 21)

Physiological Definition

2.3112 Production. The stops have complete closure followed by opening. The constrictives have incomplete closure; but the narrowing considerably reduces the contribution of the cavities behind the point of articulation. . . . (Jakobson, Fant, & Halle, 1952/1967, p. 22)

Discussion

Although when one contrasts the terminology and the definition, there is an obvious difference in the point of emphasis, a solid state or onset concept, the student of distinctive feature theory should remember that the definitions are secondary in importance to the overall model. Whereas most authors would agree that the stop/fricative dichotomy is important (Danhauer & Singh, 1975, pp. 37–48), many experimenters would debate the exact nature of the perceptual cue. In the mentalistic realm of cognitive acquisition, the fact that a child makes a certain decision has more importance than the specific manner in which the decision is made. The phonemic plane of explanation is paramount. A phonemic explanation can obviate a phonetic cue, but a phonetic cue cannot obviate the phonemic explanation—until all the cues are exhausted. In the latter case the phonemic explanation must be reformulated.

STAGE 10: STRIDENT/MELLOW CONSONANTS

The [ð = z] and [θ = s] relationships are redefined with the addition of the last distinctive feature, the strident/mellow contrast. Physiologically the strident sounds are referred to as "rough edged." In the production of [s], for instance, the lower row of teeth make contact with the upper row of teeth. This contact produces many small irregular holes between the upper and lower structure. (See Figure 5.) As the

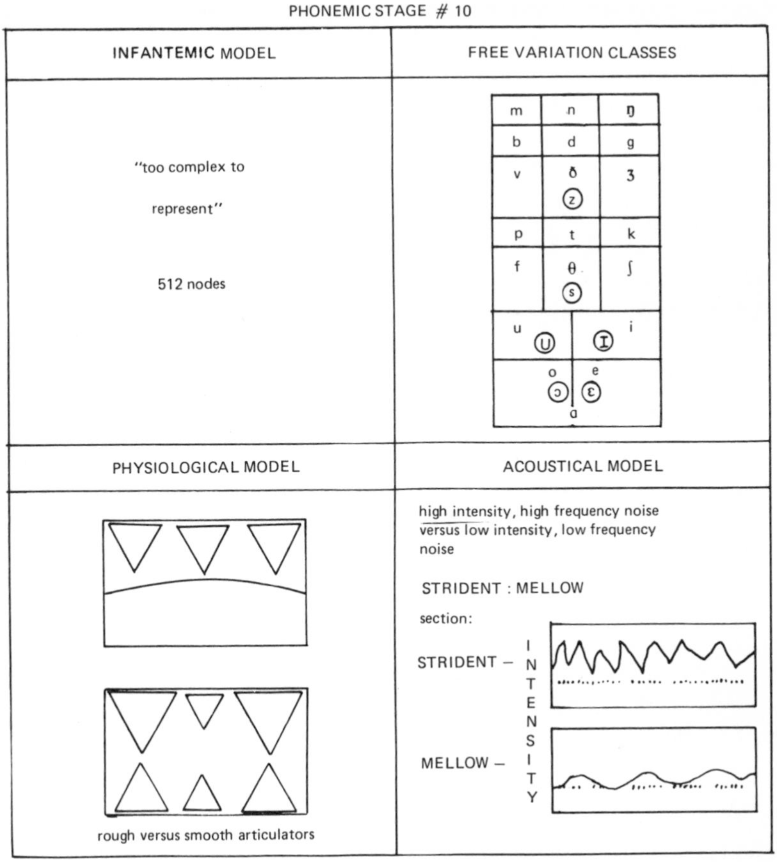
PHONEMIC STAGE # 10
INFANTEMIC MODEL
FREE VARIATION CLASSES
"too complex to
represent"
512 nodes
m n ŋ
b d g
v ð ʒ
z
p t k
f θ ʃ
s
u U I i
o e
ɔ ɛ
a
PHYSIOLOGICAL MODEL
ACOUSTICAL MODEL
high intensity, high frequency noise
versus low intensity, low frequency
noise
STRIDENT : MELLOW
section:
STRIDENT –
MELLOW –
INTENSITY
rough versus smooth articulators

Figure 5. Four different representations of strident/mellow as viewed from phonemic and phonetic perspectives.

air, which is under pressure, is forced through these structures at high intensity, high frequency noise is produced. The air molecules bounce against one another in irregular patterns and serve as a vibrating sound source. To the human ear this sound under prolonged use produces an irritating or *strident* quality. In contrast to this phonemenon, mellow sounds are referred to as "smooth edged." In the production of [θ] the tongue makes contact with the upper teeth. This has several effects. First the tongue tends to fill more holes than the lower teeth, thus reducing the total number of "sharp" edges. Second, as part of the holes are filled with the tongue, there is less turbulence, and a more mellow sound is produced.

In acoustic terms this feature may be represented on a "section" of a sound spectrograph. As previously mentioned, a section is a form of acoustic analysis in which frequency is displayed along the horizontal axis or abscissa; intensity is displayed on the vertical axis or ordinate. A section depicting stridency shows that the strident sounds are more intense and more irregular in terms of their spectrum specifications. The mellow sounds, on the other hand, are lower in intensity and smoother in terms of their display.

STAGE 10: FORMAL DEFINITIONS

Strident (versus Mellow)

Acoustic Definition

2.321 Stimulus. Sounds that have irregular waveforms are called strident. In the spectrogram such sounds are represented by a random distribution of black areas. They are opposed to sounds with more regular waveforms. The latter are called mellow and have spectrograms in which the black areas may form horizontal or vertical striations. (Jakobson, Fant, & Halle, 1952/1967, p. 23)

Physiological Definition

2.322 Production. Strident phonemes are primarily characterized by a noise which is due to turbulence at the point of articulation. This strong turbulence, in its turn, is a consequence of a more complex impediment which distinguishes the strident from the corresponding mellow consonants. (Jakobson, Fant, & Halle, 1952/1967, p. 24)

Discussion

The addition of the last distinctive feature separates [θ] and [s] as well as [ð] and [z]. This final reduction in free variation may be viewed as sufficient to place each and every linguistically significant sound into its proper category. At this point in the learning process each infanteme has acquired its adult phonemic status. It is this match, between the child's understanding and the standards of the adult culture, that is most important. Each culture can, and will, have its own acoustic specifications that are inherently related to the physiological structure:

> Nature presents nothing but an indefinite number of contingent varieties, the intervention of culture extracts opposite terms. The gross sound matter knows no opposition. It is human thought, conscious or unconscious, which draws from this sound matter binary oppositions for their phonemic use. (Jakobson, 1949, p. 54)

Table 1. Modification of the distinctive feature matrix as presented by Jakobson, Fant, & Halle (1952/1967, p. 43)

Feature	a	æ	ɛ	ʊ	ʌ	ı	l	ŋ	ʃ	ǰ	k	ʒ	ž	g	m	f	p	v	b	n	s	θ	t	z	ð	d	h	#
1. Vocalic/nonvocalic	+	+	+	+	+	+	+	-	-	-	-	-	-	-	-	-	-	-	-	-	-	-	-	-	-	-	-	-
2. Consonantal/nonconsonantal	-	-	-	-	-	-	+	+	+	+	+	+	+	+	+	+	+	+	+	+	+	+	+	+	+	+	-	-
3. Compact/diffuse	+	+	+	-	-	-	-	+	+	+	+	+	+	+	-	-	-	-	-	-	-	-	-	-	-	-		
4. Grave/acute	+	-	-	+	+	-	-	+	-	-	+	-	-	+	+	+	+	+	+	-	-	-	-	-	-	-		
5. Flat/plain	+	-	-	+	-	-																						
6. Nasal/oral								+							+					+								
7. Tense/lax									+	-	+	-	+	-		+	+	-	-		+	+	+	-	-	-		
8. Continuant/interrupted									+	-	-	+	-	-		+	-	+	-		+	+	-	+	+	-	+	
9. Strident/mellow									+	+		+	+			+		+			+	-		+	-			

THE DISTINCTIVE FEATURE MATRIX

Finally, the distinctive feature matrix as presented in *Preliminaries to Speech Analysis* (Jakobson, Fant, & Halle, 1952/1967, p. 43) is not the model of acquisition but the adult phonemic goal (see Table 1). The acquisition model as presented in *Kindersprache* (Jakobson, 1941/1968) differs from it in many significant ways. The order of acquisition of features does not follow the order of use in the matrix. This aspect of the theory is yet to be delineated. As an example, nasality, an early feature to be acquired, is used in the sixth position in the adult decision process. It may not be presumed, furthermore, that a child is merely adding a series of features, one after another, in the acquisition process. In the acquisition process the child is adding features by using representative sounds for certain sound categories, and evaluating the specific physiological and phonetic substance he or she is exposed to. Finally the matrix is a natural one. Certain distinctive features do not apply to certain sound categories and have been left blank. This neutralization strategy has not been integrated into a paradigmatic model. This model is ostensive—a point in the direction, so to speak, of phonemic acquisition.

THEORETICAL
ALTERNATIVES

chapter 19

Revision and Extensions of the Model

STRENGTHS AND DEFICIENCIES OF THE JAKOBSONIAN MODEL

Looking back over the Jakobsonian model and the structural philosophy that supports it, several conclusions may be drawn. The model, in and of itself, contains a strong, broad, and comprehensive frame to explain the acquisition process. The definition of the distinctive features as linguistic operations to be learned in a psychosocial setting, with a concomitant physiological and acoustic base, has definite intuitive strength. The general agreement that the laws of implication do predict with success the general pattern of infantemic development is another definite strength. Finally, the definitions of most features have special appeal to those versed in acoustic and/or articulatory phonetics. In all, the theory's strength is its construct validity.

From a negative viewpoint, the theory is a mixed model. Some authors point to the matrix as the acquisition process, while others point to the laws of implication. Even others point to the binary mathematical model and imply that this is the operation in an abstract, generic sense. In all, distinctive feature acquisition is a series of steps in cognitive development. These steps must be defined in a detailed and testable manner. The insufficient treatment of vowels and the poor predictive power of Stumpf's triangle, which arranges the early consonantal array, are specific areas that need improvement. The slight acoustic bias of the approach may be used to temper the theory into a receptive model that culminates in the stronger articulatory model of the American structuralists. Little discussion is devoted to the receptive, retentive, and productive aspects of the theory. This tendency has caused Sanders (1977) to refer to the model as "passive" (pp. 102–104). In terms of the derivation of the theory it was anthropologically and linguistically based with a holistic-teleological goal. The static nature of the matrix and the attempts to put limits on the genetic potential of man, the latter developments of the theory, both tended to distract from the origin of the theory. For this reason, the topic of universality, in its modern sense, has been avoided. Furthermore, the cognitive implications of the ($\pm$) code are more important than the matrix itself. Finally, the order of acquisition of the late features and their subsequent integration into the larger system have been ignored. In all, the theory's strength—its abstract and comprehensive nature—is its worst weakness: a lack of specificity for experimental purposes.

GOALS OF REVISION

Because of these deficiencies, I have attempted to develop a definitive series of steps that maintain the strengths of the abstract theory and extend and modify the theory to retain the salient implications of the matrix system. This was done by integrating the sound-class evolution concept with the binary unfolding model. In doing so, a specific strategy was worked out to relate the acoustic power of the early stages (and its construct validity) with the predictive power of the American linear model. This revision mainly requires the assumption that acoustic perception preceded articulatory production, as a two-step process. Finally, the entire series put forward for review does not purport to be universal to man. These steps represent the most probable order of acquisition that most children will follow. In other words, the "best bet" is always the fastest and strongest horse. This is no guarantee that the horse will always win; but if you must choose, that is the best choice. Theories are seldom disproved by exceptions. They are disproved when they fail to explain as well as other theories on the same subject matter.

BROAD PRINCIPLES OF ORGANIZATION AND GROWTH

In his provocative book, Miller (1967) contended that man does not systematically analyze an array of elements but partitions the matter into specific "chunks." These chunks, after they have been formed, serve as the new elements within the system:

> In order to speak more precisely, therefore, we must recognize the importance of grouping or organizing the input sequences into units or chunks. Since memory span is a fixed number of chunks [the "magic" number 7, plus or minus 2], we can increase the number of bits and information that it contains simply by building larger and larger chunks, each chunk containing more information than before.
>
> A man just beginning to learn radio-telegraphic code hears each *dit* and *dah* as a separate chunk. Soon he is able to organize these sounds into letters and then he can deal with the letters as chunks. Then the letters organize themselves as words, which are still larger chunks, and he begins to hear whole phrases. . . .
>
> In the jargon of communication theory, this process would be called *recoding*. The input is given in a code that contains many chunks with few bits per chunk. The operator recodes the input into another code that contains fewer chunks with more bits per chunk. There are many ways to do this recoding, but probably the simplest is to group the input events, apply a new name to the original group, and then remember the new name rather than the original input events. (Miller, 1967, pp. 37–38)

This strategy, delineated by Miller, shares much in common with the attempts of Jakobson, Cherry, and Halle (1953) to recode the consonantal (±) and vocalic (±) subclasses. It is this similarity in approaches that served as a catalyst for the following modifications.

The higher level chunks are made apparent to the speech scientist and the student of articulatory phonetics. Consonants are easily recognized as belonging to one of five subclasses: stops, velars, semivowels, fricatives, or sibilants. Each of these classes has marked dissimilarities when viewed sonographically. Vowels also are easily recognized as being members of three general classes: short vowels, cardinal vowels, or diphthongs. Once an a priori basis is assumed for the final goals, the specific sequence of acquisition is apparent from Jakobsonian writings. We know that in general:

1.   FRONT→ MIDDLE → BACK

Front sounds precede middle sounds, and middle sounds precede back sounds.

2.   STOPS → FRICATIVES → SIBILANTS

Stops precede fricatives, and fricatives precede sibilants.

Table 1.   Description of sound classes by age of acquisition of elements

Class	Sound	Age correctly produced				Distribution				
		Templin	Wellman et al.	Poole	Year	I	II	III	IV	V
I. Forward stops	m	3	3	3.5	7.5			2	2	2
	p	3	4	3.5	7.0				2	2
	n	3	3	4.5	6.5			2	2	2
	t	6	5	4.5	6.0	1		1	4	
II. Velars and voiced stops	ŋ	3	—a	4.5	5.5				1	
	k	4	4	4.5	5.0	1		1	2	2
	b	4	3	4.5	4.5	2	4	1	1	2
	d	4	5	4.5	4.0	1	6	3		
	g	4	4	3.5	3.5	2	1	3		
	h	3	3	3.5	3.0	5	2	4	2	
III. Semivowels	w	3	3	3.5	Age estimates:	3:1	4:0	4:7	5:9	6:1
	j	3.5	4	4.5						
	r	4	5	7.5						
	l	6	4	6.5						
IV. Fricatives and affricates	hw	—a	—a	7.5						
	f	3	3	5.5						
	tʃ	4.5	5	—b						
	θ	6	—a	7.5c						
	v	6	5	6.5c						
	ð	7	—b	6.5						
	dʒ	7	6	—b						
V. Sibilants	s	4.5	5	7.5c						
	ʃ	4.5	—b	6.5						
	z	7	5	7.5c						
	ʒ	7	—b	6.5						

Adapted from Templin, 1957, p. 53.

a Sound was tested but was not produced correctly by 75% of the subjects at the oldest age tested. In the Wellman data the "hw" reached the percentage criterion at 5 but not at 6 years, the medial "ng" reached it at 3, and the initial and medial "th" and "ʉ" at 5 years.

b Poole, in an unpublished study of 20,000 preschool and school-age children reports the following shifts: "s" and "z" appear at 5.5 years, then disappear and return later at 7.5 years or above; "th" appears at 6.5 years and "v" at 5.5 years.

c Sound not tested or not reported.

3.   NASALS → VOICED → VOICELESS

Nasal sounds precede voiced sounds, and voiced sounds precede voiceless sounds.

These dimensions of development are the Jakobsonian principles derived from the initial phase of the theory. These principles will help sequence the acquisition of the sound classes as well as the subsequent evolution of the constituent sounds. In this manner the strength of the broad frame can be retained.

An informal examination of the sound class concept does seem to organize the age of acquisition estimates of Templin (1957), Wellman et al. (1931), and Poole (1934) (see Table 1). The five sound classes were formed as follows:

Consonantal Class I   (Forward stops)   :[p, t, m, n]
Consonantal Class II (Velars and remaining stops):[k, ŋ, g, b, d]
Consonantal Class III(Semivowels)   :[w, hw, l, r, j, h]
Consonantal Class IV(Fricatives and affricates)   :[f, v, θ, ð, tʃ, dʒ]
Consonantal Class V (Sibilants)   :[s, z, ʃ, ʒ]

These classes represent an initial constituency hypothesis of the organization of the chunks. This organization of the sound classes is specified or implied by phase I of the theory and the perceptual order of the matrix, as well as by the known descriptive data available concerning the sounds themselves. Similar categorical schemes have been developed by Menn (1971, p. 227) for phonotactic acquisition, by Moskowitz (1970, passim), and Ferguson and Farwell (1975, passim) to compare case studies, and by Crocker (1969, pp. 206–210) to explain the evolution of specific sounds. The constituent elements, in and of themselves, are my conjecture based upon a research program of some seven years standing. The details and results of this program are reported in support of the revision hypotheses.

THE SYMBOL SYSTEM

$\begin{bmatrix} \\ \end{bmatrix}$ = The paradigmatic system at a given moment in time. It is an equivalent of the full matrix in its infantemic stage. Modern-day authors use this symbol syntagmatically as a sound segment. However, the former status is to be used throughout this writing.

$\begin{bmatrix} A \\ \text{---} \\ B \end{bmatrix}$ = A subsection of the system (chunk). Information conveyed in this mode is from B to A and is limited therein. The segmented line (- - - -) is the chunk marker.

$\begin{bmatrix} A \\ \text{---} \\ B \\ \underline{C} \end{bmatrix}$ = Underlining denotes the integration of a distinctive feature as it is: 1) being learned, 2) generalized, or 3) recorded.

$\begin{bmatrix} \text{- - -} \\ B \\ \underline{C} \end{bmatrix}$ = Denotes an integration series as it is evolving within the most recently discussed substructure. (An abbreviation, in essence.)

(3) $\begin{bmatrix} \\ \end{bmatrix}$ = A specific sequential stage that represents a major cognitive milestone in the child's infantemic development.

(b) $\begin{bmatrix} \text{- - -} \\ \end{bmatrix}$ = A specific developmental step in an integration series that represents the application of distinctive features to other distinctive features.

Distinctive features	*Jakobsonian binary features*
consonantal ±	Stage 1
vocalic ±	Unintegrated feature
nasal ±	Stage 2
grave ±	Stages 3 and 5
compact ±	Stages 4 and 6
complex ±	Hypothesized features
short ±	For vowels
voicing ±	Stage 8
continuation ±	Stage 9
stridency ±	Stage 10
	Linearly related features
Duration 0, 1, 2	Short, cardinal, complex
Place 0, 1, 2	Front, middle, back
Manner I: 0, 1, 2	Voiceless, voiced, nasal
Manner II: 0, 1, 2	Stop, fricative, sibilant

Operations   At any given moment in the acquisition sequence it is presumed that the child is involved in one of four basic operations:

1. *Acquiring a feature*—Denoted by '_____', an underlined feature.
2. *Class organization*—Generalization is denoted by ( ), parentheses, that surround a previously learned distinctive feature. In the subspace the nature and direction of the generalization is denoted by →, the generalization marker.
3. *Class reorganization*—Denoted by the introduction '- - - -', a segmented line, and the introduction of new terminology above the chunk marker.
4. *Feature recoding*—Denoted by '_____', an underlined feature that is new to the sequence and replaces a previously used term or terms.

VALIDATIONAL EXPERIMENTS

At various points in the explanation of the revised model, certain hypotheses will be analyzed to confirm or deny the specific sequences, generalization processes, or recoding strategies. The analysis uses post hoc techniques on two major descriptive studies of children's misarticulations (Blache, 1975; Olmsted, 1971), two large scale experiments involving adult's psychoperceptual judgments (Blache, 1970; Martin, 1973), and four small group experiments (Blache, 1972) involving college students. The results of these hypothesis tests should be viewed as independent statistical operations. Each operation is a mathematical experiment that can confirm or refute the construct validity of the revised model. Full confirmation of the results of the organization may be used to support the predictive validity of the revision.

The Olmsted Study

In 1971, D. L. Olmsted published an extensive descriptive study of children's articulatory productions entitled, *Out of the Mouth of Babes*. In this study Olmsted analyzed a spontaneous corpus of young children's speech. Each corpus was limited to 32 minutes in duration (tape length, 1200 feet at 7.5 ips). The use of 100 middle class children, ranging in age from 1:3 years to 4:6 years, produced a preschool language sample. The group was balanced for sexual status, 58 females and 42 males. The substitution pattern for the consonants and vowels (see Tables 2 and 3) served as a working statistical base. The 3133 consonantal substitutions and the 2077 vocalic substitutions were considered the phenomena to be accounted for by the theory. Each substitution served as a potential subject or data point. The general field of explanation was, in this case, preschool speech sound substitutions.

The Blache Analysis

In 1975, Blache collected and analyzed the articulatory test results of 1287 grade school children in preparation for the construction of an experimental articulation test. These children constituted a natural, unrestricted sample of the first three grades. The subjects were obtained from two Midwestern public school systems (51.8% male; 48.7% female). The structured corpus, which utilized a modification of a standard articulation test, produced 3209 consonantal substitutions to serve as a data pool (Tables 4 and 5). No vocalic analysis was performed because of a low incidence of errors in the class. The field of explanation for generalization was, and is, elementary school speech sound substitutions.

These two data pools complemented each other and served as a developmental age range sample from early acquisition, 1:3 years, through phonemic maturity, 8:11 years (Templin, 1957). More weight may be placed on the former data pool of Olmsted, for it represents the

Table 2. The speech sound substitution pattern of the consonantal production patterns of 100 children during 32-minute samples

Target sounds								Sound substitutions[a]								
	p	t	k	b	d	g	f	v	θ	ð	s	z	š	ž	l	m
p	—	1	7	56	3	1	11							1		1	2
t	6	—	36	8	135	2	13	2	13	6	6			3			1
k	9	35	—	4	17	45					4			3		1	
b	10			—	8	3	1	8									7
d	1	33	4	5	—	35	1	1		3	1	2				1	4
g		3	30	2	12	—	3	4	1						1		
f	2		1	3			—	7	2		5	2					
v		1		37	2		10	—			1						2
θ	7	9		1	7		36	2	—	1	21		3				
ð		9	1	1	753	4	1	5	2	—	4	43			3		
s	2	19	7		7		28		59	2	—	18	50				
z		3			13		3	1	25	15	67	—	17	2			1
š		2	4		3				12		85	2	—	7			
ž													3	—			
l		1		3	12	1		2							—		1
m	5			13			1									—	
n		4		2	11											2	17
ŋ				1		6										1	3
ʔ																	
r		1			2												
tš		38	3	1	7	1					6		5		9	1	
dž					24	2			8	4	6	2		7			
	42	158	94	137	1016	100	107	33	128	31	205	69	89	19	12	34

Table 3. The speech sound substitution pattern of the vocalic production pattern of 100 children during 32-minute samples

Target sounds						Sound substitutions								
	i	ɪ	ɛ	æ	ə	ʌ	a	u	ʊ	ɔ	w	y	i̯	ɪ̯
i	—	17	6			8		5		3	3			
ɪ	67	—	33	14	37	66	2	2	4	4			1	7
ɛ	7	39	—	18	2	21	19		3	2		1		
æ	2	16	22	—	6	41	28	1	2	2	3			
ə	5	7	4	—		16	1	1	2	3	2			
ʌ	9	31	19	18	3	—	35	21	4	48				
a	2	1	2	1		11	—		4	13		11		
u	2	2	4		3	35	1	—	4	3	2	2		
ʊ	1	5			4	13	5	15	—	6				
ɔ		1	1	5	1	33	63	6	7	—				
ɔw				1	2	25	1	10	3	4	1			
aw	1		3	2		3	17			2	5			
ɛy	26	9	10	6	2	7	7							
ay	13		7	6	2	11	23							
ɔy							3							
i̯	2									3		32	—	
ɪ̯		8			7	6						16		—
ɛ̣	5	5	36	4	4	6	9	1		4		44	1	6
æ̣		1				1	1					33	1	
ə̣	7	11	16	1	27	87	6	45	33	23	2	1		5
ʌ̣						1	9			3	15			
ạ				4	2	8				8	47			
ụ						4				4	4			
ʊ̣		1				3	1	2						
ʔ		2		1	2	8	10	1	2	9	31			
	149	56	163	77	106	403	249	113	67	141	237	21	7	11

n	ð	ʔ	tš	dž	x	γ	ϑ	w	y	r	V	Ɣ	~	ñ	Total
1		3					1	1							89
9		37	13					5	2						297
3	3	8	7		1										140
2		2		1				16	1						59
4		9		2				1	5						112
2	1	1					1	1							62
			1					3							26
							1								54
2															89
2			1	2				1	8						840
		2	1	1				1							197
1		1						2							151
		2	10	1	2										130
															3
5				1				238	22	1	123	17			427
10	4			1				4					2		40
—	10	4											28	11	89
175	—	3						1		1			2		193
			—												
			1					1		—					5
								2							73
		3	—					1							57
216	18	73	36	7	5	1	2	278	38	2	123	17	32	11	

Adapted from Olmsted, 1971, p. 71.
[a]V, nonretroflex vowel; Ɣ, retroflex vowel.

ɛ	æ	ə	ʌ	ạ	ụ	ʋ	ʔ	ɛy	ay	ɔw	aw	ɔy	C	Total
		1						7	2	1				54
3	3	1						4	1	5			s1	256
1								6						120
		1						2	5	4	1			138
									1	2				44
		2						1	3	14	1			211
1	1									2	2			50
	5									3				93
										2				53
1								2	16	5	3		ws	150
	1							1	—	8			1, ϑ	79
								1	1	5			av	66
	12								8	1		3		94
1				6								8		77
							3						dz, t	10
														38
1	5							5		1				48
—	8		3					12	2				dž, n	194
1	—													39
18	1	—		2						4			ʔ	304
1			—											29
		10											lz, d, ʔ	85
				•									n	9
		1	1		—				1				ʔ	11
	3	4					—		3					79
28	1	5	1	8	0	2	0	44	30	63	17	14	17	

Adapted from Olmsted, 1971, pp. 84–85.

Table 4.   Distribution of subject's ages as analyzed by Blache (1975) in preparation of norms for an experimental articulation test

| | | School system A | | | | School system B | | | |
| | | Black | | White | | Black | | White | |
Age level	Total	M	F	M	F	M	F	M	F
4:9–4:11	61	3	10	8	12	0	3	13	12
5:0–5:2	76	12	7	12	13	0	2	14	16
5:3–5:5	89	10	5	23	20	0	0	13	18
5:6–5:8	81	5	11	23	15	2	1	17	7
5:9–5:11	72	6	3	18	18	0	0	15	12
6:0–6:2	95	9	2	20	26	0	3	17	18
6:3–6:5	87	6	7	18	18	0	3	21	14
6:6–6:8	61	6	5	12	12	0	1	14	11
6:9–6:11	79	12	11	21	14	0	0	11	10
7:0–7:2	103	12	7	19	27	2	0	18	18
7:3–7:5	77	6	11	18	11	1	0	8	22
7:6–7:8	65	6	3	17	12	0	1	15	11
7:9–7:11	71	7	8	19	13	1	0	11	12
8:0–8:2	75	5	9	21	22	0	0	8	10
8:3–8:5	69	7	6	19	14	1	1	14	7
8:6–8:8	82	4	8	19	14	1	2	13	21
8:9–8:11	44	4	8	12	7	0	1	11	1

general pattern of early development whereas the latter substitution patterns may be affected by individual articulatory anomalies in the latest and oldest test groups. The former group by comparison suffers in that the examiner had to estimate the target words the children intended to say as part of the analysis paradigm. Each method of elicitation of sound substitutions, a highly controlled sample (small N) with extensive analysis versus an unrestricted sample (large N) with a limited and structured analysis, has its merits. The salient point is that the results represent the phenomenon to be accounted for: the articulatory similarity as measured by the frequency of the substitution patterns themselves. Conclusions drawn from the data pool are heuristic or exploratory in nature. It is fully expected that the derived patterns of organization will be used in predictive studies.

The Adult Studies

Throughout the time period of 1970 through 1977, several psychoperceptual experiments were carried out involving adults. In general, these experiments involved college students and required them to es-

Table 5. Speech sound substitution pattern of the consonantal production patterns of 1287 children derived from a structured articulatory sample

Sound substitutions

Target sound	m	n	p	t	f	ŋ	b	d	k	g	w	l	r	j	v	θ	ð	tʃ	dʒ	s	z	ʃ	ʒ
m		3										1											
n	28							1				1											
p				3														2					
t							1	4															
f	1		3	4			1	1	1	1	2				5	7				2			
ŋ																							
b			2					1		1		1			8		2						
d			1	67	1		1					1											
k				5																			
g								12	11														
w												1											
l			1	1			1	1			53												
r											148			4									
j																							
v					6		260		1	1	10					20				1	2		
θ			1	144	498			48		1	1	3			20		5			38	2	6	
ð				2	9		19	274		1	2	1			109	12				4	4		
tʃ				8	2				4		3								1	20	4	12	
dʒ					3			17	1	2		1			9	3	9	13		13	4	4	2
s				15				3	1	1		1				248		1					
z				2				16	4	1		1			1	31	322		23	46		12	
ʃ				6				1	3	1		2				13		13	4	94	5		6
ʒ				1	1			8		1	10				2	21	28		141	10	60	19	

From Blache (1975).

timate the similarity between two- or three-element sound combinations. Because these experiments differ in nature and intent, each is detailed at the most appropriate levels of the forthcoming discussion. In general, it may be said that, working with adults, these studies produced conclusions relevant to the adult phonemic model—the ultimate goal—rather than the evolving child pattern.

CITY-BLOCK MODEL

Finally, as part of the revision process a new explanatory model has been developed. This model, the city-block model, represents a type of mathematical logic in which multidimensional or hyperspace structures can be represented geometrically (see Torgerson, 1958, pp. 251–259). It may be observed that only the first three dimensions are capable of being represented on a piece of paper, a planar surface with perspective. To get around this problem mathematicians have suggested that one need only accept certain logical restrictions, which are commonplace, and four dimensions and more may be portrayed on a two-dimensional surface. For instance, if one asks in the city the location of a certain building, a common response is three blocks away; go down two blocks, and turn right for one more block:

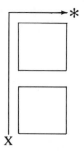

It is well known, however, that as the "crow flies" the distance is really $\sqrt{a^2 + b^2}$. From high school geometry, we will recall that the formula for the hypotenuse of a right triangle is:

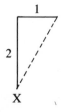

$$\sqrt{2^2 + 1^2} = \sqrt{3} = 1.73 \text{ blocks}$$

Model constructors have their option of using either model depending upon their particular bias. Distinctive feature theory has always been based upon a city-block model. Multidimensional scaling experiments, which have tried to confirm the theory, are based on the Euclidean design. Because it may be expected at the outset that more than three dimensions or features are needed to explain acquisition, the first city-block model is used here. As a working example, our original microphonemic system has city-block properties:

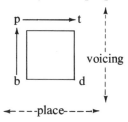

To determine the number of distinctive feature differences between [b] and [t], one simply needs to note the "streets" traveled [b/t = voicing and place]. The total distance is two differences: [b/p = voicing; p/t = place]. It may be noted that the alternate route b/d then d/t produces the same distance estimates (two features) and the same features (place and voicing). The difference between the two routes lies in the order of the features, but this is not considered significant for the explanation at hand.

As the city-block model expands, it will be adjusted to meet the specific mathematical requirements of the explanation. The final adult city-block model has all the same properties as the Miller and Nicely (1955, p. 351) distinctive feature system. Whereas some studies (Martin, 1973; Wang & Bilger, 1973) have shown that none of the major distinctive feature systems has a clear predictive superiority over the other systems, the choice of the adult model has been based on pragmatic criteria. The Miller and Nicely system is the classic linear model upon which many other theoreticians have based their systems. This model has the fewest number of sound properties and is the most parsimonious. Finally the system has sound properties and an arrangement that are clearly understandable to the layman. This adult model, the Miller and Nicely (1955) system, has no ultimate validity, but because of its simplicity future revision would tend to be more complex and harder to explain. In any case the system serves as a good initial choice.

The Most Representative Sound

In conjunction with the city-block model adult-like speech sounds can be represented. These symbols are not meant, however, to be sounds learned, but a cognitive, free-varying class. The sound symbols chosen are class representatives, and only take on adult meaning in the final stages of development. These tenets, of course, are not new and were thoroughly discussed in the Jakobsonian model. The symbols are intended to represent the most probable "phone" to be used to represent the infantemic class. In all, the revision sequence constitutes a hypothetical portrayal of cognitive development initially sketched in the Jakobsonian model. The actual sequence in its present form is felt to be more definitive and subject to additional experimentation.

THE REVISED MODEL

Stage 1–6 (The Early Jakobsonian Stages)

The first six stages of the revised model parallel the developmental sequence as described by Jakobson (see Figure 1). In stage 1, the child learns to discriminate and/or produce representative consonants in contrast to vowels. In stage 2, the actively produced consonant (coded +) is split into two classes, nasal and non-nasal. In stage 3, grave/acute is applied to the entire consonantal system. The resultant four-element infantemic structure (see Velten, 1943/1971, p. 83) is dependent upon a two-dimensional planar arrangement of four infantemes: (p), (m), (t), (n). This system, because it involves the first active integration of two features, is given a formal name: the "nascent" or "primitive" system. Because the features will no longer be used as developmental milestones, these labeled systems will serve as the monotonic guides in the acquisition sequence. Stage 4 involves the introduction of compact/diffuse to a part of the infantemic system, consonantal (−). As previously mentioned, in the Jakobsonian model compact/diffuse in stage 5 is applied to the high vowels, producing a triangular relationship. In stage 6, a collateral application of compact/diffuse is integrated with the grave (−) category (the tongue tip sounds) of both the nasal and non-nasal classes. Note that steps 5 and 6 involve generalizations of features previously learned in the alternate chunks, consonantal (±).

At this juncture it is possible to test the hypothesis that the "nascent" system is acquired before the "velars." As will be noted, if the former class is acquired before the latter, the former sounds have a higher probability of being used for the latter class. If the sequence is wrong, no difference or a difference in the opposite direction (velars replacing the nascents) will be noted. There are eight ways in which [p, m, t, n] can replace [k, ŋ], and eight ways in which [k, ŋ] can replace [p, m, t, n]. The frequency of occurrence of sound substitutions are equi-

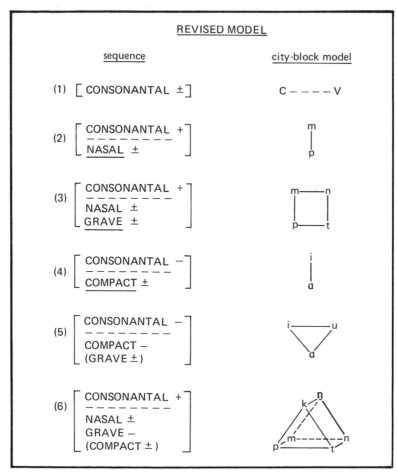

Figure 1.   Two different representations of the first six developmental stages. The lefthand configuration represents the chunks being organized whereas the righthand model represents the evolving distance metric.

probable. One-half of the 282 sound substitutions involving these sounds should fall in each category; nascents replacing velars (predicted) and velars replacing nascents (contradicting theory).

Stage 6—"Velar Hypothesis"

H_0: The rate at which [p, m, t, n] are used for [k, ŋ] is equal to the rate at which [k, ŋ] are used for [p, m, t, n].

H_1: The rate at which [p, m, t, n] are used for [k, ŋ] is greater than the rate at which [k, ŋ] are used for [p, m, t, n].

Table 6.   Stage 6: Chi-square analysis of velar hypothesis (Olmsted (1971) data)

Comparison[a]	Substitutions		
	Predicted	Not predicted	Total
f_i	225	57	282
e_i	141	141	282
$\dfrac{(f_i - e_i)^2}{e_i}$	50.04	50.04	

[a]f_i, frequencies observed; e_i, frequencies expected.

The χ^2 value of 100.08 (Table 6) was far in excess of the 10.8 value needed to reject the null hypothesis at the .001 level of significance (Courts, 1966). The null hypothesis was rejected, and the proposition was accepted that velars follow the nascent sounds developmentally. This finding was confirmed also in the alternate data pool ($\chi^2 = 30.12; p > .001$).

Stage 7 (Consonant and Vowel Recoding)

It would seem that if the vocalic ($\pm$) property is to be inserted into the acquisition sequence, it would tend to occur in or around the third year (Templin, 1957). Vowels are usually complete in this period. For this reason it was hypothesized that vocalic ($\pm$) is applied to consonantal ($\pm$) at stage 7. By integrating these two features, four developmental chunks are generated:

(7)   [CONSONANTAL $\pm$]

CONSONANTAL $\pm$
VOCALIC $\pm$

Recoding
(a) [+] = consonants
     [−]
(b) [+] = semivowels
     [+]
(c) [−] = vowels
     [+]
(d) [−] = null phoneme
     [−]

This stage, implied in Jakobson, Cherry, and Halle (1953), no doubt is involved in syntagmatic development. The null phoneme, which permits the comparison of words of unequal segments, must be an early

Table 7.   Distribution by major sound classes

Class	Proportion (%)
1. Consonants	74
2. Vowels	22
3. Semivowels/vowels	1
4. Semivowels/consonants	3

acquired phenomenon. The semivowels, which have a privilege of occurrence in the second position of the CCV syllable, would seem to require a syntagmatic chunk. Furthermore, the early completion of the vowel system also points toward the early integration of the vocalic ($\pm$) feature. For this reason it is presumed that the entire infantemic system beyond this point is recoded to handle these four subsets.

From a descriptive viewpoint it should be noted that the number of substitution errors that occur within the subclasses are disproportionately large in favor of the consonantal system. In comparing the number of consonantal errors to the number of vocalic errors in the Olmsted (1971) data, it was noted that 14.6 errors occurred per consonantal pair whereas only 9.5 errors occurred per vocalic sound pair. While it is true that 69% of the possible errors fall in the consonantal class because of their greater number in the language, the proportion of error still exceeded the adjusted value, 77% (+8%). The absence of appreciable vowel errors in the older Southern Illinois group would tend to support this finding (Tables 7 and 8).

Because one of the four subclasses of stage 7 contains one element, consonantal $(-)$/vocalic $(-)$ = /#/, the remaining classes in the

Table 8.   Stage 7: Chi-square analysis of the frequency of substitution error in consonantal versus vocalic classes (Olmsted (1971) data)

Comparison	Substitutions		
	Consonants	Vowels	Total
Pairs	171	78	249
Proportions	0.69	0.31	1.00
f_i	2502	743	3245
e_i	2239	1006	3245
$\dfrac{(f_i - e_i)^2}{e_i}$	30.89	68.76	

$\chi^2 = 99.65; p > 0.001; df = 1$ (needed 10.8).

Table 9.   Linear comparison of the proximity of the three major subclasses: consonants, vowels, and semivowels: Recoding comparisons (consonantal ±/ vocalic ±)

	Linear comparisons[a]		
	0–1:1–2	0–2	Total
Pairs	27	11	38
Proportions	0.71	0.29	1.00
f_i	451	12	463
e_i	328.7	134.3	463
$\dfrac{(f_i - e_i)^2}{e_i}$	45.48	111.34	

Computations based upon the Olmsted (1971) data.
[a]Included in 0–1 are the semivowel for vowel, as well as the semivowel for consonant substitutions. The 0–2 class includes the vowel for consonant substitutions.
$\chi^2 = 156.83; p > 0.001; df = 1$ (needed 10.6).

paradigmatic domain may be evaluated for linear relationships (Table 9). Ignoring the (=) possibility of /#/, it may be noted that the hyper-code produces the following relationship:

	Consonants	Semivowels	Vowels
Consonantal	+	+	−
Vocalic	−	+	+
Distance	0	1	2

This indicates that semivowels are more likely to be substituted for consonants and vowels (one feature difference), whereas the substitution of consonants for vowels is more unlikely. When the number of possibilities are taken into account, it can be seen that a 97% rate of substitutions involving semivowels is 16% in excess of that expected. The possibility of consonants and vowels being interchanged is much less likely than the semivowel transformations ($\chi^2 = 156.82; p > .001$).

Stages 8–12 (Later Vocalic Development)

Stage 8 involves a generalization process in which grave (±) is applied to compact (+), the low, passive vowel. This process involves the expansion of the vowel triangle into the vowel quadrilateral. Stages 9–11 involve the ambiguous distinctive feature status of the diphthongs. Because of the drastically changing phonetic character of the diphthongs, [aɪ, ɔɪ, aʊ] have a changing distinctive feature status. In stage 9 it is presumed that [aɪ] is singled out for particular inspection. This vowel begins with two formants in a central or compact domain (500 Hz–1750 Hz). The formant structure of [a__], (165 Hz and 1200

Hz), rapidly changes to a diffuse or noncentral state [___ɪ], (485 Hz and 1975 Hz) (Lehiste & Peterson, 1961; cf. Peterson & Barney, 1952; Ladefoged, 1975). The rapid shift in formant structure gives [aɪ] a transitory feature status.

In stage 10, [ɔɪ] and [aʊ] undergo a similar analysis in terms of the grave/acute feature. It should be noted that the sequence of the analysis of the diphthongs follows the same developmental pattern of stages 4 and 5. Once an operational sequence is established, such as compact/diffuse preceding grave/acute, it is presumed that it continues to have influence. Considering [ɔɪ] and [aʊ], it should be noted that their grave/acute status (F_2 below 1125 Hz) is ambiguous. [ɔɪ], which initially is considered grave because the second formant is low pitched in the region of 900 Hz, is later reevaluated as acute because of its final formant position ($F_2 = 1610$ Hz). From the opposite direction [aʊ], which begins as acute ($F_2 = 1500$ Hz), quickly changes to the low register (910 Hz) (Lehiste & Peterson, 1961; cf. Peterson & Barney, 1952; Ladefoged, 1975). This produces the unusual situation that if a compact consonant changes its status from grave to acute, it is [ɔɪ]; if it changes in the opposite direction, acute to grave, it is [aʊ]. However, this process is too sophisticated for a child at these cognitive levels. What undoubtedly happens is the child passing through stages 9 and 10 simply attends to the ambiguity. This ambiguity or complexity is the essence of stage 11. Complexity ($\pm$) is meant to be used with all diphthongs with a changing phonetic structure contained in a stable segmental and phonemic frame (see Figure 2).

To test the idea that cardinal vowels [i, æ, a, u] are learned earlier than complex vowels [aɪ, aʊ, ɔɪ, eɪ, oʊ], the following hypotheses were formulated.

Stage 11—"Complex Vowel Hypothesis"

H_0:   The rate at which [i, æ, a, u] are used for [aɪ, aʊ, ɔɪ, eɪ, oʊ] is equal to the rate at which [aɪ, aʊ, ɔɪ, eɪ, oʊ] are used for [i, æ, a, u].

H_1:   The rate at which [i, æ, a, u] are used for [aɪ, aʊ, ɔɪ, eɪ, oʊ] is greater than the rate at which [aɪ, aʊ, ɔɪ, eɪ, oʊ] are used for [i, æ, a, u].

The results of this chi-square test (Table 10) indicated a significantly higher rate of substitution of cardinal vowels for complex vowels rather than the converse. The χ^2 value of 52.2 was well beyond the 10.6 to reject the null hypothesis at the .001 level of significance.

The one remaining subclass to be added to the vowel system is the unstressed or lax vowels [ɪ, ɛ, ɔ, ʊ]. These vowels, with their short, relaxed character, are presumed to be late because they represent quick, off-target approximations of the initial cardinal points. This postulate follows the traditional Jakobsonian sequence:

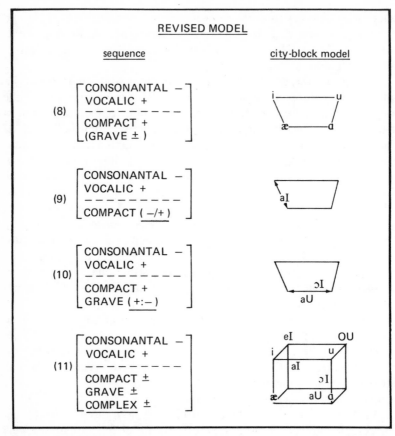

Figure 2. Two different representations of the advanced evolution of the vowel system. The lefthand configuration represents the chunks being organized whereas the righthand model represents the evolving distance metric.

Table 10. Stage 11: Chi-square analysis of complex vowel hypothesis (Olmsted (1971) data)

Comparison	Substitutions		
	Predicted	Not predicted	Total
f_i	116	29	145
e_i	72.5	72.5	145
$\dfrac{(f_i - e_i)^2}{e_i}$	26.1	26.1	

$$(12) \begin{bmatrix} \text{CONSONANTAL } - \\ \text{VOCALIC } + \\ \text{-----------} \\ \text{COMPACT } \pm \\ \text{GRAVE } \pm \\ \text{COMPLEX } \pm \\ \text{SHORT } \pm \end{bmatrix}$$

To test the monotonic sequencing of this feature, short ($\pm$), in reference to the cardinal vowels, the following hypotheses were formed.

Stage 12—"Short Vowel Hypothesis"

H_0: The rate at which [i, æ, a, u] are used for [ɪ, ɛ, ɔ, ʊ] is equal to the rate at which [ɪ, ɛ, ɔ, ʊ] are used for [i, æ, a, u].

H_1: The rate at which [i, æ, a, u] are used for [ɪ, ɛ, ɔ, ʊ] is greater than the rate at which [ɪ, ɛ, ɔ, ʊ] are used for [i, æ, a, u].

As can be seen from the chi-square analysis of the Olmsted data (Table 11), the cardinal vowels do replace the short vowels, as opposed to the converse relationship. The χ^2 value of 45.0 was significant at the .001 level of significance. It was concluded that short vowels evolve at a later stage than the cardinal vowels.

Phases of Feature Alignment   As two features are being interrelated, a city-block solution would seem to indicate three definite stages of interaction: an orthogonal phase, a potential phase, and a pragmatic phase. In the first stage the child must see a distinctive feature as being truly different from other features learned. Regardless of the mathematical model these phases of alignment are represented by an orthogonal configuration or relationship:

Table 11.   Stage 12: Chi-square analysis of short vowel hypothesis (Olmsted (1971) data)

	Substitutions		
Comparison	Predicted	Not predicted	Total
f_i	220	100	320
e_i	160	160	320
$\dfrac{(f_i - e_i)^2}{e_i}$	22.50	22.50	

(1a) $[\pm] = \underline{A \quad B}$ (1b) $\begin{matrix} [\pm] \\ [\pm] \end{matrix}$ =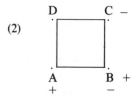

As the second feature is applied to the first feature (1b), the initial phase is conceived as orthogonal because feature 2 is perpendicular to feature 1. Irrespective of the point of orientation +, −, or ±, the following relationship holds true:

$$AC = 1, \; BC = 1, \; AB = 1$$

As feature 2 is applied to *both* + and − of feature 1, a quadrilateral array is formed:

(2)

```
D          C  −
 ┌──────┐
 │      │
 │      │
 └──────┘
A          B  +
+          −
```

At this stage the following relationships hold true:

$$AB = 1, \quad AD = 1, \quad AC = 2$$
$$DC = 1, \quad BC = 1, \quad BD = 2$$

This phase represents the full potential of the interaction space. To see this type of expansion, compare stage 5 with stage 8. This alignment phase is ideal and is inherent in all symmetrical expansions, such as Platonic solids (Holden, 1971). In many cases this full structure is used. In some cases, however, the potential is unused. If the point for element D is unused in a particular system, a simple adjustment can be made:

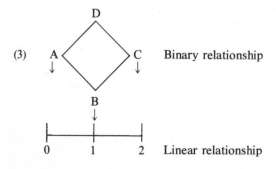

(3)   Binary relationship

        Linear relationship

If the point for an element becomes irrelevant through repeated disuse, it tends to be ignored. While the second binary feature is essential to the decision process, areas AD, DC, and BD cease to be significant in the decision process. Points A, B, and C and distances AB = 1, BC = 1, and AC = 2 are a simple linear relationship. In the city-block model for stage 11 all the dimensions that can be used have been used. The city-block model and the linear resolution of features can solve the pictorial problem of adding the fourth dimension. As previously noted in stage 12, the + complex and + short features are incompatible in American English. In other words, a certain amount of potential is unused. It is assumed that this produces a linear resolution of the two features. The + complex node and the + short node serve as fixed end points on a dimension referred to as DURATION 0, 1, 2. The one dimension may be used to represent two distinctive feature properties.

DURATION: 0–1 = short
DURATION: 1–2 = complex
DURATION: 0–2 = short + complex

This strategy permits a four-dimensional configuration to be presented in three dimensions (Figure 3). With this in mind it is proposed that certain feature combinations may be viewed as transitional when particular perceptual points are not used in the space. For this discussion three phases are postulated:

1. *Orthogonal phase* (new feature)—triangulates the structure with a perpendicular projection

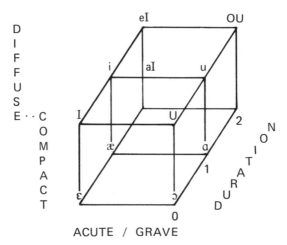

Figure 3.   Four-dimensional configuration presented in three dimensions.

2. *Potential phase* (where the full implications are realized)—creates a quadrilateral structure
3. *Pragmatic phase* (where the use of the potential space is evaluated)—creates a linear structure

With two features the substructures possible are a point, a line, a triangle, and a quadrilateral.

Stage 13 (Full Vocalic System)

$$(13) \quad \begin{bmatrix} \text{CONSONANTAL } - \\ \text{VOCALIC } + \\ \text{-----------------} \\ \text{COMPACT } \pm \\ \text{GRAVE } \pm \\ \text{DURATION } 0, 1, 2 \end{bmatrix}$$

The linear recoding of the vowels along the time dimension was tested using the Olmsted data (Table 12). It was reasoned that a true linear relationship existed if the cardinal vowels [i, æ, a, u] replaced the less complex dipthongs [eɪ, oʊ] at a greater rate than the short vowels [ɪ, ɛ, ɔ, ʊ] for the same dipthongs. Although there were only 77 substitutions to test the hypothesis with, the chi-square values were encouraging ($\chi^2 = 8.12; p > .01$ [needed 6.6]).

For those who would like to monitor the affects of the previous 13 stages on the matrix itself, charts have been prepared (Figures 4 and 5).

Table 12.   Stage 13: Linear comparison of the proximities of three major vowel subclasses: short, cardinal, complex (computations based upon the Olmsted (1971) data)

Comparison	Linear comparisons		
	0–1.	0–2	Total
f_i	51	26	77
e_i	38.5	38.5	77
$\dfrac{(f_i - e_i)^2}{e_i}$	4.06	4.06	

Note: The 0–1 category includes the primary vowels [i, æ, a, u] for [eɪ, oʊ]; the 0–2 category contains the short vowels [ɪ, ɛ, ɔ, ʊ] for [eɪ, oʊ].

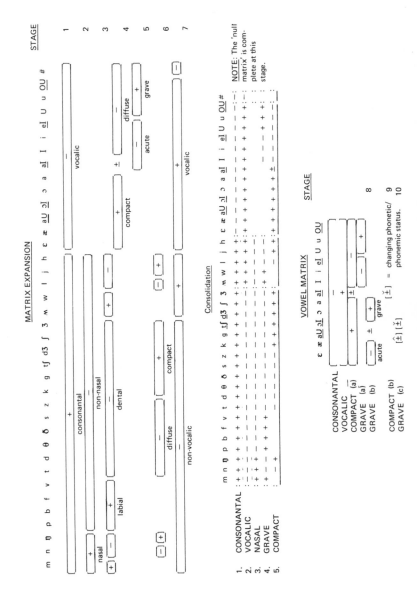

Figure 4.   Matrix expansion, stages 1–10.

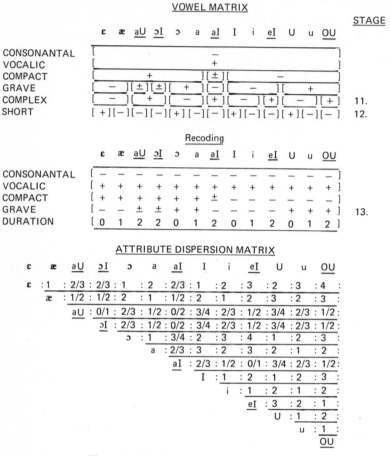

Figure 5.   Matrix expansion, stages 11–13.

These charts represent the organic growth in the matrix as the child integrates one feature after another. For the initial seven stages the matrix makes use of all the major sounds of English. At the end of stage 7, the matrix is consolidated to show the recoding effects of the consonantal (±) and vocalic (±) properties, which are indicated by the consolidation. This is followed by concentrated efforts to organize the vowel system with stages 8 through 10. Stages 11 and 12, which introduce the features complex (±) and short (±), are shown in their binary form. This is subsequently followed by the recoding of the previous two features by the DURATION; 0, 1, 2 feature. This serves as the final matrix form for vowels.

The full vowel matrix is used to determine the number of distinctive feature differences throughout the entire system. This is indicated by the attribute dispersion matrix. As can be seen in Figure 5, some features vary in terms of the number of distinctive feature differences that separate them. This is because of the diphthongs, which are variable. For instance, at any given moment in time [æ] may be 1 to 2 distinctive feature differences removed from [aʊ]. If one were forced to estimate the best point value it would be 1.5 differences; this seems a little illogical, but it is practical.

To test the validity of the attribute dispersion matrix, all the relevant vowel substitutions were placed into a monotonically increasing feature scale system. All substitutions that involved 0/1 to 1 distinctive feature errors fell in the first category. All substitutions that involved 1/2 to 2 differences fell in the second category. This was repeated until four categories were evolved. It was presumed that the vowel metrics as pictured by the city-block model and the attribute dispersion matrix would predict a monotonic function. As the number of features increased on the scale the possibility of error decreased. Sounds that are closer or are more similar have a higher chance of substitution; sounds that are more dissimilar are presumed to be less likely to be interchanged. The results were very strong. The chi-square value of *each* category exceeded the value needed at the .001 level for the entire comparison (16.3, with $df = 3$). This indicated that each feature step was a legitimate scale point. (See Table 13.)

Table 13.   Stage 13: Predictions of similarity (vowels)

| Comparison | Number of feature differences | | | | |
	0/1 + 1	1/2 + 2	2/3 + 3	3/4 + 4	Total
Pairs	19	29	22	8	78
Proportions	0.243	0.372	0.282	0.103	1.00
f_i	428	204	109	2	743
e_i	180.5	276.4	209.5	76.5	742.9
$(f_i - e_i)^2$	339.4	18.9	48.2	72.5	
e_i					
$\overline{X}$	22.52	7.03	4.95	.25	

$\chi^2 = 479.0; p > 0.001; df = 3$ (needed 16.3).

Stages 14–18 (Basic Consonants)

Linear Resolution 2 (Stages 14–16)   Returning to the consonantal class it may be noted that the existing structure is triangular in nature from stage 6. In stage 14 this triangle undergoes a transformation similar to that of the vowels. The compact (±) as of this stage has not been applied to the grave (+) class.

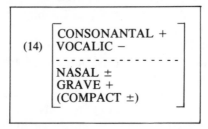

Considering the phases of alignment (see Figure 6), the starting point is Stumpf's triangle in the orthogonal orientation of stage 6. The potential of compact, however, is not used as it was with the vowels. In American English grave (+) and compact (+) are not possible (see Figure 7). As indicated in the figure the grave (+)/compact (+) node is deleted. This of course resolves into the linear system of the American psychometric matrices. In cognitive terms this indicates a stronger

(a) Orthogonal and (b) Potential Phase

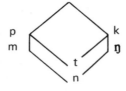

(c) Pragmatic Phase

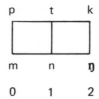

Figure 6.   Orthogonal, potential, and pragmatic phases.

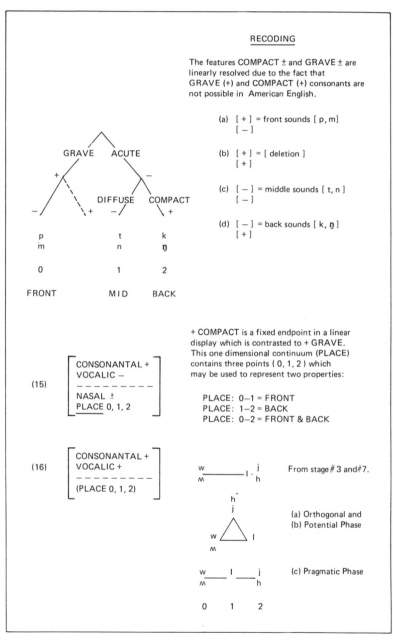

The features COMPACT ± and GRAVE ± are linearly resolved due to the fact that GRAVE (+) and COMPACT (+) consonants are not possible in American English.

RECODING

(a) [+] = front sounds [p, m]
     [−]

(b) [+] = [deletion]
     [+]

(c) [−] = middle sounds [t, n]
     [−]

(d) [−] = back sounds [k, ŋ]
     [+]

+ COMPACT is a fixed endpoint in a linear display which is contrasted to + GRAVE. This one dimensional continuum (PLACE) contains three points (0, 1, 2) which may be used to represent two properties:

PLACE: 0−1 = FRONT
PLACE: 1−2 = BACK
PLACE: 0−2 = FRONT & BACK

(15)   CONSONANTAL +
       VOCALIC −
       − − − − − − − − −
       NASAL ±
       PLACE 0, 1, 2

(16)   CONSONANTAL +
       VOCALIC +
       − − − − − − − − −
       (PLACE 0, 1, 2)

From stage # 3 and#7.

(a) Orthogonal and
(b) Potential Phase

(c) Pragmatic Phase

Figure 7. Representations of stages 14, 15, and 16. The superior figure indicates the recoding strategy using a decision diagram.

Table 14. Stage 15: Recoding comparisons (primary consonants—place) (based on Olmsted (1971) data)

	Linear comparisons		
Comparison	1–2	0–2	Total
f_i	213	12	225
e_i	112.5	112.5	225
$\dfrac{(f_i - e_i)^2}{e_i}$	89.78	89.78	

articulatory emphasis, as opposed to the triangular acoustic paradigm. Stage 15 indicates the recoding process. PLACE: 0, 1, 2 is the common coding scheme for place found in the Miller and Nicely (1955) system. The (0–1) contrast is the front place (grave) feature. The (1–2) contrast is the back place (compact) feature.

To test the linear relationship, the number of times the lingua-alveolar nascent consonants were compared to the number of times the bilabial nascents were substituted for the velars. As might be expected both data pools (Olmsted, 1971; Blache, 1975) indicated the proper linear model (see Table 14) ($\chi^2 = 179.56, p > .001; \chi^2 = 33.0, p > .001$, respectively).

Stage 16 involves the generalization of the PLACE feature to the semivowel subsystem. From stage 3 the labial semivowels are identified as being different from the lingual sounds. As the PLACE feature is integrated into the semivowel system, the front tongue (grave) consonants are contrasted to the back tongue (compact) consonants. This linear relationship was also examined statistically (Table 15). Although

Table 15. Stage 16: Generalization hypothesis (based on Olmsted (1971) data)

	Linear comparisons		
Comparison	0–1	0–2	Total
f_i	238	22	260
e_i	130	130	260
$\dfrac{(f_i - e_i)^2}{e_i}$	89.72	89.72	

the number of sounds in the semivowel system are few, it was possible to compare the proximity of [w] to [l] a middle consonant and [j] a back tongue consonant. The results indicated that [w] is much closer to [l] than [j]. This observation should come as no surprise to the speech therapist who commonly refers to this condition as "lalling," a specific articulatory condition. The chi-square value of 179.45 was greater than the .001 level of significance for the Olmsted substitution pattern. This finding was also confirmed in the Southern Illinois data ($\chi^2 = 53.0, p > .001$).

Linear Resolution 3 (Stages 17–18)   Once the nascent consonants have been expanded into a linear model it is assumed that the voicing feature is introduced. This is indicated in stage 17 with the addition of the voicing ($\pm$) binary feature. Voicing ($\pm$) and nasality ($\pm$) are related in an unusual way. Under normal circumstances nasality ($+$) requires an ancillary vibrator in order to be activated. The nasal cavity is a passive type of structure that requires vibration from an outside

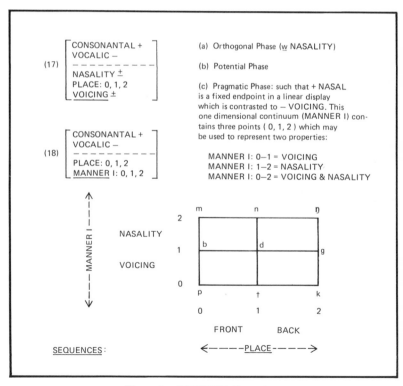

Figure 8.   MANNER dimension.

source, much like the box of a guitar needing a vibrating string. If there is no vibrator there is no resonance. This implies that nasality is interrelated with voicing, which involves the active vibrator, the larynx. For this reason voicing (−)/nasality (+) combination is an unused potential. This relationship permits a linear resolution. This dimension is referred to as MANNER I: 0, 1, 2; where 0–1 = voicing and 1–2 = nasality. (See Figure 8.)

With the introduction of the voicing (±) feature and its recoding, the second major class has been evolved. This class in its entirety is called the "back-nine system." This is not a golfing term. At the completion of the adult model these nine sounds will be located at the back of the city-block model, hence the name. In stages 17 and 18 three ways exist to add voicing minimally: [p/b, t/d, k/g]. In addition to these, five contrastive pairs [b/m, d/n, g/ŋ, b/d, d/g] must be sequenced as part of a generalization strategy.

Generalization Priorities   To sequence the integration and generalization process three simple priorities were established. Each priority is an estimate of the most logical way of attacking the problem. To begin:

1. New features are introduced first

(a)
$$
\begin{array}{|l}
\hline
\text{- - - - - - - - - - -} \\
\text{PLACE: } 0 \rightarrow 2 \\
\text{MANNER I: } \underline{0\text{–}1} \\
\text{i.e., voicing} \\
\hline
\end{array}
$$

This notation indicates that 0–1 (voicing) is introduced throughout the PLACE dimension in front to back direction (0 → 2). The generalization operator is simply an abbreviation here for Jakobson's principle that front sounds are learned before back sounds. This operation results in the following learning sequence: 1) p/b, 2) t/d, and 3) k/g. The second principle of generalization is:

2. Remain in feature dimension for additional features:

(b)
$$
\begin{array}{|l}
\hline
\text{- - - - - - - - - - -} \\
\text{PLACE: } 0 \rightarrow 2 \\
\text{MANNER I: } \underline{1\text{–}2} \\
\text{i.e., nasality} \\
\hline
\end{array}
$$

The dimension that has been linearly coded MANNER I represents a continuum of learning. As part of the recoding process it is understood that the two features are being associated as part of the reorganization. The final order of learning should represent this phenomenon. Following the same front to back direction, nasality (MANNER I: 1–2) is learned in the following order: 1) b/m, 2) d/n, and 3) g/ŋ. Once the full dimension has been integrated into the subsystem, the previously learned features must be integrated into the newly created substructure. Because the structures for integration are of two types, two-dimensional and three-dimensional, their expansion principles should be general enough to serve as collateral modulators. The general modulator for both structures is simply that which has gone on before.

> 3a. Within a two-dimensional space the generalization follows a linear progression established by the *order of acquisition* (in this case 0–1 precedes 1–2 because the front contrast was learned before the back contrast):

(c) $\left\lceil \begin{array}{l} \text{- - - - - - - - - - -} \\ \text{PLACE: } \underline{0\text{–}1} \\ \text{MANNER I: } 1 \end{array} \right.$

(d) $\left\lceil \begin{array}{l} \text{- - - - - - - - - - -} \\ \text{PLACE: } \underline{1\text{–}2} \\ \text{MANNER I: } 1 \end{array} \right.$

Note that in the arrays the new feature MANNER I: 1 is held constant with the change occurring at the previous (first learned) level. To simplify the discussion, principle 3b is explained in conjunction with stage 20, where it is first applied.

The introduction of voicing into the nascent system was tested using both the Olmsted (1971) and Blache (1975) data. The following hypotheses were formulated.

Stage 17—"Voiced Stops Hypothesis"

H_0: The rate at which [m, n, ŋ, p, t, k] are used for [b, d, g] is equal to the rate at which [b, d, g] are used for [m, n, ŋ, p, t, k].

H_1: The rate at which [m, n, ŋ, p, t, k] are used for [b, d, g] is greater than the rate at which [b, d, g] are used for [m, n, ŋ, p, t, k].

Unfortunately the results are ambiguous. The Olmsted substitution patterns indicate that voiced sounds replaced voiceless and nasal sounds at a greater rate than the converse relationship ($\chi^2 = 106.86, p > .001$). The Southern Illinois data indicated the opposite ($\chi^2 = 62.69, p > .001$). Although this finding is a definite deficiency in the model, it must be weighed against the model's overall construct validity. Whatever the reason for the Olmsted results, I feel that the explanation will not be found in the inadequacy of the model but in an artifact that is extraneous to the learning process. The linear comparisons that tested

Table 16. Stage 18: Recoding comparisons (MANNER I)

	Linear comparisons		
Comparison	0–1	0–2	Total
f_i	33	9	42
e_i	21	21	42
$\dfrac{(f_i - e_i)^2}{e_i}$	6.86	6.86	

the idea that voiced sounds [b, d, g] are closer and more easily substituted for nasal sounds [m, n, ŋ], as opposed to the voiceless sounds [p, t, k], revealed a positive finding. Although the error rate within this part of the subsystem is low, 42 substitutions, the distribution is convincing (Table 16).

The chi-square value of 13.71 exceeds the .001 level of significance. It was concluded that the linear relationship specified by MANNER I is worthy of further consideration. The back-nine system, which integrates four distinctive features on a two-dimensional plane, contains all the proper mathematical relationships found in the Miller and Nicely (1955) system. Using a city-block approach with the configuration in stage 18, the number and type of distinctive feature differences between two sounds can be determined by merely noting the "streets."

Stages 19–22 (Later Consonants)

Semivowel Chunk (Stage 19)   With the establishment of voicing (±) in the back-nine system, it is assumed that the same feature MANNER I: 0–1 is incorporated into the semivowel system. This chunk evolved at a later date than the consonants and it is assumed that voicing is also applied here at a later sequential step. (See Figure 9.) The [h] sound has been coded in the original Jakobson, Fant, and Halle (1952, p. 43) matrix as consonantal −/vocalic −. Stage 19 and previous stages, however, place this sound in the consonantal +/vocalic + (semivowel) class. Without the structural orientation, with its mentalistic and linguistic slant, the double negative code would have had to have been supported by the /#/, null, phoneme. The [h] symbol seems a good one to also place in this class because it had phonetic substance that is unused. However, I believe the symbol should read [ʰ], the aspiration marker, rather than the /h/ phoneme. Furthermore, the use of voicing

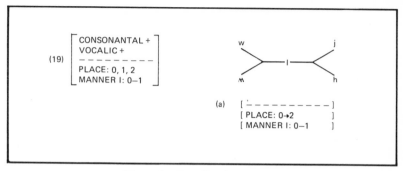

Figure 9.   Recoding for stage 19.

(−) as a property of /#/ confuses silence with air turbulence. In any case, in this paradigm, the phoneme /h/ is evolved as distinct from /j/, the y-like semivowel, in conjunction with the voicing property. Syntagmatic theoreticians may make better use of this sound as a member of the semivowel chunk than if it is coded in another part of the system.

Continuation (Stage 20)   In 1970, 40 college students were asked to judge the similarity between [p, b, m, f, v, θ, ð, t, d, n, k, g] (Blache, 1970, pp. 60–61). Thirteen male and twenty-seven female students enrolled in a hearing and speech science program were asked to evaluate sounds presented three at a time, triadically. The 660 stimulus items were presented in a prerecorded series in a sound-treated room that could accommodate five subjects per session. The results of the one hour, 45 minute task were analyzed by means of a multidimensional scaling technique.

The multidimensional scaling technique employed was a modification of the original Torgerson (1958; 1965, pp. 247–297) technique. This is one technique that can be used without the aid of a computer and permits the experimenter to monitor each assumption of the technique. Three major decisions have to be made in using the Torgerson method: 1) Will the original scores be transformed [P · normal deviate · √2]? (p. 281); 2) What number will be used as the communality figure (an artifact of the centroid solution)? (p. 288; cf. Fruchter, 1954, pp. 51–52); and 3) Will a generalized solution be the ultimate goal? Because the centroid method of factor analysis is mainly a mathematical technique for resolving scalar values into their complex roots, it was decided that there was no advantage in transforming the scale scores. The factor analysis program was used to re-create the original scale estimates of the group. This had the advantage of avoiding the determination of the "additive-constant" (Torgerson, 1958; 1965, pp. 268–277) problem. Second, it was decided that the largest row and column value would

Table 17.   Stage 20: Results of factor analysis

Sound	Factor	
	I	II
p	0.72	−0.26
b	0.74	−0.30
m	0.73	−0.20
t	0.72	−0.14
d	0.75	−0.26
n	0.71	−0.17
k	0.69	−0.21
g	0.70	−0.27
f	0.71	0.48
v	0.75	0.39
θ	0.70	0.50
ð	0.74	0.45

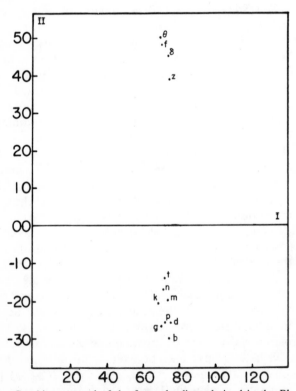

Figure 10.   Graphic portrayal of the factor loadings derived in the Blache (1970) experiment. Factor II is reclassified as the first general factor.

serve as the communality estimate. Third, it was decided that a general solution would be the ultimate goal.

The results of the factor analysis were very exciting (Table 17). The values indicated that adults found continuation to be a very important sound property (see Figure 10). Factor I did not separate the sounds at all, but factor II showed that the fricatives have a strong affinity for each other and that the stops and nasals are closely associated. Remaining attempts to derive features with this method were judged instructive although ultimately unsatisfactory (Blache, 1970, 80–95).

Guilford (1967, pp. 46–60) pointed out that various factor analytic interpretation strategies made use of general and specific solutions. With this in mind, the question was asked: What is the general factor and specific factors associated with the two subsets: the stop/nasals and the fricatives? The two separate factor analyses of the subspaces were again exciting. The factor loadings for both subspaces are shown in Table 18.

Plotting the stop/nasal class was most revealing. Remembering that the first factor derived tends to adjust the internal relationships so that the subsequent stages may be unfolded, the first factor was ignored. The second and third factors were then plotted. The results revealed the back-nine system derived earlier by Miller and Nicely in 1955. However, this configuration was not readily apparent (see Figure 11). With a 30° rotation of the factors the internal relationships became apparent. Factor II held place of articulation characteristics. Low

Table 18.   Stage 20: Factor loadings

Sound	Subspace			Rotation 30°	
	I	II	III	II	III
p	0.77	−0.18	−0.30	−0.34	−0.09
b	0.80	−0.22	−0.25	−0.27	0.04
m	0.75	−0.53	0.23	−0.23	0.53
t	0.73	0.31	−0.26	0.04	−0.40
d	0.79	0.12	−0.20	−0.06	−0.23
n	0.73	−0.23	0.31	0.04	0.38
k	0.72	0.42	0.20	0.42	−0.14
g	0.75	0.34	0.26	0.43	−0.05
f	0.86	−0.17	−0.18		
v	0.84	−0.23	0.14		
θ	0.86	0.20	−0.18		
ð	0.86	0.20	0.14		

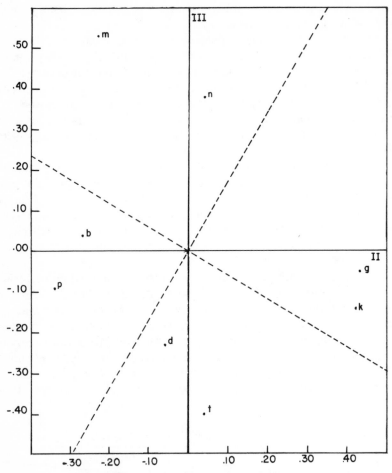

Figure 11.   Graphic portrayal of the factor loadings derived from the subspaces of factor II of the original analysis.

numbers indicated bilabial; no factor loadings (midpoint of the scale) were lingua-alveolar sounds; high loadings on factor II were used for velars. The dimension was (0–1–2), a front-middle-back arrangement. Factor III gave high loadings to nasal sounds. All three voiced sounds on the average had center point loadings on factor III. The voiceless sounds always had lower loadings on factor III; this is most apparent when the cognates are compared to each other. It appeared that factor III entailed a (0–1–2) dimension, which related the laryngeal activity and the resonance system. In the city-block model this is MANNER I:

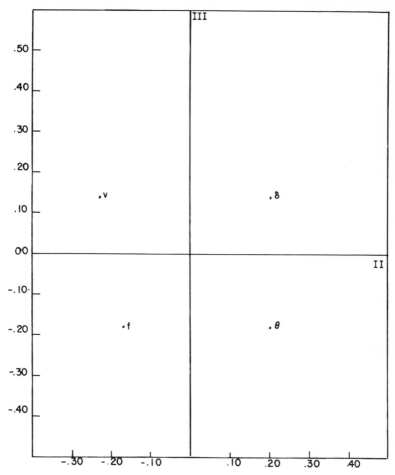

Figure 12. Graphic portrayal of the factor loadings derived from the subspaces of factor II of the original analysis.

0, 1, 2. It was from this configuration that the city-block model was derived. In a sense this study was the key to unlocking the acquisition sequence. The study provided the model. The model was readily available in mathematical terms in the Miller and Nicely study. The remaining problem was to relate the Jakobsonian model to the city-block model.

When the fricatives were plotted in the same manner as the stop/nasal class certain similarities were apparent (see Figure 12). Factor II again contained place information. Sounds made by the lips had nega-

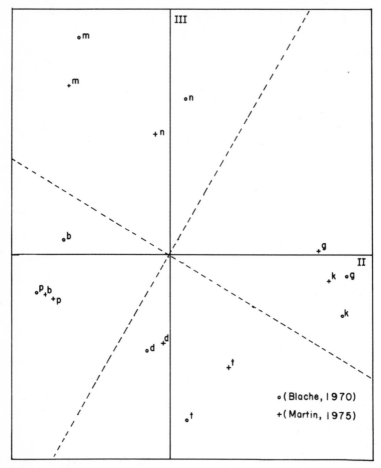

Figure 13.   Graphic representation of the factor loadings for stops and nasals as derived from two different samples.

tive loadings whereas sounds made by the tongue tip had high positive loadings. Factor II again involved voicing. Voiced sounds were given a high positive loading whereas voiceless sounds were given low or negative loadings. The dimensions of the subspaces seemed to be related to each other. Factor II coded place; factor III coded manner properties.

Because the subjects in this study had had training in phonetics the entire experiment was replicated 5 years later. A group of 40 untrained college students were tested with a different speaker. Both speaker and subjects came from new parts of the country. In addition to these variations the randomization list was re-randomized. The results of this

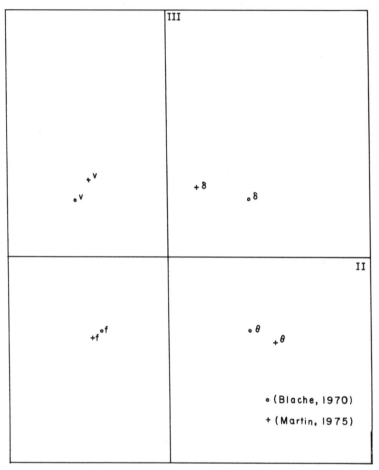

Figure 14. Graphic representation of the factor loadings for fricatives as derived from two different samples.

study (Martin, 1975) matched the original model almost perfectly. The only adjustment needed was a 90° rotation of the fricative class (see Figures 13 and 14).

Stage 20 shows the hypothesized structure as it evolves in the child (see Figure 15). The continuation feature is orthogonal to the back-nine plane. This perpendicular relationship places the feature on the perspective lines in the third dimension. The [p/f, b/v, t/θ, d/ð, k/tʃ, g/dʒ] contrasts each contain continuation (±) as the significant differential property. In addition, the introduction of this feature creates a class [f, v, θ, ð, tʃ, dʒ] that has to be differentiated internally. The

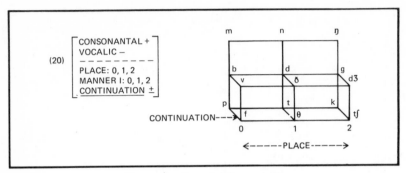

Figure 15.   Recoding for stage 20.

voicing contrasts [f/v, θ/ð, tʃ/dʒ], the front place contrasts [f/θ, v/ð], and the back place contrasts [θ/tʃ, ð/dʒ] all must be learned in a prescribed sequence. Note that in the later stages the integration and generalization process is more complex than feature acquisition. This was observed from the simple fact that the process involves a geometric progression.

The actual order of learning at this stage of development is similar to the generalization principles established at stage 17, and so we can present the final generalization priority:

> 3b. Within a three-dimensional space, expansion follows a quadrilateral structure—"double binary model." The internal sequence within the quadrilateral structure establishes a progression in which the *order of acquisition of organization* (as opposed to feature) has priority. Dimensions that were organized first are varied first before the other dimensions. Thus, the generalization order for stage 20 is as follows:

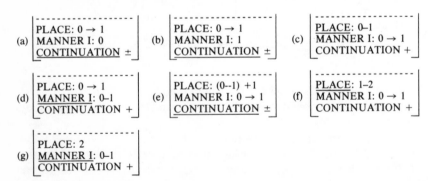

Without commenting on each individual phase, the contrast order is as follows: [p/f, t/θ], [b/v, d/ð], [f/θ, v/ð], ff/v, θ/ð], [k/tʃ, g/dʒ], [θ/tʃ, ð/dʒ] and [tʃ/dʒ]. To many, the position of the affricates [tʃ, dʒ] will seem

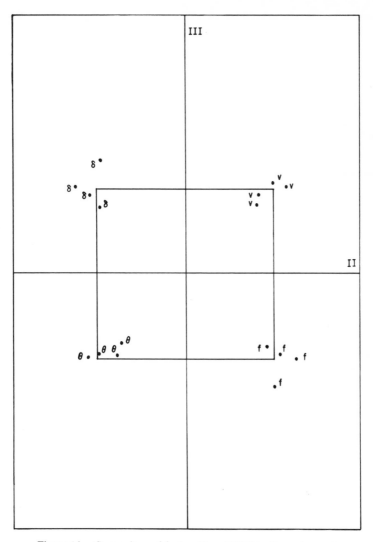

Figure 16.   Comparison of factors II and III (fricative subspace).

strange. In the original Miller and Nicely (1955) experiment, although they had a feature named "affrication" they did not test affricates. On the original city-block model these spaces were empty. However, when young children are asked to approximate a [k] sound in contrast to [t] they often produced [tʃ]. After this phenomenon happened repeatedly it became apparent that the velars and affricates are quite

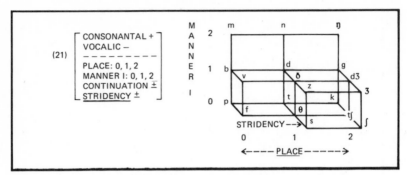

Figure 17.   Recoding for stage 21.

close. For this reason the affricates have been inserted into the Miller and Nicely paradigm. (See Figures 16 and 17.)

Stage 20—"Continuant Hypothesis"

H_0:   The rate at which [p t k b d g m n ŋ] are used for [f v θ ð tʃ dʒ] is equal to the rate at which [f v θ ð tʃ dʒ] are used for [p t k b d g m n ŋ].

H_1:   The rate at which [p t k b d g m n ŋ] are used for [f v θ ð tʃ dʒ] is greater than the rate at which [f v θ ð tʃ dʒ] are used for [p t k b d g m n ŋ].

The validity of the continuant subsystem was evaluated by means of a chi-square analysis. Sounds from the back-nine system replace the continuants at a much greater rate than the converse. The resultant value ($\chi^2 = 696.11$) was well above the value needed to reject the null hypothesis at the .001 level of significance.

This value was confirmed with the Southern Illinois data ($\chi^2 = 762.83$). (See Table 19.) The resultant value was also significant at the .001 level of significance. The fact that continuation is such a dominant factor in adult perception, plus the very high chi-square values found with children's substitution patterns and the almost 2 year, 9 month delay in the completion of this system (see Table 1), points toward the significance of this distinctive feature. In retrospect it is hard to equate the features from the various stages. The child trying to understand the speaking game with the first word faces a tremendous qualitative task; the older child trying to work out all the manifestations of continuation ($\pm$) has a tremendous quantitative task.

Stridency (Stage 21)   Stridency, the last major distinctive feature, helps in the creation of the sibilant class [s, z, ʃ, ʒ]. Each of these sounds requires air forced through the vocal tract at a high rate of speed. This air is then passed through the teeth, which serve as an obstruction for air turbulence. (See Jakobson's stage 10: strident/

Table 19. Stage 20: Chi-square analysis of continuation hypothesis

Comparison	Substitutions		
	Predicted	Not predicted	Total
f_i	920	84	1004
e_i	502	502	1004
$\dfrac{(f_i - e_i)^2}{e_i}$	348.06	348.06	

mellow.) This feature is pictured on the city-block model as an extension along the same dimension as continuation ($\pm$).

During the time period between 1968 and 1972, four small-group experiments were done to examine the predictive adequacy of the distinctive feature scale. In these experiments eight sounds [p, b, f, v, θ, ð, s, z] were presented to college students dyadically in the manner of the Greenberg and Jenkins (1964) study. Students heard two sounds and were asked to rate them as to their degree of dissimilarity using a Mohr and Wang (1968) scale. Each group contained 9–11 subjects. The eight sounds differed from each other throughout a range of one to four distinctive features. It was hypothesized that a treatment-by-subjects analysis of variance design (Bruning & Kintz, 1968, pp. 43–47) and subsequent post hoc testing would show four independent distinctive feature steps when the group's scale values were analyzed. In general, the matrix of Jakobson, Fant, and Halle (1952/1967, p. 43) was found to be a successful predictor of scaled dissimilarity. In light of the current discussion, however, the results are presented using the Miller and Nicely (1955, p. 351) matrix estimates. In all cases this matrix was superior in prediction to the Jakobsonian model. The values for r were as follows: experiment 6: .78 versus .63; experiment 7: .74 versus .53; experiment 10: .77 versus .71; and experiment 11: .73 versus .67. The Miller and Nicely code for these eight sounds is equivalent to that of Singh and Black (1966, p. 384), Voiers (1967, p. 11), and Wickelgren (1966, p. 390). The results of the Halle (1961, p. 90) and Chomsky and Halle (1968, pp. 176–177) matrix were poorer than the Jakobsonian predictions. In three experiments the predictions were no better than chance. This occurred only once in the Jakobson, Fant, and Halle coding, and it never happened with the linear models.

In the first experiment (6) (the number seemed more important to the students), 11 college students with a live voice presentation of the stimulus and a record of phonetic training were asked to judge the eight sounds in all their various combinations. The 56 items (N · N − 1) were presented to the listeners three times for judgment and the first list discarded. The results of the first experiment did confirm four feature steps.

This experiment was then replicated with a new group of subjects with no experience in phonetics. The results again confirmed four significantly different feature steps (see Table 20). All post hoc testing was done by a Duncan's Multiple-Range test (Bruning & Kintz, 1968, pp. 115–117). Each distinctive feature step was significant at the .01 level of significance.

Because both of the previous experiments had been done with live voice, it was decided that visual cues might be affecting the results. For this reason the stimuli were recorded and the experiments were replicated using two different groups: one with phonetic training, the other without. The results of the mean scale scores for all four experiments are presented in Figure 18. As can be seen, the monotonic function of the scale steps was maintained in experiment 10 (no phonetics and no visual cues) and experiment 11 (phonetics and no visual cues). The differences between the third and fourth feature steps in both groups were not significant, but all other steps maintained their independence.

To resolve the question of the effects of the visual cues and the phonetic experience, a two-factor mixed design with a repeated measure on one factor (Bruning & Kintz, 1968, pp. 54–61) was used to test each factor independently. When the affects of visual cues were examined with the feature scale steps, it was found that the number of

Table 20.   Results of replication experiment

Source	SS	df	ms	F	p
Experiment 6					
Total	50.441	43	—	—	—
Subjects	18.565	10	—	—	—
Treatments	27.763	3	9.254	67.498	0.001
Error	4.113	30	0.137	—	—
Experiment 7					
Total	36.288	43	—	—	—
Subjects	15.579	10	—	—	—
Treatments	16.506	3	5.502	39.272	0.001
Error	4.203	30	0.1401	—	—

MEAN VALUES

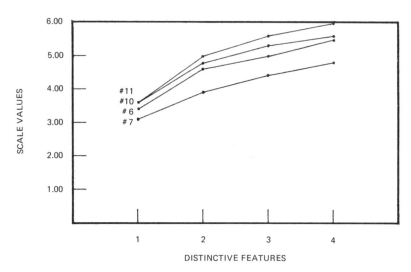

Figure 18. Comparison of mean scale score values for four experiments involving students with phonetic training (experiment 6—visual cues; experiment 11—no visual cues) and without phonetic training (experiment 7—visual cues; experiment 12—no visual cues).

features was significant, but the fact that one group or the other had visual cues (conditions) was not significant (see Table 21).

In a subsequent statistical test the effect of the phonetic training was examined. The results of the two-factor mixed design indicated that there was no difference between those with phonetic training as opposed to those without phonetic training. The scale steps generated by the number of distinctive feature differences were still significant.

The test-retest reliability scores for the four experiments were computed to examine stability. The results indicated significantly stable scores but relatively low levels of prediction (60–70%). As a final strategy the scale scores were factor-analyzed to see the internal relationships between the speech sounds. The results seemed to indicate the problem with the missing feature step (see Figure 19). In each multidimensional array a basic categorical pattern can be seen. The stops [p, b] occur to the upper left (low factor I loadings–high factor II loadings); the sibilants [s, z] occupy the lower lefthand quadrant (low factor I loadings–low or negative factor II loadings); and the fricatives [f, v, θ, ð] always occur to the right of the stops and nasals (high factor I loadings). [θ, ð] seem to be very variable on factor II.

Table 21.   Two-factor mixed design for experiments 6, 7, 10, and 11

Source	SS	df	ms	F	p
Visual cues					
Total	183.134	143	—	—	—
Between subjects	81.029	35	—	—	—
Conditions	9.734	1	9.734	4.642	NS
Error	71.294	34	2.097	—	—
Within subjects	102.105	108	—	—	—
Trials	83.839	3	27.946	168.349	0.001
Trials × conditions	1.322	3	0.441	2.657	NS
Error	16.944	102	0.166	—	—
Phonetic experience					
Total	183.134	143	—	—	—
Between subjects	81.029	35	—	—	—
Conditions	5.570	1	5.570	2.510	NS
Error	75.459	34	2.219	—	—
Within subjects	102.105	108	—	—	—
Trials	83.839	3	27.946	167.341	0.001
Trials × conditions	1.255	3	0.418	2.503	NS
Error	17.011	102	0.167	—	—

The stimulus set [p, b, f, v, θ, ð, s, z] was deficient in that it contained two sounds from each of two categories and four sounds from a third category. This was accidental and an artifact. The original selection was based upon the desire to select phones that would represent at least four distinctive feature differences. However the sound-class nature of distinctive feature judgments was not yet hypothesized. The categorical artifact and its effects upon the binary system were not yet known.

The consistent overall placement of [s, z] helped in the theoretical placement of the sibilants. If the stops and fricatives are so close and the sibilants are so far removed, stridency must be acquired after continuation. Features such as voicing and place appeared to be working within major subclasses. This was the final key in the sequence.

When the fricative subspaces were factor-analyzed, the binary feature orientation was very apparent (see Figure 16). The front fricatives [f, v] received high factor II loadings, and [θ, ð], the tongue-tip fricatives, received a low or negative loading. The place of articulation information was still coded on factor II as in Blache (1970) and Martin (1975). However the front-back orientation was reversed. The voicing relationship of factor III remained identical.

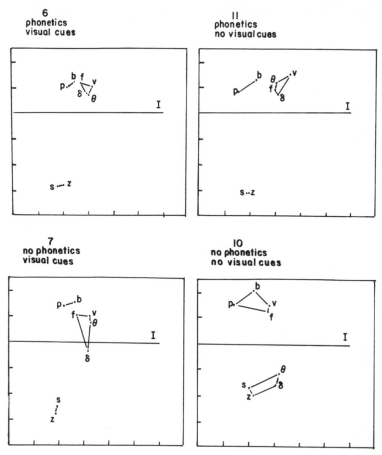

Figure 19. Comparison of the factor analysis charts of the first two dimensions of the scale scores from the four experiments.

The overall results of the factor analysis studies indicated the same general principles. Early factors tend to categorize. Later subspace analyses tend to produce binary features. Perhaps this was the essence of Miller's (1967) chunks. Although these experiments cannot be used to prove a theory, they did serve as the foundation of the sequences and the hypotheses that were formed with the children's substitution patterns. It is the substitution pattern that reaffirms the construct validity of the overall paradigm.

Returning to the stridency feature of stage 21 and the city-block model, it will be noted that four stridency comparisons must be learned in a minimal context: [θ/s, ð/z, tʃ/ʃ, dʒ/ʒ]. Also, two place (back) feature contrasts must be learned, [s/ʃ, z/ʒ], and two voicing feature contrasts, [s/z, ʃ/ʒ], must be integrated. The sequence (generalization order for stage 21) is generated as follows:

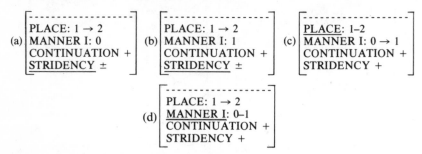

(a)
```
PLACE: 1 → 2
MANNER I: 0
CONTINUATION +
STRIDENCY ±
```

(b)
```
PLACE: 1 → 2
MANNER I: 1
CONTINUATION +
STRIDENCY ±
```

(c)
```
PLACE: 1–2
MANNER I: 0 → 1
CONTINUATION +
STRIDENCY +
```

(d)
```
PLACE: 1 → 2
MANNER I: 0–1
CONTINUATION +
STRIDENCY +
```

These rules produce the following sound contrast order: [θ/s, tʃ/ʃ], [ð/z, dʒ/ʒ], [s/ʃ, z/ʒ], and [s/z, ʃ/ʒ]. This sequence is produced by using the same principles established in previous stages.

The validity of this stage was tested using, again, the sound substitution data pools. The hypotheses formed were as follows.

Stage 21—"Sibilant Hypothesis"

H_0: The rate at which [p t k b d g m n ŋ f v θ ð tʃ dʒ] are used for [s z ʃ ʒ] is equal to the rate at which [s z ʃ ʒ] are used for [p t k b d g m n ŋ f v θ ð tʃ dʒ]

H_1: The rate at which [p t k b d g m n ŋ f v θ ð tʃ dʒ] are used for [s z ʃ ʒ] is greater than the rate at which [s z ʃ ʒ] are used for [p t k b d g m n ŋ f v θ ð tʃ dʒ].

The results of the chi-square test were supportive. The value derived from the Olmsted (1971) data was 22.56. This value is greater than that needed for a .001 level of significance. The value from the Southern Illinois data was even more supportive ($\chi^2 = 607.88, p > .001$). (See Table 22.)

The features continuation (±) and stridency (±) are linearly resolved because continuant (−) and strident (+) are not possible, due to disuse in American English. This pragmatic resolution of unused potential creates a new dimension, MANNER II. The fixed end points of continuant (−) and strident (+) produce a dimension such as that found in Figure 20.

To test the concept of this linear resolution, it was hypothesized that fricatives and affricates would have to be substituted for sibilants at a greater rate than the stop-nasal class. In the substitution patterns of both samples this idea was confirmed (Olmsted: $\chi^2 = 92.80$; Blache: $\chi^2 = 413.87$; both: $p > .001$).

Table 22.   Stage 21: Chi-square analysis of sibilant
hypothesis (Olmsted (1971) data)

Comparison	Substitutions		
	Predicted	Not predicted	Total
f_i	220	131	351
e_i	175.5	175.5	351
$(f_i - e_i)^2$	11.28	11.28	
e_i			

Stage 22 represents the final evolution of the consonants. The place and manner (with voicing) should be familiar to the American phonetician. The city-block model has all the working characteristics of the Miller and Nicely system. If the affricates are not included, as in the original, the spaces merely remain blank; but the space remains the same, for the interdistances are meaningful mathematically.

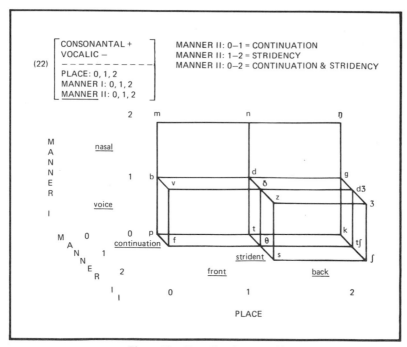

Figure 20.   Recoding for stage 22.

The city-block model for consonants (stage 22), the city-block model for semivowels (stage 19), the city-block model for vowels (stage 13), and the null phoneme /#/ constitute the four chunks of phonemic information that have been recoded. The arrangement of these larger chunks in the syntagmatic domain would seem feasible. A structural examination of the 26 rules of Smith (1973) reveals that there are only five agents that affect the syntagmatic domain: consonants, vowels, features, classes, or phonemes. These rules may occur in progressive or regressive orders, and the number of interacting elements may change, but the deletion, harmonization, and transformational rules may easily be integrated into the previous paradigmatic chunks. (See Appendix H.)

It is assumed that the chunks are related and interfaced. The semivowel system that lies between the consonantal chunk and the vocalic chunk is arranged in such a way that it may be compared to either subsystem; it has both a linear and an equivalent binary code depending upon the use of the semivowel. As noted earlier, speech sound substitutions tend to occur within the class as opposed to across

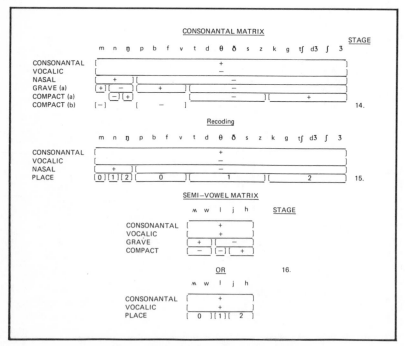

Figure 21.   Consonantal matrix, stages 14–16.

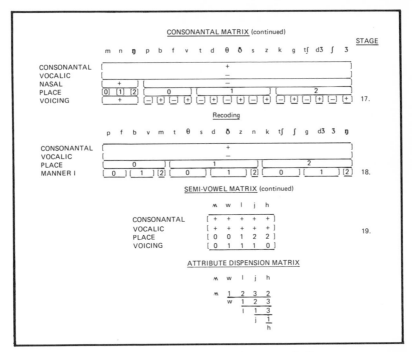

Figure 22.   Consonantal matrix, stages 17–19.

the subsystems. The matrix evolution of stages 14–22 is pictured as in Figures 21–23.

To test the adequacy of the attribute dispersion matrices, the monotonic function of the number of feature differences was examined for both the consonants and the semivowels. The total number of distinctive feature differences possible with the consonants varies from one to six. The six differences could be nasality ($\pm$), voicing ($\pm$), continuation ($\pm$), stridency ($\pm$), front ($\pm$), and/or back ($\pm$). The results of the Olmsted (1971) data are shown in Table 23. The chi-square value exceeded the figure needed to reject the null hypothesis of no monotonic function. The chi-square value for each step was higher than that value. This indicates that each step was unique as a predictor. There are 171 internal substitutions possible using the city-block model of stage 22. Reviewing the type of feature errors (1–6), it may be noted that 81% of the errors were one distinctive feature difference apart. By including those of the two-feature type, 97% of the errors were accounted for. By adding the three-feature errors, 99.9% of the errors were accounted for. The city-block model, just as a working repre-

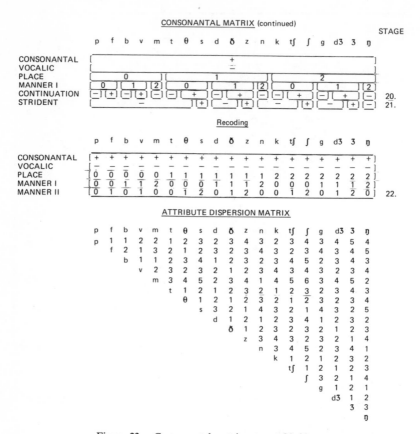

Figure 23.   Consonantal matrix, stages 20–22.

sentation of the nature of the substitution pattern, is a strong and powerful arrangement. Most substitutions are one-feature different in nature. By including the two-feature differences, almost all the substitutions are accounted for.

The Southern Illinois data with older children supported the same findings. A chi-square value for the monotonic function was significant at the .001 level ($\chi^2 = 6985.92$). The proportion of substitutions accounted for were as follows: 1 feature = 85%, 2 features = 97%, and 3 features = 99.9%. If one were asked to give an overall explanation of the nature of speech sound substitutions, the city-block model would be a good starting point.

Table 23.   Predictions of similarity (consonants) (Olmsted (1971) data)

Comparison							
	Number of feature differences						
	1	2	3	4	5	6	Total
Pairs	33	53	49	27	8	1	171
Proportions	0.193	0.310	0.287	0.158	0.047	0.006	1.001
f_i	2023	402	70	7	0	0	2502
e_i	482.8	775.5	716.9	395.1	117.1	14.6	2502
$\dfrac{(f_i - e_i)^2}{e_i}$	4913.5	179.9	583.7	381.2	117.1	14.6	
$\overline{X}$	61.3	7.6	1.4	0.26	0.0	0.0	

$\chi^2 = 6190.0$; $p > 0.001$; $df = 5$ (needed 20.5).

The interfacing of the semivowels and the vowels was also examined. Only 31 errors were found between the two classes. Because this is so small, less than 1% of the total sample, the question was considered untestable. The semivowel for consonant substitutions were slightly higher, 3% of the sample. Although there were only 94 errors, the chi-square value was significant ($\chi^2 = 27.67$). As the number of features increased across the two subsystems the number of sound substitutions decreased.

In all, the model seems to be a well founded one worthy of further testing. The 22 stages and the subsequent generalizations are a very large scale to work with conceptually. The infantemes and the features are disproportionate as scale points. To solve this problem it is suggested that the nature of the expansion series be viewed as a series of six steps. These six steps represent a rough scale of acquisition based upon the percentage of the system completed. These six basic stages are as follows: primitive stage = 2%, vocalic stage = 24%, back-nine stage = 44%, semivowel stage = 52%, continuant stage = 79%, and sibilant stage = 99%. (See Figure 24 for expansion scale values.) It is recommended that these six stages be used as the major developmental milestones of phonemic development.

As one final test of the adequacy of the sequences, the Dewey (1923) data of the frequency of occurrence of the sounds of English were analyzed. It was felt that the expanding binary nodes of development might be influenced by the frequency of occurrence of the fea-

EXPANSION SCALE VALUES

Acoustic Foundation

Stage:	Name:	Infantemes (potential)	Interdistances (potential)	Infantemes (actual)	Interdistances (actual)	Proportion Development	label:
1	consonantal	$2 = 2^1$	1	2	1	–1%	
2	nasal	$4 = 2^2$	6	3	3	–1%	
3	grave (c)	$8 = 2^3$	28	5	10	2%	"primitive stage"
4	compact (v)	$16 = 2^4$	120	6	15	2%	
5	grave (v)	$16 = 2^4$	120	7	21	3%	
6	compact (c)	$16 = 2^4$	120	9	36	6%	
7	vocalic	$32 = 2^5$	496				

phonemes per class: (c) $\overset{+}{-}$ (6)   (d) $\overset{+}{-}$ (0)   (b) $\overset{+}{-}$ (3)   (a) $\left[\overset{+}{\underset{-}{=}}(1)\right]$ ⟶

consonants   semi-vowels   vowels   'null'

Recoding Phase I   syntagmatic complication

Vocalic Organization

Stage:	Name:	Infantemes (added)	Infantemes (total)	Interdistances	Proportion Development	label:
8	'quadrilateral reorganization'	1	10	45	7%	
9/10/11	complex	4	14	91	14%	
12	short	4	18	153	24%	"vocalic system"

Consonantal Organization

Stage:	Name:	Infantemes Added: consonantals	semi-vowels	Total:	Interdistances:	Proportion Development	label:
14 & 15	'linear reorganization'						
16	3–point semivowel system		(3)	21	210	33%	
17/18	voicing (c)	(3)		24	276	44%	"back-nine"
19	voicing (s–v)		(2)	26	325	52%	"semi-vowel"
20	continuation	(6)		32	496	79%	"continuant"
21	strident	(4)		36	630	99% +	"sibilant"

BASIC STAGING SYSTEMS

Stage	System	Proportion
3	Primitive I	2%
13	Vocalic	24%
17/18	Back-Nine II	44%
19	Semi-vowel III	52%
20	Continuant IV	79%
21	Sibilant V	99%

Figure 24.   Expansion scale values.

tures. Although this analysis is only partially complete, the proportion of sounds occurring within a set does seem to parallel the order of acquisition. (See Appendix I.)

In all, this sequence integrates the Jakobsonian model, the descriptive information of the major speech sound acquisition studies, and the structural philosophy that generated the theory. It is hoped that the specificity of the approach will stimulate research, discussion, and new theoretical modifications of the basic theory.

chapter 20

Applying Distinctive Feature Theory

The revision of distinctive feature theory in the preceding chapter has definite implications for the remediation process. The basic structural assumptions of the theory, the prescribed features and their sequential development, should be integrated into *both* diagnosis and therapy. However, before this topic is developed another factor must be taken into consideration. Distinctive feature theory, although widely viewed as an acoustic theory, is not meant to have its full impact at the phonetic level of language (Walsh, 1974, p. 42). In its inception distinctive feature theory was developed to explain cognitive growth. This means that its greatest impact is meant for the learning disabled, or the functional articulation problem. Although acoustic and physiological definitions may be used with success to help the poor phonetic productions of the organically impaired, it is the higher phonemic levels of the theory that have the most importance (q.v. Leonard, 1973; Parker, 1976).

PHONOLOGICAL PROBLEMS

Retarded Phonemic Development

At its most abstract levels the theory is based upon the fact that there is an ideal order of feature development. As with any other basic skill, some children will not keep up with their peers. While allowing for individual differences, it may be presumed that some children will not develop the basic phonemic subsystems—primitive, vowel, back-nine, semivowel, continuant, and sibilant—at the same rate as other children. The etiology of such problems are often simply accepted as unknown. The causes are sometimes referred to generically as "central." In general, the child is viewed as delayed.

The confirmation of a true phonemic problem, however, should be based on a thorough differential diagnosis. This diagnosis should eliminate all possible environmental and constitutional causes of the problem. Therapy based solely on the articulatory performance of the child should have at its foundation no sustaining etiological agents, and ideally no etiological precursors. If etiological agents are known to exist, the remediation process must be shaped to account for them.

Deviant Phonemic Development

In many cases a young child may have an adequate capacity for the phonemic demands of his/her native language, but the child's output is considered impaired as a result of environmental causes. The child who has had to "change" native languages because of geographical movement on an international scale may be presumed to have learned his/her language model in an atypical way. A child who has moved from one region to another, within a nation, may have sound or word selection difficulties in the new environment. The "idioglossia," unique language, found between siblings or twins, as well as a poor parental model, represent a familially influenced type of mis-learning. This is opposed to retarded phonemic development. The phonological system the child has learned is culturally unacceptable. In essence it deviates from the master model. In the case of deviancy, it cannot be presumed that there is "slow" development; it must be presumed that the capacity is adequate to acquire the model but the potential has been, in pragmatic terms, misdirected.

Deviant Phonetic Development

The cerebral palsied child, the motorically deficient, and the structurally impaired are presumed to have phonetic problems. The lack of a productive component from the learning sequence does not impair the understanding or learning of language. The significance of the features is comprehended and discriminated but the total acquisition is incomplete. In the types of disorders mentioned above, the models are poorly developed or mismatched; but in an organically impaired child the model is presumed to exist and needs to be activated productively.

Mixed Problems

Several types of etiologies produce mixed problems, both phonetic and phonemic. The mentally retarded child, with an overall skill deficiency, is presumed to lack the cognitive skills to decode and integrate features or to increase vocabulary at the same rate as other children. In conjunction with this, the child may lack the cognitive skills necessary to control the articulators at will. The overall slowness of development affects phonemic as well as phonetic skills.

The deaf child suffers, in turn, from the same type of problem. Although the capacity to learn is potentially adequate in pragmatic terms, barring a miracle the child cannot decode; therefore, the child cannot integrate and will not, ultimately, produce phonetically. Alternate modalities, of course, will be used, but an acoustically controlled sequence will no longer be of value as a predictor. The optic pathway will carry greater weight in terms of maximal contrast, and when problems occur the tactile pathways will be called upon. In this case the entire learning model is different.

The emotionally deficient child, specifically the autistic, is presumed to have a mixed problem, for he or she can contend neither with the cultural model nor the phonetic requirements of production. The desire to speak and understand is a prerequisite to the learning process in its entirety.

In summary, the functionally or phonemically problematic child is presumed to *lack* the following etiological agents:

A. Environmental
    1. Foreign language model
    2. Regional dialect model
    3. Deficient parental model
    4. Idioglossal model
B. Sensory
    1. Deficient auditory pathway
C. Constitutional
    1. Lack of emotional desire
    2. Lack of intellectual capacity

3. Deficient articulatory structure
4. Lack of motoric control

Although many of these etiologies may cause deviant phonological growth, it is presumed that they represent unique deviations, in their own right, in the acquisition process. The abstract model of conceptual development implied by the model is the paramount discussion point. The ramifications of the above-mentioned factors for the abstract model need to be developed in detail in subsequent discussions and research. At present it is presumed that throughout the subsequent discussion, the topic is restricted to the phonemically disabled (i.e., the developmentally delayed child).

DIAGNOSIS

Patterning

Once the child has been given an exhaustive battery of tests to determine the sustaining or contributing etiologies, and none have been found, the therapist must turn to the symptoms themselves: the defective infantemes, features, and subsystems. Various diagnostic strategies for therapy have been developed (Compton, 1976; Lorentz, 1976; McReynolds, 1972; McReynolds & Huston, 1971; Oller, 1974; Pollack & Rees, 1972). However, these strategies have lacked developmental paradigms. The idea that one static distinctive feature matrix may be used in all stages of development may not be the best working assumption.

In 1970, Jo Ann Higgs, from the University of Edinburgh, published an in-depth discussion of the advantages and disadvantages of the articulation test, as opposed to the linguistic corpus. She concluded that the "test," with certain deficiencies, is a valid measuring technique. In truth, an articulation test is nothing more than a structured corpus (as opposed to spontaneous). The structured corpus permits the comparison of the results of one child to be compared to another. In the past it was presumed that the production of a speech sound in the initial, medial, and final positions in a word constituted an ideal test. This was true only if every articulation problem was physiological in nature, or at least organically consistent. It was not until the time of McDonald (1964) that the idea that a sound could be partially correct was widely accepted. This concept presumed a coarticulatory paradigm. The psycholinguistic approach, which includes non-organic problems, is difficult to contend with because it presumes that, even though a child says a sound, he or she may not know its full meaning, as in the free variation form. In light of modern theory, as Higgs (1970) pointed out, an articulation test applies only to the phonetic levels (p. 262) of language. The phonemic levels have been presumed to be equivalent to the phonetic. This, of course, from our modern perspective, is inaccurate. To solve this problem speech pathologists will have to reorient themselves to the entire testing process or remain locked into a phonetic domain, the world of the speech physiotherapist, so to speak.

An alternate approach to diagnosis has been underway in recent years. This approach, commonly referred to as "patterning," stipulates that the diagnostician should review the overall phonetic output of the child and then hypothesize the pattern of the existing phonological system (Haas, 1963; Weber, 1970). This system-approximation, a conceptual model, can become quite complicated using modern distinctive feature strategies (q.v. Compton, 1970; Oller, 1974; Pollack & Rees, 1972). For a diagnostic system to be clinically useful, it must be easily determined and specific enough to specify therapeutic goals.

The revised distinctive feature acquisition model, with its developmental milestones, can serve as the basic hypotheses to be established. If the six stages—primitive, vowel, back-nine, semivowel, continuant, and sibilant—represent relatively equal intervals in the acquisition process, the diagnostic task is to estimate which stage the child is in. The earliest defective stage serves as a guidepoint for the stage that precedes it. It marks the presumed level of attainment. But how can these hypotheses be formed?

In Table 1 are the percentile scores representing the number of times a sound was misarticulated using a standard pictorial word list (see Appendix J). The results of five age groups are presented (4:9–4:11, 5:0–5:11, 6:0–6:11, 7:0–7:11, 8:0–8:11). These grouped percentiles show whether a sound was misarticulated 3, 2, or 1 times on the test, irrespective of the position in the words. Children who do not misarticulate the words (i.e., 0) are scored cumulatively at the 100th percentile. The performance of each of the 25 consonant and semivowel sounds is plotted on a graph referred to as a developmental profile (see Figure 1). These sounds have been arranged serially from left to right in their developmental order (i.e., by class). The back-nine system is first; it is then followed by the semivowel system, the front fricatives, the affricates, and finally the sibilants. Once the percentile performance for each sound has been plotted on the profile, the diagnostician simply determines which is the earliest system that *may* be learned. An error of two or more sounds in any subsystem discounts it as being learned.

Table 1. Percentile scores for five age groups

Phoneme	Age groups[a]														
	4:9–4:11			5:0–5:11			6:0–6:11			7:0–7:11			8:0–8:11		
	3	2	1	3	2	1	3	2	1	3	2	1	3	2	1
[m]	0.00	0.00	0.05	0.00	0.00	0.01	0.00	0.00	0.01	0.00	0.00	0.01	0.00	0.00	0.01
[n]	0.00	0.00	0.03	0.00	0.00	0.02	0.00	0.00	0.02	0.00	0.00	0.01	0.00	0.00	0.01
[ŋ]	—	0.11	0.21	—	0.06	0.13	—	0.04	0.10	—	0.04	0.10	—	0.01	0.07
[p]	0.00	0.01	0.03	0.00	0.01	0.02	0.00	0.00	0.01	0.00	0.00	0.01	0.00	0.00	0.01
[t]	0.00	0.02	0.13	0.00	0.01	0.07	0.00	0.00	0.07	0.00	0.00	0.06	0.00	0.00	0.06
[k]	0.00	0.01	0.05	0.00	0.01	0.05	0.00	0.00	0.01	0.00	0.00	0.01	0.00	0.00	0.01
[b]	0.00	0.00	0.06	0.00	0.00	0.06	0.00	0.00	0.05	0.00	0.00	0.03	0.00	0.00	0.02
[d]	0.00	0.01	0.15	0.00	0.01	0.11	0.00	0.00	0.07	0.00	0.00	0.07	0.00	0.00	0.07
[g]	0.00	0.02	0.08	0.00	0.01	0.06	0.00	0.00	0.03	0.00	0.00	0.03	0.00	0.00	0.01
[ʍ]	—	—	0.39	—	—	0.24	—	—	0.20	—	—	0.20	—	—	0.08
[w]	—	0.02	0.20	—	0.01	0.10	—	0.00	0.05	—	0.01	0.03	—	0.00	0.03
[l]	0.06	0.12	0.24	0.05	0.09	0.16	0.00	0.01	0.03	0.00	0.01	0.03	0.00	0.00	0.01
[r]	0.17	0.29	0.38	0.09	0.11	0.19	0.06	0.08	0.13	0.04	0.06	0.10	0.01	0.01	0.04
[j]	—	0.02	0.08	—	0.01	0.03	—	0.01	0.02	—	0.00	0.00	—	0.00	0.00
[h]	—	—	0.00	—	—	0.00	—	—	0.00	—	—	0.00	—	—	0.00
[f]	0.01	0.03	0.05	0.01	0.03	0.05	0.00	0.01	0.01	0.01	0.00	0.01	0.00	0.00	0.01
[v]	0.08	0.18	0.41	0.05	0.18	0.28	0.01	0.16	0.19	0.01	0.03	0.11	0.00	0.01	0.03
[θ]	0.39	0.51	0.60	0.25	0.46	0.60	0.14	0.26	0.36	0.10	0.17	0.27	0.05	0.15	0.26
[ð]	0.10	0.33	0.47	0.08	0.18	0.34	0.02	0.05	0.19	0.00	0.03	0.11	0.00	0.03	0.11
[tʃ]	0.07	0.13	0.21	0.06	0.09	0.19	0.02	0.03	0.06	0.02	0.03	0.06	0.01	0.01	0.04
[dʒ]	0.08	0.15	0.26	0.04	0.06	0.12	0.02	0.03	0.07	0.01	0.01	0.05	0.00	0.00	0.03
[s]	0.20	0.26	0.38	0.17	0.21	0.26	0.11	0.15	0.19	0.09	0.12	0.15	0.08	0.09	0.13
[z]	0.21	0.23	0.32	0.16	0.21	0.30	0.11	0.14	0.24	0.10	0.12	0.18	0.06	0.09	0.16
[ʃ]	0.07	0.11	0.18	0.07	0.10	0.15	0.03	0.04	0.08	0.03	0.04	0.07	0.01	0.02	0.04
[ʒ]	—	0.13	0.30	—	0.13	0.30	—	0.07	0.19	—	0.05	0.12	—	0.04	0.11

[a]All positions marked (—) indicate that the sound was only tested in restricted contexts. Sounds which cannot occur in all positions in a word were tested a fewer number of times.

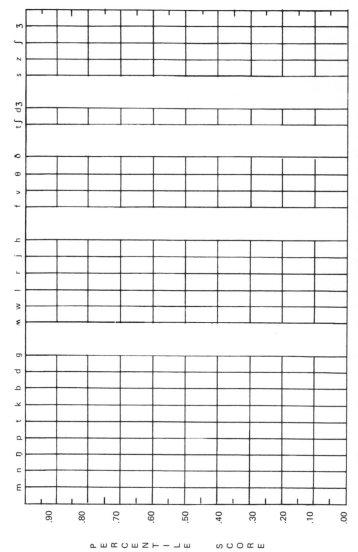

Figure 1.   Basic graph used to portray the level of infantemic development.

Later developing systems (to the right in Figure 1) that lie above a defective system are not guaranteed to be stable. Experience has shown that these sounds tend to become defective as earlier subsystems become more stable. The newly stabilized sounds tend to be used for righthand classes. (Each of the chi-square hypotheses proved this.)

To confirm the stage, the diagnostician transfers the developmental hypothesis to the city-block model (Figure 2). Using any type of marking device (colored pencils, pens, etc.), the hypothesized stage can be enhanced and outlined. This produces a configuration similar to stages 3, 18, 20, or 21. If the child is severely impaired and does not have a back-nine system, the primitive consonants should be evaluated [p, t, m, n]. If these sounds are properly produced, the intervening vowels and semivowels should be evaluated in terms of their respective models, stage 12 or stage 19.

The enhanced images that the diagnostician hypothesizes are evaluated by means of the substitution pattern. Each individual substitution is drawn onto the model by means of arrows that parallel the master model. The arrows originate from the sound substituted and point toward the target sound. With substitutions that involve more than one feature, it is suggested that the same "streets" be used to develop an overall pattern of substitution.

The general patterning, the hypothesized stage of development, and the substitution pattern can be pictured in a conceptual sense. When there is a need for a highly stable analysis, as in research, or the substitution pattern is complicated by the fact that the child has too

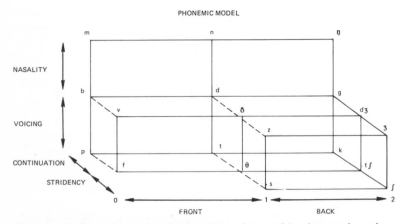

PHONEMIC MODEL

Figure 2.   Configuration used to plot hypothesized stage of development in conjunction with the derived substitution pattern.

many errors, the technique of McReynolds (McReynolds, 1972; McReynolds & Engmann, 1975) may be used. This technique requires the full administration of the McDonald (1964) Deep Test of Articulation, which augments the structured stimulus set by an approximate factor of six. Subsequently the proportion of error is computed for each speech sound on the model.

To compute the total contribution of each of the six features— nasality, voicing, front place, back place, continuation, and stridency—to the misarticulation pattern the following operations are performed:

1. Insert each sound substitution onto a "sound property analysis" chart (see Figure 3).
2. Determine the number of features in error for each substitution (use Appendix K). Insert the coded features onto the analysis chart.
3. Indicate the number of times each substitution occurred directly beneath the substitution.
4. Once each substitution has been analyzed, total the number of times each feature has been found in error and insert into chart.
5. After all six features have been accounted for, and all the substitutions counted, add all the features for the grand total.
6. Finally, divide the number of times each feature was in error by the grand total. Insert this figure under column titled "percent." These figures indicate the contribution made by each feature to the total misarticulation process and should total 100%.

This form of analysis is optional and is used only in cases of severe articulation difficulties or for research. It carries with it the assumption that a feature may be studied independently of the system. The previous discussion and revision, of course, contradict this basic assumption. A distinctive feature must be, in the ultimate case, studied in its developmental and systemic context.

The ultimate diagnostic question is, "What is the earliest stage that could be considered fully developed?" The infantemic stage becomes the working therapeutic hypothesis. The selection of the feature depends upon the level of infantemic development. The voicing feature [θ/ð] may be appropriate if the child is developing the continuant system, but it may be inappropriate if the child is only beginning to organize the stops and nasals. For this reason more emphasis is placed on the developmental profile (Figure 1) and the phonemic model (Figure 2) than on the sound property analysis (Figure 3).

SOUND PROPERTY ANALYSIS

SUBSTITUTIONS: __/ __ ,__/ __ ,__/ __ ,__/ __ ,__/ __ ,__/ __ ,__/ __ ,__/ __ ,

PROPERTIES:

NUMBER: ___ ___ ___ ___ ___ ___ ___

SUBSTITUTIONS: __/ __ ,__/ __ ,__/ __ ,__/ __ ,__/ __ ,__/ __ ,__/ __ ,

PROPERTIES:

NUMBER: ___ ___ ___ ___ ___ ___ ___

SUBSTITUTIONS: __/ __ ,__/ __ ,__/ __ ,__/ __ ,__/ __ ,__/ __ ,__/ __ ,

PROPERTIES:

NUMBER: ___ ___ ___ ___ ___ ___ ___

SUBSTITUTIONS: __/ __ ,__/ __ ,__/ __ ,__/ __ ,__/ __ ,__/ __ ,__/ __ ,

PROPERTIES:

NUMBER: ___ ___ ___ ___ ___ ___ ___

SUBSTITUTIONS: __/ __ ,__/ __ ,__/ __ ,__/ __ ,__/ __ ,__/ __ ,__/ __ ,

PROPERTIES:

NUMBER: ___ ___ ___ ___ ___ ___ ___

	NUMBER	PER CENT
NASALITY	_____	_____
FRONT PLACE	_____	_____
BACK PLACE	_____	_____
VOICING	_____	_____
CONTINUATION	_____	_____
STRIDENCY	_____	_____
TOTAL	_____	_____

Figure 3. Configuration used to plot the contribution of each feature to the misarticulation pattern.

To return to the developmental profile, to determine the level of infantemic development the following operations are performed:

1. Stimulate the child to produce the 89 words of Appendix J using pictures.
2. Transfer the percentile equivalence scores for each sound to the developmental profile (Figure 1).
3. Estimate the earliest stage that could be fully developed (having less than two errors).
4. Transfer this hypothesis to the phonemic model (Figure 2).
5. Indicate the substitutions, distortions, and omissions on the model.
6. Confirm or reject the initial functional hypothesis.

If differences are noted in the back-nine system (more than two errors), the primitive infantemes [p, t, m, n] should be evaluated. If there are no problems with these sounds examine the vowel and semivowel systems. Children with specific etiologies, organic or environmental, will have specific patterns of their own. Unfortunately, space does not permit expansion on these topics here, but I hope to do so in the near future.

Severity Index

Once the diagnostician has established the infantemic level of development, he or she may establish the severity of the misarticulation pattern. Given any array of substitutions, the examiner may establish a child's overall performance in reference to the appropriate age group. This comparison is done by means of a value termed the "severity index." Given any fixed number of sound substitutions, the child will make a certain number of distinctive feature errors (see Table 2). A minimum of one feature has to be made per substitution, but the average number of features missed may be greater than this figure. The greater the number of distinctive features missed per substitution, the more severe the misarticulation pattern. The severity index represents the average number of features or sound properties missed per substitution. To derive the average number of features missed per substitution, the following procedure is recommended. Referring to a display such as that in Figure 4, perform each of the following steps:

1. Insert *all* substitutions.
2. Directly beneath each substitution indicate the number of features in error (use Table 2).
3. Count the number of one-feature errors and insert in summary table.

Table 2. Table for determining the number of distinctive feature differences between any two sounds

Allophone used	Target phoneme																		
	m	n	ŋ	p	t	k	b	d	g	f	v	θ	ð	tʃ	dʒ	s	z	ʃ	ʒ
m	—	1	2	2	3	4	1	2	3	3	2	4	3	5	4	5	4	6	5
n	1	—	1	3	2	3	2	1	2	4	3	3	2	4	3	4	3	5	4
ŋ	2	1	—	4	3	2	3	2	1	5	4	4	3	3	2	5	4	4	3
p	2	3	4	—	1	2	1	2	3	1	2	2	3	3	4	3	4	4	5
t	3	2	3	1	—	1	2	1	2	2	3	1	2	2	3	2	3	3	4
k	4	3	2	2	1	—	3	2	1	3	4	2	3	1	2	3	4	2	3
b	1	2	3	1	2	3	—	1	2	2	1	3	2	4	3	4	3	5	4
d	2	1	2	2	1	2	1	—	1	2	2	2	1	3	2	3	2	4	3
g	3	2	1	3	2	1	2	1	—	4	3	3	2	2	1	4	3	3	2
f	3	4	5	1	2	3	2	2	4	—	1	1	2	2	3	2	3	3	4
v	2	3	4	2	3	4	1	2	3	1	—	2	1	3	2	3	2	4	3
θ	4	3	4	2	1	2	3	2	3	1	2	—	1	1	2	1	2	2	3
ð	3	2	3	3	2	3	2	1	2	2	1	1	—	2	1	2	1	3	2
tʃ	5	4	3	3	2	1	4	3	2	2	3	1	2	—	1	2	3	1	2
dʒ	4	3	2	4	3	2	3	2	1	3	2	2	1	1	—	3	2	2	1
s	5	4	5	3	2	3	4	3	4	2	3	1	2	2	3	—	1	1	2
z	4	3	4	4	3	4	3	2	3	3	2	2	1	3	2	1	—	2	1
ʃ	6	5	4	4	3	2	5	4	3	3	4	2	3	1	2	1	2	—	1
ʒ	5	4	3	5	4	4	3	2	4	3	3	2	2	1	2	1	1	1	—

SEVERITY INDEX ANALYSIS

SUBSTITUTION: __/__,__/__,__/__,__/__,__/__,__/__,__/__,__/__,
NUMBER: ___ ___ ___ ___ ___ ___ ___

SUBSTITUTION: __/__,__/__,__/__,__/__,__/__,__/__,__/__,__/__,
NUMBER: ___ ___ ___ ___ ___ ___ ___

SUBSTITUTION: __/__,__/__,__/__,__/__,__/__,__/__,__/__,__/__,
NUMBER: ___ ___ ___ ___ ___ ___ ___

SUBSTITUTION: __/__,__/__,__/__,__/__,__/__,__/__,__/__,__/__,
NUMBER: ___ ___ ___ ___ ___ ___ ___

SUBSTITUTION: __/__,__/__,__/__,__/__,__/__,__/__,__/__,__/__,
NUMBER: ___ ___ ___ ___ ___ ___ ___

SUMMARY TABLE

NUMBER OF FEATURES		NUMBER OF SUBSTITUTIONS		F_p	F_s
1	X	___	=	___	
2	X	___	=	___	
3	X	___	=	___	
4	X	___	=	___	
5	X	___	=	___	
6	X	___	=	___	
TOTAL:		[ ] S		[ ] P	

$$INDEX = \frac{P}{S} = \underline{\qquad}$$

Figure 4. Configuration used to plot the severity index of the misarticulation pattern.

4. Count the number of two-feature errors and insert in summary table.
5. Repeat operation through the three- to six-feature errors.
6. Total the number of substitutions (S) and record.
7. Total the number of properties (P) or features and record.

8. Divide the number of properties (P) by the number of substitutions (S).

This results in the severity index. To translate this figure into meaningful terms use Table 3. These figures represent the equivalent percentile scores for the index for the appropriate age groups. By comparing the child's misarticulation pattern to that of his or her peers, the diagnostician can estimate the child's performance qualitatively as well as quantitatively.

The semivowel responses, as well as vowel performance, are generally not included. Errors in the former class have a latent syntagmatic component. The latter errors place the child in the pre-4:9–4:11 age level. Omissions are not used in this analysis. The advantages and disadvantages of including the omissions in the misarticulation analysis are equally balanced. The major advantage lies in the fact that it raises few questions from standard analysis procedures. Omissions are highly regarded as indicators of severe articulatory difficulty, possibly because of their sensitivity to structural and organic problems or severe cases of articulatory underdevelopment. However, to include this type of misarticulation into the paradigm a basic assumption would also have to be made. Scoring an omission presumes that the child misarticulates all six features, and, furthermore, the child is in error on

Table 3. Percentile scores for the severity index as determined for five different age groups

Severity index	Age groups				
	4:9–4:11	5:0–5:11	6:0–6:11	7:0–7:11	8:0–8:11
1.0	0.43	0.32	0.11	0.04	0.02
1.1	0.36	0.26	0.11	0.03	0.01
1.2	0.32	0.19	0.08	0.02	0.01
1.3	0.14	0.13	0.05	0.01	0.01
1.4	0.11	0.09	0.02	0.01	0.01
1.5	0.08[a]	0.05	0.02	0.01	0.01
1.6	0.08[a]	0.05	0.02	0.01	0.01
1.7	0.05[a]	0.03	0.02	0.01	0.01
1.8	0.03[a]	0.02	0.02	0.01	0.01
1.9	0.03[a]	0.02	0.02	0.01	0.01
2.0	0.02[a]	0.01	0.00	0.00	0.00

[a]Estimates established by interpolation.

one-half of a feature (the half not articulated). This option reorients the theory from its cognitive-oppositional base to a phonetic-tag theory. The price payed, a phonetic theory rather than a phonemic theory, seems too high. For this reason omissions are simply accounted for on the city-block model. They usually occur in the undeveloped phonemic areas and can be easily accounted for on the developmental information at hand. Distortions are not used because they usually indicate phonemic understanding of the target but poor phonetic approximation. These options of discounting the omission and distortion are not meant to indicate they are not of importance. The reason a child omits may be phonetic or phonemic. The procedures are meant to elicit phonemic development alone. Distortions are more properly included in a phonetic analysis. In all, the severity index is meant to serve as a single figure of overall peer performance, and it is not an intelligibility index. It is expected that there is a relationship between the two figures, but the current bias is developmental adequacy in preference to social adequacy.

Evaluating Features

Under the revised sequence of acquisition the type of feature in error is not as important as the subsystem in which it occurs. [p/b] is more severe than [f/v], and [s/z] is less severe than the former two. Although voicing is in error in each case, most therapists would agree that [s/z] is a poor therapeutic objective with a 4-year-old child. In fact the sonographic displays would indicate gross differences in the property within the subclasses themselves. For this reason it is suggested that feature decisions be confined to the subsystem in question. The overall system analysis of a feature takes on more meaning with the organically impaired. For instance, the goal of laryngeal adequacy is a different therapeutic goal than teaching its linguistic significance.

THERAPY

Minimal-Pairs Orientation

Traditional articulation therapy has not made a distinction between phonemic and phonetic problems. The terms "delayed speech" and "delayed language" have tended to intimate that speech sounds were not a significant part of language delay. Whitacre, Luper, and Pollio (1970) have disputed this contention and shown that children with defective articulation have concomitant problems with vocabulary, syntagmatic sequencing, and sentence repetition tasks. Phonological development is a linguistic skill. The dichotomy between "speech" and "language" has allowed phonology to fall between the cracks.

The basic assumptions of the structural linguistic movement concerning the phoneme have reawakened our understanding of the importance of the speech sound. A speech sound is meant to *make words different*. This is what a phoneme is. There are many ways to make words different, but there is only one basic requirement for distinctiveness: the child must obtain a certain physiological position in order to produce an acoustic signal that the culture recognizes as significant. If the child does not understand this basic concept, therapy becomes a form of blindman's buff. Current techniques of articulation therapy are well adapted to trigger the specific physiological postures (Bacus & Beasley, 1951; Berry & Eisenson, 1956; Van Riper, 1954/1972; Van Riper & Irwin, 1958; Young & Hawk, 1955). Techniques to provide the significant "cues" of production are well known (Van Riper, 1954/ 1972, pp. 199–243; 1963, pp. 242–300). But these cues, such as teaching the sound in isolation, are not the phoneme. The sound in isolation is the substance and not the function. Children with phonemic problems need therapy directed to the importance of their productions.

In order to organize existing therapeutic techniques, a new therapeutic paradigm has been developed. This paradigm is called a "minimal-pairs orientation." This technique has been developed not to replace existing techniques but to emphasize the linguistic, cultural, psychological, acoustic, and physiological components into an organized protocol. The protocol procedure was established to teach the child how to make words different, that is, distinctive.

Differential Function and Smallest Unit

Distinctive feature theory presumes that a phoneme cannot be taught all at once. The smallest unit of language is the distinctive feature or sound property. It is this unit that therapy should be directed at. The subsystem establishes the strategy, or plan of action; the feature establishes the tactic, or method of implementation. The differential function of the smallest unit is taught by means of a minimal-pair contrast. If the child is presented with two pictures, one of a "pin" and another of a "fin," and the child indicates that knowledge of the difference between an object that can be stuck into something and the dorsal appendage of a fish, and subsequently indicates that he/she can hear the difference between the two words while touching each card in response to the pronunciation of each word, it may be presumed that the child can discriminate continuation ($\pm$). When the roles are reversed and the child is asked to pronounce the words while the therapist indicates the word he or she hears, the child is indicating a functional phonemic ability. The minimal pair crystalizes the task for the child; the child must make the words different. The therapist represents the culture and its requirements as he/she moves a finger from word to word.

Cultural Component

The therapist represents the culture in several ways. In the most abstract sense the therapist stipulates the best sequence for therapy by means of the working therapeutic hypothesis and the diagnostic decisions (see Figure 5). The therapist controls not only the presentation phase of therapy but the preparation phase as well.

Preparation Phase   During the preparation phase the therapist determines if the problem is phonetic or phonemic as the ultimate culmination of step 1. The etiology and symptoms must clearly indicate a learning problem. If they do not, the following procedures must be modified. A common modification, for instance, with the hearing-impaired child is to amplify the signals and evaluate the importance of visual cues. With a child having a developmental problem, a specific subsystem is selected for development (strategy). The feature must then be selected. Those who understand the generating principles of the developmental sequence will have little difficulty selecting the feature (tactic). However, for those who find the steps obtuse Appendix L has been prepared. This appendix lists the stage, feature, sound-pair, and sample words in the developmental sequence. Those who choose this approach exclusively will not be able to retain a flexibility to treat individual differences.

Once the feature (step 3) and system (step 2) have been selected, the feature must be put into an infantemic context. Representative adult sounds are used and embedded into culturally significant words. These steps (4 and 5) depend upon the level of phonemic development of the child and the lexical background that he or she has been exposed to. The last step (6) in the preparation stage involves the construction of the picture cards themselves. Appendix L may be used for representative lexical items which may be pictured with relative ease.

Presentation Phase   Not only does the therapist represent the culture in terms of the direction of therapy, he or she serves as its representative in the learning task at hand. In the first face-to-face contact (step B: 1), the therapist presents words of significance for the child. These words should be ones that the child can use in everyday conversational speech. As the therapist talks to the child about the words, he or she ascertains that the child's general cognitive development is ad-

MINIMAL-PARTS ORIENTATION

A. PREPARATION PHASE:

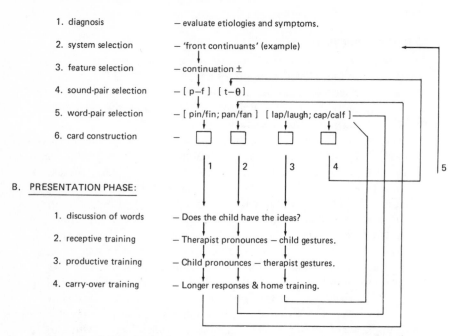

1. diagnosis	— evaluate etiologies and symptoms.
2. system selection	— 'front continuants' (example)
3. feature selection	— continuation ±
4. sound-pair selection	— [p–f] [t–θ]
5. word-pair selection	— [pin/fin; pan/fan] [lap/laugh; cap/calf]
6. card construction	— □ □ □ □

B. PRESENTATION PHASE:

1. discussion of words	— Does the child have the ideas?
2. receptive training	— Therapist pronounces — child gestures.
3. productive training	— Child pronounces — therapist gestures.
4. carry-over training	— Longer responses & home training.

Figure 5.   Protocol procedure for organizing a minimal-pairs therapy program.

vanced enough to benefit from the addition of these words. In some cases the child will know the words and merely needs to learn how to make them different physiologically.

With the establishment of rapport and a general understanding that the child understands the *ideas* to be expressed, the therapist says:

> I am going to say the names of both words. I want to see if you can hear the difference between the two words. Please touch the word I say and then put your hand back in your lap. Are you ready?

No further instructions are needed at this level. Verbosity, although it sometimes implies knowledge, reduces important practice time for the child. The therapist randomly repeats the words until the child indicates that he/she can hear the difference between the two words. With reinforcement schedules so popular today, there is a tendency to want to establish a percentage criterion. This however is wasteful here. The therapist must determine whether a child's responses are merely chance behavior. This is done by means of the binomial expansion series. When a child can pick one of two words in a task, by chance he/she will get a certain number correct. What is needed is a certain number of correct responses that would indicate that the performance is too unlikely to have occurred using guessing behavior. If the child succeeds in getting four words correct in a row, the probability is 6 in 100; five words correct, 3 in 100; 6 correct, 2 in 100; and 7 correct, 1 in 100. These levels constitute levels of significance using a nonparametric base. It is suggested that 6 correct ($p = .03$) responses be used. Absolute certainty sometimes has to be weighed against the danger of boring the child. This necessitates reinforcement schedules to build motivation. Once the child indicates he/she knows the difference between the two words proceed to the next step; it is the most important.

In step B: 3 the situational roles are reversed. The therapist instructs the child as follows:

> Alright, now you're going to be the teacher. You say the words and I'll touch the words I hear. Are you ready?

The instructions do not need to be any more complicated than this. Experience has shown that the child will respond in the following way. First the child will say the word he/she can say. This is the word that contains the infanteme from the previous system that has been determined to be developed. If the therapist is sitting directly across from the child, the child's eyes may be noted to shift to the opposite part of the card. The child will attempt to say the other word but repeats the first word. For instance, the child who does not understand continuation generally can say "pin" but not "fin." After saying "pin" and receiving situational reinforcement from the therapist's gesture, the child will attempt "fin." Not being able to produce continuation (+) produces [pɪn] as the approximation of "fin." The therapist immediately puts a finger on the "wrong" (in the child's eyes) card. The child wanted you to touch "fin" but you indicated that you heard "pin." Say nothing, for the moment is "pregnant." The child undoubtably will repeat an attempt at "fin." As it is misarticulated a second time say:

> Were you trying to say this word (indicate "fin")?

As the child indicates that he or she was trying to say that word, demonstrate how the word is said, stressing the feature of significance. Any traditional cue used to teach the sound in isolation may be used at this *moment,* but the cue should not detract from the task at hand— making the words different. As soon as the child says the word praise him or her. For any attempt to make the words different, reinforce.

Because the task at hand has been isolated, producing continuation, the child can attack it unambiguously. Asking the child to make the "f" sound is too ambiguous: It is a labiodental, it is voiceless, it is a continuant, it is low pitched, it is mellow. Furthermore, from the systemic view it is not a tongue tip sound, it is not a back tongue sound, it is not a nasal, it is not voiced, etc. The "f" sound, even in isolation, is a complex entity. Only by working at the word level, in a minimal-pairs context, can the situation be simplified. The equivalent parts of the words, in this case [-ɪn], are ignored in the discrimination training and the production training. The therapist, much like the child, must keep the specific goal in mind and not be distracted by later syntagmatic factors. Working from the initial position to the final position protects against aberrant developments in this domain.

Carryover training (step B: 4) is begun by delaying the target words in the productive task of step B: 3. The child is instructed to say:

Level 2—"the [target word]" = Two-element phrase
Level 3—"touch the [target word]" = Three-element sentence
Level 4—"point to the [target word]" = Four-element sentence

By repeating the task of being the teacher and using longer and longer lexical segments, the child can build a spontaneous component into a phrase structure. This is, of course, not complete until the words are used in everyday speech. As soon as the child can pronounce a word, inform the parents of this accomplishment and tell them to be ready to positively reinforce any occurrence of the word in the home situation. Specific times of the day should be set aside in which the child can recite the words accomplished. Errors should be noted by the parents and brought to the attention of the therapist. However, the parents should be encouraged only to reinforce general attempts to improve speech and specific lexical accomplishments.

Once a child has progressed through one learning sequence from feature selection to carryover, he or she is recycled through the protocol procedure into other words, other positions, other sound pairs, other features, and other systems. As noted earlier, 87% of American English makes use of very simple syllable structures: CV, VC, V, CVC. This finding tends to de-emphasize the importance of the medial position.

The tactical reorganization paradigm of the preparation program is only in skeletal form. It is presumed that normal carryover monitoring of the "substitution pattern" will suffice at present. However, this statement should not be used to indicate that the protocol procedure is a system of substitution eradication. Without the developmental undergirding for the substitution selection, the protocol is reduced from a strategy to a tactic in a phonetic world.

Psychological Component

At step B: 3 in the presentation phase, when the therapist asks the child if he/she is attempting to say the target word, the therapist enjoys a delightful social position of friend and helper. Creating a situation in which you can say, "Oh! That's what your trying to say. Let's see if I can help you," is far superior to the normal pedantic relationship in which the child is being socially manipulated. This social manipulation often detracts from the psychological task at hand.

Asking a child to verbalize the fact that he or she has difficulty with other words may emphasize the importance of therapy as a helpful interchange. Simply asking the child, "Do you have trouble saying other words? Well, I'm going to help you make words different," does much in establishing a collateral working relationship. Peer pressure often is enough to motivate therapy. During a particularly unsuccessful attempt to teach sounds in isolation a 4-year-old once blurted out, "Sticks and stones will break your bones but words will never hurt you!" This statement out of context seemed to indicate social pressure on my little friend. After moralizing a bit over ignoring negative comments the child resumed work only to interrupt the therapy group 20 minutes later. "You know," she said, "words do hurt!" This kind of spontaneous recognition of the importance of speaking properly seemed to be related to very significant therapeutic success. Not only do words hurt, they have power and they are fun to use. Children know this as they play word games. When a child is not making words different, it is the therapist's job to create a situation in which this fact is obvious. This situation becomes the challenge. Trying to be like mother and father may be too much of a jump; it may be a problem that can only be handled one word at a time.

Acoustic Component

Difficulties in receptive training should immediately call to mind, again, the possibility of a hearing problem. If none exists, there is a linguistic discrimination problem. Even though no hearing problem exists, amplification of the acoustic model is wise. Many different gadgets used in therapy merely make the signal louder. Tape recorders may be driven by reels, cassettes, loops, index cards, or push buttons. In themselves they represent a surface type of contrast. By increasing the signal the property will be magnified for reexamination. Rolled-up tubes, paper, or hands can serve the same purpose. If amplification does not bring immediate success, a reinforcement schedule may be considered on a short trial basis. If success is not forthcoming, the therapist should reexamine the previous stages in sequential order. Does the child have the ideas? Are the words well represented? If the answers to these questions are "yes," alternate word pairs should be selected (step A: 5). If several words pairs are unsuccessful, vary the sound pair (step A: 4). If several sound pairs are not shown to be leading to progress, the feature should be reevaluated (step A: 3). If an alternate feature within a subsystem is not shown to produce success, reevaluate the system hypothesized (step A: 2). If the previous system reveals little progress from a tactical viewpoint, reevaluate the diagnostic process for intervening variables (step A: 1). If success is not immediate the tactical options must be constantly reevaluated. This makes the system organic or responsive in nature. Although the system is highly structured, it has been made flexible enough to constantly adapt goal behavior.

Physiological Component

The vast amount of writing available for teaching the proper placement of the speech sounds need not be repeated here. However, certain points should be made. The cues for production should be as natural as possible. They should be similar to the basic acquisition process. Modeling the production of the word phonetically as a cue is superior to "mirror work." However, the mirror may be the only way in which some children can be taught. Tongue exercises are sometimes frowned upon with some justification. But the total lack of this option when a motoric component is an outstanding etiology would be negligent, especially if it works. In any case the first option should be the most natural cue, preferably a simple statement of what is required. The feature system presented has very simple cues:

1. Front place = Use your lip(s)
2. Back place = Use your tongue (tip or back)
3. Continuation = Make it longer or slower (versus shorter or faster)
4. Stridency = Make sure you get your teeth together
5. Nasality = Do not explain; rely on acoustic cues, or tactile monitoring of nares
6. Voiced = Utilize concepts of singing versus whispering; use tactile monitoring of lateral neck area, avoiding thyroid gland

These concepts, though simple, must fit a simple mind. The vocabulary level of the cues should be appropriate to the child and as brief as possible. For instance a tongue depressor restraining the front tongue tip often causes an immediate raise in the back tongue in the attempt for the velars. Simply saying, "Use the back of your tongue," may not be enough, and explaining the internal structure of the oral cavity may be too much.

Special Problems

Evaluating Responses   Two major types of responses, besides correct approximation, should be discussed. As a child begins to alter the phonetic approximations of a sound he or she may overestimate or underestimate the response at hand. In the first case, overestimation, the child gives more than one sound property. The child is asked to produce back place, "tea" versus "key." In moving from [t] to [k], many times a child will say [tʃi]. The [tʃ] does represent back placement, but it also differs in terms of continuation. The child has given too much. In such cases the therapist is encouraged to look at the positive aspects of the response and ignore, for the moment, the negative aspects. Doing something different is the most abstract goal and the child is trying. Negative comments here lower motivation, and in fairness to the child he/she did produce the correct property. In subsequent minimal-pairs the importance of continuation may be illustrated with such pairs as "keys" and "cheese" or "kick" and "chick." This protocol procedure permits the child to indicate to the therapist the point of misunderstanding. In the previous example the child would appear not to know which feature to work on—continuation or back place. Underestimation is a phenomenon that occurs mainly with the continuant class. With a three-point place system [f] and [v] are taught simply as sounds that are longer than [p] and [b]. At times the child will produce [Φ] and [β]. These sounds represent continuation but lack the proper lingua-alveolar placement familiar to American English. For situations such as these the [Φ] and [β] are looked on as intervening phonetic steps in phonemic production.

Reinforcement   To keep the protocol procedure as natural as possible, reinforcement is structured to be as unobstrusive as possible. The task, getting the therapist to move his or her finger, is the basic reinforcer from both the positive and negative domain. Smiles, gestures, and praise are used to encourage task approximation and are not scheduled on the rate of success. The reinforcer is used to motivate, not to teach. If motivation lags because of a lack of success, token reinforcers may be used. These reinforcers, however, tend to distract from the task at hand, making words different. Tangible reinforcers must be used, however, with some children. Although they are somewhat slower aŋd cumbersome, their use should be for motivation to make the words different (as an abstract goal) and not for the word contrasts (the specific goal). This latter format represents an inferior cognitive response, that is, conditioning. The use of appetitive reinforcers not only slows the process, it obstructs the oral cavity, impairing production. This format, however, may have to be used with the most severe cases. Delayed reinforcers, latent money systems, again are not considered a good first choice with all children. The reinforcers should be selected to fit the task at hand. Is the appropriate reinforcer being used or is one being used just to satisfy current therapy styles? It is commonly understood that the therapeutic task should be structured to maximize the number of attempts at the goal behavior for a given period of time. Deviation from this goal must be supported by the lasting effects of the reinforcement technique.

SUMMARY

Space does not permit any more than a cursory outline of the implications of the revised model for diagnosis and therapy. It would seem that the skeletal outline developed to date will serve as adequate specification for research in the clinical setting. Initial testing and experience in the clinical setting have indicated that the theory developed to date is well founded and worthy of further testing and modification. One final comment should be made. The application of distinctive feature theory is not meant to replace existing therapeutic programs. Distinctive feature theory, in its fullest implications, forces the therapist to work in a highly exact and scientific way. In the past the therapist has had the luxury of assuming that he or she could teach what a speech sound is. Distinctive feature theory presumes that you must teach what a speech sound is *not*. No sound can exist alone. It must be contrasted to another sound. What a speech sound *is not* is the distinctive component of the phonemic system. If a language chooses not to use voicing, as in Arabic, its spontaneous production is no guarantee of acquisition. It is the integration of the child and the child's own culture, along with the child's unique ability to think, that is of paramount importance. The shift from the phonetic world to the child's mind is a radical one. It is much like moving into a mirror-image world. Relativity theory that has shaped the theories of physics may be on the verge of reshaping the world of paradigmatic phonemics.

References

Abbs, M., & Minifie, F. D. Effect of acoustic fricatives on perceptual confusions in preschool children. J. Acoust. Soc. Amer., 1969, 46, 1535–1542.

Abbs, J., & Sussman, H. Neurophysiological feature detectors and speech perception: A discussion of theoretical implications. J. Sp. Hear. Res., 1971, 14, 23–36.

Ahmed, R., & Agrawal, S. S. Significant features in the perception of (Hindi) consonants. J. Acoust. Soc. Amer., 1969, 45, 758–763.

Akhmanova, O. Phonology, Morphonology, Morphology. The Hague: Mouton, 1971.

Albright, R. W. The International Phonetic Alphabet: Its background and development. Int. J. Amer. Ling., 1958, 24, 1–78.

Allers, R. Sigmund Freud: The Origin and Development of Psychoanalysis. Chicago: Henry Regnery, 1955.

Ament, W. The development of speech and thought in children. In A. Bar-Adon & W. Leopold (Eds. and trans.), Child Language: A Book of Readings. Englewood Cliffs, N.J.: Prentice-Hall, 1971. (Originally published in German, 1899.)

Ames, L. Predictive value of infant behavior examinations. In J. Hellmuth (Ed.), Exceptional Infant (Vol. 1): The Normal Infant. New York: Bruner/Mazel, 1967.

Bacus, O., & Beasley, J. Speech Therapy with Children. Boston: Houghton-Mifflin, 1951.

Bally, C., & Sechehaye, A. Course in General Linguistics: Ferdinand de Saussure. New York: McGraw-Hill, 1966.

Baltaxe, C. (trans.). N. S. Trubetzkoy: Principles of Phonology. Berkeley: University of California Press, 1969.

Baltaxe, C. Foundation of Distinctive Feature Theory. Baltimore: University Park Press, in press.

Bar-Adon, A. S., & Leopold, W. Child Language: A Book of Readings. Englewood Cliffs, N.J.: Prentice-Hall, 1971.

Baudouin de Courtenay, J. Aspects of a theory of historical phonetics. In G. Lepschy (Ed. and trans.), A Survey of Structural Linguistics. London: Faber & Faber, 1970. (Originally published in German, 1881.)

Bayley, N. Mental growth during the first three years. Genet. Psychol. Monogr., 1933, 14, 92.

van Bergeijk, W., Pierce, J., & David, E. Waves and the Ear. Garden City, New York: Doubleday Anchor, 1960.

Berry, M., & Eisenson, J. Speech Disorders. New York: Appleton-Century-Crofts, 1956.

Bever, T. Pre-linguistic Behavior. Unpublished honors thesis, Department of Linguistics, Harvard University, 1961.

Blache, S. An exploratory investigation of the use of multidimensional scaling in the perception of phonemic stimuli. Doctoral dissertation, Ohio University, 1970. (Dissertation Abstracts International, 1971, 31, 5014-B; University Microfilms No. 71-4783, 229.)

Blache, S. Some current research findings in distinctive feature theory. Paper presented to the Southern Illinois Linguistics Association, Carbondale, Ill., fall, 1972.

Blache, S. Sound Properties Production Test. Test in preparation, 1975.

Black, J. W. Relative Perceptual Similarity of Sixty Initial Consonants. Columbus: Ohio State University Research Foundation, 1969.

Blesser, B. Speech perception under conditions of spectral transformation: I. Phonetic characteristics. J. Sp. Hear. Res., 1972, 15, 5–41.

Bloomfield, L. A set of postulates for the science of language. Language, 1926, 2, 153–164.

Bosma, J. F., & Fletcher, S. G. The upper pharynx: A review. Part I: Embryology and anatomy. Ann. Otol. Rhinol. Laryngol., 1961, 70, 953–973.

Braislin, W. C. A study of some casts of the infantile pharynx with special reference to the eustachian tubes. Ann. Otol. Rhinol. Laryngol., 1919, 21, 36–74.

Brill, A. A. Basic Principles of Psychoanalysis. New York: Washington Square Press, 1960.

Brosnahan, L. The Sounds of Language. Cambridge, England: Heffer & Sons, 1961.

Brown, R. Words and Things: An Introduction to Language. New York: The Free Press, 1958/1968.

Bruning, J., & Kintz, B. Computational Handbook of Statistics. Glenville, Ill.: Scott, Foresman, 1968.

Bühler, C. The First Year of Life (P. Greenberg & R. Ripin, Eds. and trans.). New York: Day, 1930. (Originally published in German as three separate articles, 1927, 1928, 1930.)

Bühler, C., & Hetzer, H. Testing Children's Development from Birth to School-age. New York: Farrar & Rinehart, 1935.

Bush, C. N. Phonetic Variation and Acoustic Distinctive Features. The Hague: Mouton, 1964.

Carmichael, L. The early growth of language capacity. In E. Lenneberg (Ed.), New Directions in the Study of Language. Cambridge, Mass.: MIT Press, 1969.

Carrell, J., & Tiffany, W. Phonetics: Theory and Application to Speech Improvement. New York: McGraw-Hill, 1960.

Cattell, P. The Measurement of Intelligence of Infants and Young Children. New York: The Psychological Corporation, 1940.

Chapanis, A. Men, models and machines. In M. Marx (Ed.), Theories in Contemporary Psychology. New York: Macmillan, 1963.

Chase, R. Evolutionary Aspects of Language Development and Function. Baltimore: Neurocommunications Laboratory, Johns Hopkins, 1965a.

Chase, R. Verbal Behavior: Some Points of Reference. Baltimore: Neurocommunications Laboratory, Johns Hopkins, 1965b.

Chen, H., & Irwin, O. Infant speech: Vowel and consonant types. J. Sp. Hear. Dis., 1946, 11, 27–29.

Cherry, E. C. R. Jakobson's "distinctive features" as the normal coordinates of a language. In M. Halle, H. G. Lunt, H. McClean, & C. H. van Schooneveld (Eds.), For Roman Jakobson. The Hague: Mouton, 1956.

Cherry, E. C. On Human Communication: A Review, A Survey and a Criticism. Cambridge, Mass.: MIT Press, 1966.

Chiba, T., & Kajiyama, M. The Vowel: Its Nature and Structure. Tokyo: Tokyo-Kaiseikan Co., 1941.

Chomsky, N. Aspects of the Theory of Syntax. Cambridge, Mass.: MIT Press, 1965.

Chomsky, N., & Halle, M. The Sound Pattern of English. New York: Harper & Row, 1968.

Cohen, A., Slis, I. H., & Hart, J. On tolerance and intolerance in vowel perception. Phonetica, 1967, 16, 65–70.

Compton, A. Generative studies of children's phonological disorders. J. Sp. Hear. Dis., 1970, 35, 315–337.

Compton, A. Generative studies of children's phonological disorders: Clinical ramifications. In D. Morehead and A. Morehead (Eds.), Normal and Deficient Child Language. Baltimore: University Park Press, 1976.

Conant, J. On Understanding Science. New York: Macmillan, 1947.

Cooper, F., Delattre, P., Liberman, A., Borst, J., & Gerstman, L. Some experiments on the perception of synthetic speech sounds. J. Acoust. Soc. Amer., 1952, 24, 597–606.

Courts, F. Psychological Statistics. Homewood, Ill.: Dorsey Press, 1966.

Crocker, J. R. A phonological model of children's articulation competence. J. Sp. Hear. Dis., 1969, 34, 203–213.

Danhauer, J., & Singh, S. Multidimensional Speech Perception by the Hearing Impaired. Baltimore: University Park Press, 1975.

Darley, F., & Winitz, H. Age of the first word: Review of research. J. Sp. Hear. Dis., 1961, 26, 271–290.

DeGeorge, R., & DeGeorge, F. The Structuralists from Marx to Lévi-Strauss. Garden City, N.Y.: Doubleday Anchor, 1972.

Delattre, P. Un triangle acoustique des voyelles orales du français. The French Review, 1948, 21, 477ff.

Delattre, P., Liberman, A., & Cooper, F. Acoustic loci and transitional cues for consonants. J. Acoust. Soc. Amer., 1955, 27, 769–773.

Delattre, P., Liberman, A., Cooper, F., & Gerstman, J. An experimental study of the acoustic determinants of vowel color; Observations on one- and two-formant transitions. Word, 1952, 8, 195–210.

Denes, P., & Pinson, E. The Speech Chain. Bell Telephone Laboratories, 1963, 1969.

Dewey, G. Relative Frequency of English Speech Sounds. Cambridge, Mass.: Harvard University Press, 1923.

Dorf, R. C. Matrix Algebra. New York: John Wiley & Sons, 1969.

Durkheim, E. Le Suicide. Paris: Presses Universitaires de France, 1969.

Edwards, M. Perception and production in child phonology: The testing of four hypotheses. J. Child Lang., 1974, 1, 205–219.

Eimas, P. D., & Corbit, J. D. Selective adaptation of linguistic feature detectors. Cognitive Psychology, 1973, 4, 99–109.

Fairbanks, G., House, A., & Stevens, E. An experimental study of vowel intensities. J. Acoust. Soc. Amer., 1950, 22, 457–459.

Faircloth, S., & Faircloth, M. Phonetic Science. Englewood Cliffs, N.J.: Prentice-Hall, 1973.

Fant, C. G. On the predictability of formant levels and spectrum envelopes from formant frequencies. In M. Halle, H. Lunt, & H. MacLean (Eds.), For Roman Jakobson. The Hague: Mouton, 1956.

Fant, G. On the predictability of formant levels and spectrum envelopes from formant frequencies. In I. Lehiste (Ed.), Readings in Acoustic Phonetics. Cambridge, Mass.: MIT Press, 1967. (Originally published, 1961.)

Fant, G. Analysis and synthesis of speech processes. In B. Malmberg (Ed.), Manual of Phonetics. Amsterdam: North-Holland, 1968.

Fant, G. Speech Sounds and Features. Cambridge, Mass.: MIT Press, 1973.
Farnsworth, P. R. Review of B. Faddegon, Phonetics and Phonology. Amer. J. Psychol., 1940, 53, 169.
Ferguson, C. Baby talk in six languages. Amer. Anthropol., 1964, 66, 103–114.
Ferguson, C., & Farwell, C. Words and sounds in early language acquisition. Language, 1975, 51, 419–439.
Ferguson, C., & Garnica, O. Theories of phonological development. In E. Lenneberg (Ed.), Foundations of Language Development (Vol. 1). New York: Academic Press, 1975.
Ferguson, C., Peizer, D., & Weeks, T. Model-and-replica phonological grammar of a child's first words. Lingua, 1973, 31, 35–65.
Fischer-Jørgensen, E. The commutation test and its application to phonemic analysis. In M. Halle, H. G. Lunt, H. McLean, & C. H. van Schooneveld (Eds.), For Roman Jakobson. The Hague: Mouton, 1956.
Flanagan, J. L. Speech Analysis, Synthesis and Perception. Berlin: Springer Verlag, 1965.
Foulkes, J. D. Computer identification of vowel types. J. Acoust. Soc. Amer., 1961, 33, 7–11.
Francis, W. N. The Structure of American English. New York: Ronald Press, 1958.
Franke, C. Early speech development. In A. Bar-Adon & W. Leopold (Eds. and trans.), Child Language: A Book of Readings. Englewood Cliffs, N.J.: Prentice-Hall, 1971. (Originally published in German, 1912.)
Fruchter, B. Introduction to Factor Analysis. New York: Van Nostrand, 1954.
Fry, D. The development of the phonological system in the normal and the deaf child. In F. Smith & G. Miller (Eds.), The Genesis of Language. Cambridge, Mass.: MIT Press, 1967.
Gerstman, L. Classification of self-normalized vowels. IEEE Trans. Audio Electro Acoust., 1968, 16, 78–80.
Gesell, A. The Mental Growth of the Preschool Child. New York: Macmillan, 1925.
Gesell, A., & Thompson, H. Infant Behavior: Its Genesis and Growth. New York: McGraw-Hill, 1934.
Gesell, A., Thompson, H., & Armatruda, C. The Psychology of Early Growth. New York: Macmillan, 1938.
Graham, M. Intra-uterine crying. Brit. Med. J., 1919, 1, 675.
Gray, G. The great ravelled knot. Scientific American, 1948, Oct., 1–15.
Gray, G., & Wise, C. The Bases of Speech. New York: Harper & Brothers, 1959, 1969.
Greenberg, J. The first (and perhaps only) non-linguistic distinctive feature analysis. Word, 1967, 23, 214–220.
Greenberg, J., & Jenkins, J. Studies in the psychological correlates to the sound system of American English. Word, 1964, 20, 157–177.
Guilford, J. The Nature of Human Intelligence. New York: McGraw-Hill, 1967.
Haas, W. Phonological analysis of a case of dyslalia. J. Sp. Hear. Dis., 1963, 28, 239–246.
Hála, B. Akusticka podstata Samohlásek, Prague, 1941.
Halle, M. On the role of simplicity in linguistic descriptions. In Structure of Language and Its Mathematical Aspects: Proceedings of Symposia on

Applied Mathematics (Vol. 12). Providence: American Mathematical Society, 1961, 89–94.

Halle, M. On the bases of phonology. In J. Fodor & J. Katz (Eds.), The Structure of Language: Readings in the Philosophy of Language. Englewood Cliffs, N.J.: Prentice-Hall, 1964.

Halle, M., & Stevens, K. Speech recognition: A model and a program for research. In J. Fodor & J. Katz (Eds.), The Structure of Language: Readings in the Philosophy of Language. Englewood Cliffs, N.J.: Prentice-Hall, 1964.

Heidbreder, E. Seven Psychologies. New York: Appleton-Century-Crofts, 1933, 1961.

Higgs, J. The articulation test as a linguistic technique. Language and Speech, 1970, 13, 262–270.

Hirst, P. Q. Durkheim, Bernard, and Epistomology. London: Routledge & Kegan Paul, 1975.

Holden, A. Shapes, Space, and Symmetry. New York: Columbia University Press, 1971.

House, A., & Fairbanks, G. The influence of consonant environment upon the secondary acoustical characteristics of vowels. J. Acoust. Soc. Amer., 1953, 25, 105–113.

Hultzen, L. S. Degrees of difference of English consonants. In Proceedings of the 5th International Congress of Phonetic Science. Basal: S. Karger, 1965, 367–370.

Ingram, D. Fronting in child phonology. J. Child Lang., 1974a, 1, 233–241.

Ingram, D. Phonological rules in young children. J. Child Lang., 1974b, 1, 49–64.

Ingram, D. Surface contrast in children's speech. J. Child Lang., 1975, 2, 287–292.

Ingram, D. Current issues in child phonology. In D. Morehead & A. Morehead (Eds.), Normal and Deficient Child Language. Baltimore: University Park Press, 1976a.

Ingram, D. Phonological Disability in Children. New York: Elsevier, 1976b.

Irwin, O. Infant speech: Consonant sounds according to manner of articulation. J. Sp. Dis., 1947a, 12, 402–404.

Irwin, O. Infant speech: Consonantal sounds according to place of articulation. J. Sp. Dis., 1947b, 12, 397–401.

Irwin, O. Infant speech: Development of vowel sounds. J. Sp. Hear. Dis., 1948, 13, 31–34.

Irwin, O. Infant speech: Consonantal position. J. Sp. Hear. Dis., 1951, 16, 159–161.

Ishiki, M. A comparative analysis of the English and Japanese consonant phonemes. In Phonetic Society of Japan, Study of Sounds. Tokyo: Tiyoda, 1957.

Jaensch, E. Über Schichtenstenstruktur und Entwicklungsgeschichte der psychphysichen Organisation. Z. Psychol., 1928, 106, 457ff.

Jakobson, R. The concept of the sound law and the teleological criterion. In R. Jakobson (Ed. and trans.), Selected Writings (Vol. 1): Phonological Studies. The Hague: Mouton, 1962. (Originally published in Czechoslovakian, 1928a.)

Jakobson, R. Proposition au premier congrés international de linguistes. In R.

Jakobson (Ed.), Selected Writings (Vol. 1): Phonological Studies. The Hague: Mouton, 1962. (Originally published, 1928b.)

Jakobson, R. Remarques sur l'évolution phonologique du Russe comparée à celle des autre langues slaves. In R. Jakobson (Ed.), Selected Writings (Vol. 1): Phonological Studies. The Hague: Mouton, 1962. (Originally published, 1929).

Jakobson, R. Phonemic notes on standard Slovak. In R. Jakobson (Ed. and trans.), Selected Writings (Vol. 1): Phonological Studies. The Hague: Mouton, 1962. (Originally published in Czechoslovakian, 1931a.)

Jakobson, R. Principes de phonologie historique. In R. Jakobson (Ed.), Selected Writings (Vol. 1): Phonological Studies. The Hague: Mouton, 1962. (Originally published, 1931b.)

Jakobson, R. Phoneme and phonology. In R. Jakobson (Ed. and trans.), Selected Writings (Vol. 1): Phonological Studies. The Hague: Mouton, 1962. (Originally published in Czechoslovakian, 1932.)

Jakobson, R. On ancient Greek prosody. In R. Jakobson (Ed. and trans.), Selected Writings (Vol. 1): Phonological Studies. The Hague: Mouton, 1962. (Originally published in Polish, 1937.)

Jakobson, R. Sur la theorie des affinites phonologiques entre les langues. In R. Jakobson (Ed.), Selected Writings (Vol. 1): Phonological Studies. The Hague: Mouton, 1962. (Originally published, 1938.)

Jakobson, R. Un manuel de phonologie générale. In R. Jakobson (Ed.), Selected Writings (Vol. 1): Phonological Studies. The Hague: Mouton, 1962. (Originally published, 1939a.)

Jakobson, R. Observations sur le classement phonologique des consonnes. In R. Jakobson (Ed.), Selected Writings (Vol. 1): Phonological Studies. The Hague: Mouton, 1962. (Originally published, 1939b.)

Jakobson, R. The sound laws of child language and their place in general phonology. In A. S. Bar-Adon & W. Leopold (Eds. and trans.), Child Language: A Book of Readings. Englewood Cliffs, N.J.: Prentice-Hall, 1971. (Originally presented, 1939c; first published in N.S. Trubetzkoy's Grundzüge der Phonologie, 1949, as an appendix, "Les lois phoniques du langage enfantin et leur place dans la phonologie générale.")

Jakobson, R. Child Language, Aphasia and Phonological Universals (A. Keiler, trans.). The Hague: Mouton, 1968. (Originally published, 1941, as Kindersprache, Aphasie und allgemeine Lautgesetze.)

Jakobson, R. On the identification of phonemic entities. In R. Jakobson (Ed. and trans.), Selected Writings (Vol. 1): Phonological Studies. The Hague: Mouton, 1962. (Originally published, 1949.)

Jakobson, R. For the correct presentation of phonemic problems. In R. Jakobson (Ed.), Selected Writings (Vol. 1): Phonological Studies. The Hague: Mouton, 1962. (Originally published, 1951.)

Jakobson, R. Typological studies and their contribution to historical comparative linguistics. In R. Jakobson (Ed.), Selected Writings (Vol. 1): Phonological Studies. The Hague: Mouton, 1962. (Originally published, 1958.)

Jakobson, R. Why "mama" and "papa." In A. Bar-Adon & W. Leopold (Eds.), Child Language: A Book of Readings. Englewood Cliffs, N.J.: Prentice-Hall, 1971. (Also published, 1962, in Selected Writings.)

Jakobson, R. Retrospect. In R. Jakobson (Ed.), Selected Writings (Vol. 1): Phonological Studies. The Hague: Mouton, 1962.

Jakobson, R. Aphasia as a linguistic problem. In A. de Reuck & M. O'Connor (Eds.), Disorders of Language. Boston: Little, Brown, 1964.

Jakobson, R. Implications of language universals for linguistics. In J. Greenberg (Ed.), Universals of Language. Cambridge, Mass.: MIT Press, 1966.

Jakobson, R. Verbal communication. Sci. Amer. 1972, 227, 73–79.

Jakobson, R. Main Trends in the Science of Language. London: George Allen & Unwin, 1973.

Jakobson, R., Cherry, E. C., & Halle, M. Toward the logical description of languages in their phonemic aspect. Language, 1953, 29, 34–46.

Jakobson, R., Fant, G., & Halle, M. Preliminaries to Speech Analysis: The Distinctive Features and Their Correlates. Cambridge, Mass.: MIT Press, 1952/1963/1967.

Jakobson, R., & Halle, M. Fundamentals of Language. The Hague: Mouton, 1956a.

Jakobson, R., & Halle, M. Phonology and phonetics. In R. Jakobson (Ed.), Selected Writings (Vol. 1): Phonological Studies. The Hague: Mouton, 1962. (Originally published 1956b.)

Jakobson, R., & Halle, M. Phonology in relation to phonetics. In L. Kaiser (Ed.), Manual of Phonetics. Amsterdam: North-Holland, 1957.

Jakobson, R., & Halle, M. Phonemic patterning. In S. Saporta (Ed.), Psycholinguistics. New York: Holt, Rinehart and Winston, 1961.

Jakobson, R., & Halle, M. Phonology in relation to phonetics. In B. Malmberg (Ed.), Manual of Phonetics. Amsterdam: North-Holland, 1968.

Jakobson, R., & Halle, M. Phonemic patterns. In A. Bar-Adon & W. Leopold (Eds.), Child Language: A Book of Readings. Englewood Cliffs, N.J.: Prentice-Hall, 1971.

Jakobson, R., & Lotz, J. Notes on the French phonemic pattern. In R. Jakobson (Ed.), Selected Writings (Vol. 1): Phonological Studies. The Hague: Mouton, 1962. (Originally published, 1949.)

Johnson, W., Darley, F., & Spriestersbach, D. Diagnostic Methods in Speech Pathology. New York: Harper & Row, 1963.

Jones, D. The Phoneme. Cambridge, England: Heffer & Sons, 1967. (Originally published, 1950.)

Jones, D. The History and Meaning of the Term "Phoneme". London: International Phonetic Association, 1957/1967.

Joos, M. Acoustic phonetics. Language, 1948, 24 (Supplement).

Kagan, J. The growth of the "face" schema: Theoretical significance and methodological issues. In J. Hellmuth (Ed.), Exceptional Infant (Vol. 1): The Normal Infant. New York: Brunner/Mazel, 1967.

Kaiser, L. Manual of Phonetics. Amsterdam: North-Holland, 1957.

Kant, I. Introduction to the "Critique of Pure Reason". In P. Edwards and A. Pap (Eds.), A Modern Introduction to Philosophy. New York: The Free Press, 1973. (Originally published, 1781—Norman Kemp Smith translation.)

Kantner, C., & West, R. Phonetics. New York: Harper & Brothers, 1960.

Karlgren, H. Statistical methods in phonetics. In B. Malmberg (Ed.), Manual of Phonetics. Amsterdam: North-Holland, 1968.

Kessen, W., Haith, M., & Salapatek, P. Infancy. In P. Mussen (Ed.), Manual of Psychology (3rd ed.). New York: John Wiley & Sons, 1970.

Koenig, W., Dunn, H., & Lacy, L. The sound spectrograph. J. Acoust. Soc. Amer., 1946, 17, 19–49.

Kornfeld, J. Theoretical issues in child phonology. PCLS, 1971 (7th Regional Meeting), 454–468.

Kruskal, J. B. Multidimensional scaling by optimizing goodness of fit to a nonmetric hypothesis. Psychometrika, 1964a, 29, 1–27.

Kruskal, J. B. Nonmetric multidimensional scaling: A numerical method. Psychometrika, 1964b, 29, 115–129.

Ladefoged, P. A Course in Phonetics. New York: Harcourt Brace Javanovich, 1975.

Lafon, J. Auditory basis of phonetics. In B. Malmberg (Ed.), Manual of Phonetics. Amsterdam: North-Holland, 1968.

Lehiste, I., & Peterson, G. Transitions, glides and diphthongs. J. Acoust. Soc. Amer., 1961, 33, 268–277.

Leonard, L. Some limitations in the clinical application of distinctive features. J. Sp. Hear. Dis., 1973, 38, 141–143.

Leopold, W. The study of child language and infant bilingualism. In A. Bar-Adon & W. Leopold (Eds.), Child Language: A Book of Readings. Englewood Cliffs, N.J.: Prentice-Hall, 1971. (Originally published, 1948.)

Leopold, W. Patterning in children's language learning. In A. Bar-Adon & W. Leopold (Eds.), Child Language: A Book of Readings. Englewood Cliffs, N.J.: Prentice-Hall, 1971. (Originally published, 1953.)

Lepschy, G. A Survey of Structural Linguistics. London: Faber & Faber, 1970.

Leutenegger, R. The Sounds of American English. Milwaukee: Scott, Foresman, 1963.

Lévi-Strauss, C. The structural study of myth. In R. DeGeorge & F. DeGeorge (Eds.), The Structuralists from Marx to Lévi-Strauss. Garden City, N.Y.: Doubleday Anchor, 1972a.

Lévi-Strauss, C. Four Winnebago myths. In R. DeGeorge & F. DeGeorge (Eds.), The Structuralists from Marx to Lévi-Strauss. Garden City, N.Y.: Doubleday Anchor, 1972b.

Liberman, A., Cooper, F., Shankweiler, D., & Studdert-Kennedy, M. Perception of the speech code. Psychol. Rev., 1967, 74, 431–457.

Liberman, A., Delattre, P., Gerstman, L., & Cooper, F. Tempo of frequency change as a cue for distinguishing classes of speech sounds. J. Exper. Psychol., 1956, 52, 127–137.

Liberman, A., Ingemann, F., Lisker, L., Delattre, P., & Cooper, F. Minimal rules for synthesizing speech. J. Acoust. Soc. Amer., 1959, 31, 1490–1499.

Lieberman, P., Harris, K., Wolff, P., & Russell, L. Newborn infant cry and nonhuman primate vocalizations. J. Sp. Hear. Res., 1971, 14, 718–727.

Lisker, L., & Abramson, A. A cross-language study of voicing initial stops: Acoustical measurements. Word, 1964, 20, 383–427.

Locke, J. Experimentally elicited articulatory behavior. Lang. Sp., 1969, 12, 187–191.

Lorentz, J. An analysis of some deviant phonological rules of English. In D. Morehead & A. Morehead (Eds.), Normal and Deficient Child Language. Baltimore: University Park Press, 1976.

Lynip, A. The use of magnetic devices in the collection and analysis of the preverbal utterances of an infant. Genet. Psychol. Monogr., 1951, 44, 221–262.

Malmberg, B. Phonetics. New York: Dover, 1963.

Malmberg, B. Manual of Phonetics. Amsterdam: North-Holland, 1968.

Martin, C. The prediction of similarity judgments with a distinctive feature system and the relative frequency of occurrence of distinctive features in the English language. Unpublished doctoral dissertation, Southern Illinois University, 1973. (Data reexamined, 1975.)

Martinet, A. Structure and language. In J. Ehrmann (Ed.), Structuralism (T. Penchoen, trans.). Garden City, N.Y.: Doubleday Anchor, 1970. (Originally published in French, 1965, as Structure et langue.)

Marx, M. The general nature of theory construction. In M. Marx (Ed.), Theories in Contemporary Psychology. New York: Macmillan, 1963.

McCarthy, D. Language development in children. In L. Carmichael (Ed.), Manual of Child Psychology. New York: John Wiley & Sons, 1946/1954/1966.

McDonald, E. Articulation Testing and Treatment: A Sensory-Motor Approach. Pittsburgh: Stanwix House, 1964.

McNeill, D. The development of language. In P. Mussen (Ed.), Manual of Child Psychology (3rd ed.). New York: John Wiley & Sons, 1970.

McReynolds, L. Phonological Analysis of Articulation Errors. Workshop presented, Burlington, Iowa, April 13–14, 1972.

McReynolds, L., & Engmann, D. Distinctive Feature Analysis of Misarticulations. Baltimore: University Park Press, 1975.

McReynolds, L., & Huston, K. A distinctive feature analysis of children's misarticulations. J. Sp. Hear. Dis., 1971, 36, 155–166.

Menn, L. Phonotactic rules in beginning speech. Lingua, 1971, 26, 225–251.

Menn, L. Counter example to "fronting" as a universal of child phonology. J. Child Lang., 1975, 2, 293–296.

Menyuk, P. The role of distinctive features in children's acquisition of phonology. J. Sp. Hear. Res., 1968, 11, 138–146.

Miller, G. The Psychology of Communication. New York: Basic Books, 1967.

Miller, G., & Nicely, P. Analysis of perceptual confusions among some English consonants. J. Acoust. Soc. Amer., 1955, 27, 338–353.

Minkowski, M. Ueber fruhzeitige Bewegungen. Schweiz. med. Wschr., 1922, 52, 721, 751.

Mohr, B., & Wang, W. Perceptual distances and the specification of phonological features. Phonetica, 1968, 18, 31–45.

Moser, H., & Dreher, J. Phonetic confusion vectors. J. Acoust. Soc. Amer., 1955, 27, 874–881.

Moskowitz, A. The two-year-old stage in the acquisition of English phonology. Language, 1970, 46, 426–441.

Murdock, G. P. World ethnographic sample. Anthropol. Ling., 1959, 1, 1–5.

Nakazima, S. Phonemicization and symbolization in language development. In E. Lennenberg (Ed.), Foundations of Language Development (Vol. 1). New York: Academic Press, 1975.

Oller, D. Regularities in abnormal child phonology. J. Sp. Hear. Dis., 1974, 38, 36–47.

Oller, D., & Kelly, C. Phonological substitution processes of a hard-of-hearing child. J. Sp. Hear. Dis., 1975, 39, 65–74.

Oller, D., Wieman, L., Doyle, J., & Ross, C. Infant babbling and speech. J. Child Lang., 1976, 3, 1–11.

Olmsted, D. A theory of the child's learning of phonology. In A. Bar-Adon &

W. Leopold (Eds.), Child Language: A Book of Readings. Englewood Cliffs, N.J.: Prentice-Hall, 1971. (Originally published, 1966.)

Olmsted, D. Out of the Mouth of Babes. The Hague: Mouton, 1971.

Olney, R., & Scholnick, E. Adult judgments of age and linguistic differences in infant vocalizations. J. Child Lang., 1976, 3, 145–155.

Parker, F. Distinctive features in speech pathology: Phonology or phonemics? J. Sp. Hear. Dis., 1976, 41, 23–39.

Pei, M. Glossary of Linguistic Terminology. Garden City, N.Y.: Doubleday Anchor, 1966.

Peterson, G., & Barney, H. Control methods used in a study of vowels. J. Acoust. Soc. Amer., 1952, 24, 175–184.

Peterson, G., & Lehiste, I. Duration of syllable nuclei in English. J. Acoust. Soc. Amer., 1960, 32, 693–703.

Peterson, G., & Shoup, J. A physiological theory of phonetics. J. Sp. Hear. Res., 1966a, 9, 5–67.

Peterson, G., & Shoup, J. The elements of an acoustic phonetic theory. J. Sp. Hear. Res., 1966b, 9, 68–99.

Peterson, G., & Shoup, J. Glossary of terms from the physiological and acoustic theories. J. Sp. Hear. Res., 1966c, 9, 100–120.

Pickett, J. Perception of vowels heard in noises of various spectra. J. Acoust. Soc. Amer., 1957, 29, 613–620.

Pierce, J. R. Symbols, Signals and Noise. New York: Harper & Row, 1965.

Pike, K. Phonemics. Ann Arbor: University of Michigan Press, 1964.

Plomp, R., Pols, L. C., & van de Geer, J. P. Dimensional analysis of vowel spectra. J. Acoust. Soc. Amer., 1967, 41, 707–712.

Polanyi, M. The Tacit Dimension. Garden City, N.Y.: Doubleday Anchor, 1967.

Pollack, E., & Rees, N. Disorders of articulation: Some clinical applications of distinctive feature theory. J. Sp. Hear. Dis., 1972, 37, 451–461.

Pols, L. C., van de Kamp, L. J., & Plomp, R. Perceptual and physical space of vowel sounds. J. Acoust. Soc. Amer., 1969, 46, 458–467.

Poole, I. Genetic development of articulation of consonant sounds in speech. Elem. Eng. Rev., 1934, 11, 159–161.

Potter, R., Kopp, G., & Kopp, H. Visible Speech. New York: Dover, 1966. (Originally published, 1947.)

Potter, R., & Steinberg, J. Toward the specification of speech. J. Acoust. Soc. Amer., 1950, 22, 807–820.

Rūķe-Draviņa, V. "Mama" and "papa" in child language. J. Child Lang., 1976, 3, 157–166.

Russell, G. O. The Vowel. Columbus: Ohio State University, 1928.

Sander, E. K. When are speech sounds learned? J. Sp. Hear. Dis., 1972, 37, 55–63.

Sanders, D. Auditory Perception of Speech. Englewood Cliffs, N.J.: Prentice-Hall, 1977.

Sapir, E. Language. New York: Harcourt & World, 1921/1949.

Saporta, S. Frequency of consonant clusters. Language, 1955, 31, 25–30.

Saporta, S. Psycholinguistics: A Book of Readings. New York: Holt, Rinehart and Winston, 1961.

de Saussure, F. Course in General Linguistics (C. Bally & A. Sechehaye, Eds.; W. Baskin, trans.). New York: McGraw-Hill, 1966. (Lectures presented, 1906–1907, 1908–1909, 1910–1911; originally presented, 1915.)

Ščerba, L. Quantitative and qualitative relationships among Russian vowels. In G. Lepschy (Ed. and trans.), A Survey of Structural Linguistics. London: Faber & Faber, 1970. (Originally published in Russian, 1912.)

Schleicher, A. Some observations made on children. In A. Bar-Adon & W. Leopold (Eds. and trans.), Child Language: A Book of Readings. Englewood Cliffs, N.J.: Prentice-Hall, 1971. (Originally published in German, 1861, as Beiträge zur vergleichenden Sprachforschung.)

Schultze, F. The speech of the child. In A. Bar-Adon & W. Leopold (Eds. and trans.), Child Language: A Book of Readings. Englewood Cliffs, N.J.: Prentice-Hall, 1971. (Originally published in German, 1880, as Die Sprache die Kindes.)

Shannon, C., & Weaver, W. The Mathematical Theory of Communication. Urbana: University of Illinois Press, 1949/1963.

Shirley, M. M. The First Two Years: A Study of Twenty-five Babies (Vol. 2): Intellectual Development. Minneapolis: University of Minnesota Press, 1933a.

Shirley, M. M. The First Two Years: A Study of Twenty-five Babies (Vol. 3): Personality Manifestations. Minneapolis: University of Minnesota Press, 1933b.

Singh, J. Great Ideas in Information Theory, Language and Cybernetics. New York: Dover, 1966.

Singh, S. Perceptual Correlates of Distinctive Feature Systems. Washington, D.C.: Howard University Press, 1968.

Singh, S. A Step Toward a Theory of Speech Perception. Paper presented to the American Speech and Hearing Association, Detroit, 1972.

Singh, S. Distinctive Features: Theory and Validation. Baltimore: University Park Press, 1976.

Singh, S., & Black, J. Study of twenty-six intervocalic consonants as spoken and recognized by four language groups. J. Acoust. Soc. Amer., 1966, 39, 372–387.

Singh, S., & Woods, D. Perceptual structure of 12 American English vowels. J. Acoust. Soc. Amer., 1971, 49, 1861–1866.

Singh, S., Woods, D., & Becker, G. Perceptual structure of 22 prevocalic English consonants. J. Acoust. Soc. Amer., 1972, 52, 1698–1713.

Smith, M. E. An investigation of the development of the sentence in preschool children. J. Genet. Psychol., 1926, 3.

Smith, N. The Acquisition of Phonology. Cambridge, England: Cambridge University Press, 1973.

Staats, A. Learning, Language and Cognition. New York: Holt, Rinehart & Winston, 1968.

Stampe, D. The acquisition of phonetic representations. PCLS, 1969 (5th Regional Meeting), 443–454.

Stampe, D. On the natural history of diphthongs. PCLS, 1972 (8th Regional Meeting), 578–589.

Stampe, D. A dissertation on natural phonology. Unpublished doctoral dissertation, The University of Chicago, 1973.

Stevens, K., & House, A. An acoustical theory of vowel production and some of its implications. J. Sp. Hear. Res., 1961, 4, 303–320.

Strachey, J. Sigmund Freud: Three Essays on the Theory of Sexuality. New York: Avon, 1965.

Stumpf, C. Die Sprachlante. Berlin, 1926.

Taft, L. & Cohen, H. Neonatal and infant reflexology. In J. Hellmuth (Ed.), Exceptional Infant (Vol. 1): The Normal Infant. New York: Brunner/Mazel, 1967.

Templin, M. Certain Language Skills in Children. Minneapolis: University of Minnesota Press, 1957.

Tiffany, W. The threshold reliability of recorded sustained vowels. J. Sp. Hear. Dis., 1953a, 18, 379–385.

Tiffany, W. Vowel recognition as a function of duration, frequency modulation and phonetic context. J. Sp. Hear. Dis., 1953b, 18, 289–301.

Tomkins, W. Indian Sign Language. New York: Dover, 1969.

Torgerson, W. S. Theory and Methods of Scaling. New York: John Wiley & Sons, 1958.

Torgerson, W. S. Multidimensional scaling of similarity. Psychometrika, 1965, 30, 379–393.

Tracy, F. The first six months. In A. Bar-Adon & W. Leopold (Eds.), Child Language: A Book of Readings. Englewood Cliffs, N.J.: Prentice-Hall, 1971. (Originally published, 1909.)

Trubetzkoy, N. S. Principles of Phonology (C. Baltaxe, trans.). Berkeley: University of California Press, 1969. (Originally published in German, 1939, as Grundzüge der Phonologie.)

Twaddel, W. F. On defining the phoneme. Language, 1935, 16 (Supplement).

Van Riper, C. Speech Correction. Englewood Cliffs, N.J.: Prentice-Hall, 1954/1963/1972.

Van Riper, C., & Irwin, J. Voice and Articulation. Englewood Cliffs, N.J.: Prentice-Hall, 1958.

Velten, H. The growth of phonemic and lexical patterns in infant language. In A. Bar-Adon & W. Leopold (Eds.), Child Language: A Book of Readings. Englewood Cliffs, N.J.: Prentice-Hall, 1971. (Originally published, 1943.)

Voiers, W. D. Performance Evaluation of Speech Processing Devices (Vol. 3): Diagnostic Evaluation of Speech Intelligibility. Bedford, Mass.: Air Force Research Laboratories, 1967.

Walsh, H. On certain practical inadequacies of distinctive feature systems. J. Sp. Hear. Dis., 1974, 39, 32–43.

Wang, W. Mandarin phonology. Sci. Amer., 1973, 228, 50–60.

Wang, M., & Bilger, R. Consonant confusion in noise: A study of perceptual features. J. Acoust. Soc. Amer., 1973, 54, 1248–1266.

WSSD. Deaf Sign: An Introduction to Manual English. Vancouver, Wash.: Washington State School for the Deaf, 1972.

Waterson, N. Child phonology: A prosodic view. J. Ling., 1971, 7, 179–211.

Weber, J. Patterning of deviant articulation behavior. J. Sp. Hear. Dis., 1970, 35, 135–141.

Welch, P. D., & Wimpress, R. S. Two multivariate statistical computer programs and their application to the vowel recognition problem. J. Acoust. Soc. Amer., 1961, 33, 426–434.

Wellman, B., Case, I., Mengert, I., & Bradbury, D. Speech sounds of young children. Univ. Iowa Stud. Child Welf., 1931, 5, 1–82.

West, R. An historical review of the American literature in speech pathology. In R. W. Rieber & R. S. Brubaker (Eds.), Speech Pathology. Philadelphia: J. B. Lippincott, 1966.

Whitacre, J. Luper, H., & Pollio, H. General language deficits in children with articulation problems. Lang. Sp., 1970, 13, 231–239.

Wickelgren, W. Distinctive features and errors in short-term memory for English consonants. J. Acoust. Soc. Amer., 1966, 39, 388–398.

Wicker, F. W. Mapping the intersensory regions of perceptual space. Amer. J. Psychol., 1968, 81, 178–188.

Winitz, H. Articulatory Acquisition and Behavior. New York: Appleton-Century-Crofts, 1969.

Winitz, H., & Lawrence, M. Certain articulation errors and sound learning ability. J. Sp. Hear. Res., 1961, 4, 259–268.

Wundt, W. Exchanges and mutilations of sounds in child language. In A. Bar-Adon & W. Leopold (Eds. and trans.), Child Language: A Book of Readings. Englewood Cliffs, N.J.: Prentice-Hall, 1971. (Originally published in German, 1900, in Völkerpsychologie [Human Thought].)

Young, E., & Hawk, S. Moto-kinesthetic Speech Training. Stanford, Calif.: Stanford University Press, 1955.

APPENDICES

appendix A:

Jakobson, Fant, and Halle

	[ŋ]	[ʃ]	[tʃ]	[k]	[ʒ]	[dʒ]	[g]	[m]	[f]	[p]	[v]	[b]	[n]	[s]	[θ]	[t]	[z]	[ð]	[d]
[ŋ]	[ŋ]	1-NN	1-NN	1-NN	1-NN	1-NN	1-NN	1-CD	2-CD NN	2-CD NN	2-CD NN	2-CD NN	1-CD	2-CD NN	2-CD NN	2-CD NN	2-CD NN	2-CD NN	2-CD NN
[ʃ]		[ʃ]	1-CI	1-CI	1-TL	2-TL CI	2-TL CI	2-CD NN	1-CD	2-CD CI	2-CD TL	3-CD TL CI	2-CD NN	1-CD	1-CD	2-CD CI	2-CD TL	2-CD TL	3-CD TL CI
[tʃ]			[tʃ]	1-SM	2-TL CI	1-TL	2-TL SM	2-CD NN	2-CD CI	1-CD	3-CD TL CI	2-CD TL	2-CD NN	2-CD CI	3-CD CI SM	2-CD TL	3-CD TL CI	3-CD TL CI SM	3-CD TL
[k]				[k]	2-TL CI	2-TL SM	1-TL	2-NN CD	2-TL CD	3-CI CD TL	2-TL CD	2-CD TL	2-NN CD	2-TL CD	2-CD CI	3-CD TL CI	3-CD TL CI	3-CD TL	2-CD TL
[ʒ]					[ʒ]	1-CI	2-TL SM	2-CD NN	3-CD TL CI	2-CD TL	3-CD TL CI	3-CD TL CI	2-CD NN	3-CD CI SM	4-CD TL CI SM	2-CD TL	1-CD	3-CD CI SM	2-CD TL
[dʒ]						[dʒ]	1-SM	2-CD NN	3-CD TL CI	2-CD TL	2-CD CI	1-CD	2-CD NN	4-CD TL CI SM	3-CD TL	2-CD TL	3-CD CI SM	3-CD CI	1-CD
[g]							[g]	2-CD NN	3-CD TL CI	2-CD TL	2-CD CI	1-CD	2-CD NN	3-CD TL CI	3-CD TL	3-CD TL	3-CD CI	2-CD CI	1-CD

Features:

Vocalic	- V
Consonantal	- C
Compact	- CD
Grave	- GA
Flat	- FP
Nasal	- NN
Tense	- TL
Continuant	- CI
Strident	- SM

(continued)

appendix A (continued)

	[ŋ]	[ʃ]	[tʃ]	[k]	[ʒ]	[dʒ]	[g]	[m]	[f]	[p]	[v]	[b]	[n]	[s]	[θ]	[t]	[z]	[ð]	[d]
[ŋ]																			
[ʃ]																			
[tʃ]																			
[k]																			
[ʒ]																			
[dʒ]																			
[g]																			
[m]								[m]	1-NN	1-NN	1-NN	1-NN	1-GA	2-GA/NN	2-GA/NN	2-GA/NN	2-GA/NN	2-GA/NN	2-GA/NN
[f]									[f]	1-CI	1-TL	2-TL/CI	2-GA/NN	1-GA	1-GA	2-GA/CI	2-GA/TL	2-GA/TL	3-GA/TL/CI
[p]										[p]	2-TL/CI	1-TL	2-GA/NN	2-GA/CI	2-GA	1-GA	3-GA/CI	3-GA/TL/CI	2-GA/TL
[v]											[v]	1-CI	2-GA/NN	2-GA/TL	2-GA/TL	3-GA/TL/CI	1-GA	1-GA	2-GA/CI
[b]												[b]	2-GA/NN	3-GA/TL/CI	3-GA/TL/CI	2-GA/TL	2-GA/CI	2-GA/CI	1-GA
[n]													[n]	1-NN	1-NN	1-NN	1-NN	1-NN	1-NN
[s]														[s]	1-SM	1-CI	1-TL	2-TL/SM	2-TL/CI
[θ]															[θ]	1-CI	2-TL/SM	1-TL	2-TL/CI
[t]																[t]	2-TL/CI	2-TL/CI	1-TL
[z]																	[z]	1-SM	1-CI
[ð]																		[ð]	1-CI
[d]																			

Features:

Vocalic	- V
Consonantal	- C
Compact	- CD
Grave	- GA
Flat	- FP
Nasal	- NN
Tense	- TL
Continuant	- CI
Strident	- SM

appendix B:

Halle

	[ʃ]	[tʃ]	[k]	[ʒ]	[dʒ]	[g]	[m]	[f]	[p]	[v]	[b]	[n]	[s]	[θ]	[t]	[z]	[ð]	[d]
[ʃ]		1-CI	3-GA, CI, SM	1-TL	2-TL, CI	4-GA, TL, CI, SM	6-CD, GA, NN, TL, CI, SM	2-CD, GA	4-CD, GA, CI, SM	3-CD, GA, TL	5-CD, GA, TL, CI, SM	5-CD, NN, TL, CI, SM	1-CD	2-CD, SM	3-CD, CI, SM	2-CD, TL	3-CD, TL, SM	4-CD, TL, CI, SM
[tʃ]			2-GA, SM	2-TL, CI	1-TL	3-GA, TL, SM	5-CD, GA, NN, TL, SM	3-CD, GA, CI	3-CD, GA, SM	4-CD, GA, TL, CI	4-CD, GA, TL, SM	4-CD, NN, TL, SM	2-CD, CI	3-CD, CI, SM	2-CD, SM	3-CD, TL, CI	4-CD, TL, CI, SM	3-CD, TL, SM
[k]				4-TL, GA, CI, SM	3-GA, TL, SM	1-TL	3-CD, NN, TL	3-CD, CI, SM	1-CD	4-CD, TL, CI, SM	2-CD, TL	4-CD, GA, NN, TL	4-CD, GA, CI, SM	3-CD, GA, CI	2-CD, GA	5-CD, GA, TL, CI, SM	4-CD, GA, TL, CI	3-CD, GA, TL
[ʒ]					1-CI	3-GA, CI, SM	5-CD, GA, NN, CI, SM	3-CD, GA, TL	5-CD, GA, TL, CI, SM	2-GA, CD	4-CD, GA, CI, SM	4-CD, NN, CI, SM	2-CD, TL	3-CD, TL, SM	4-CD, TL, CI, SM	1-CD	2-CD, SM	3-CD, CI, SM

[k]

[ʒ]

Features:
Vocalic — V
Consonantal — C
Grave — GA
Compact — CD
Strident — SM
Nasal — NN
Continuant — CI
Voiced — TL

(continued)

appendix B (continued)

[ʃ]	[tʃ]	[k]	[ʒ]	[dʒ]	[g]	[m]	[f]	[p]	[v]	[b]	[n]	[s]	[θ]	[t]	[z]	[ð]	[d]
				[dʒ]	2-GA SM	4-CD GA NN SM	4-CD GA TL CI SM	4-CD GA TL SM	3-CD GA CI	3-CD GA SM	3-CD NN SM	3-CD TL CI	4-CD TL CI SM	3-CD TL SM	2-CD CI	3-CD CI SM	2-CD SM
					[g]	2-CD NN	4-CD TL CI SM	2-CD TL	3-CD CI SM	1-CD	3-CD GA NN	5-CD GA TL CI SM	4-CD GA TL CI	3-CD GA TL	4-CD GA CI SM	3-CD GA CI	2-CD GA
						[m]	4-NN TL CI SM	2-NN TL	3-NN CI SM	1-NN	1-GA	5-GA NN TL CI SM	4-GA NN TL CI	3-GA NN TL	4-GA NN CI SM	3-GA NN CI	2-GA NN
							[f]	2-CI SM	1-TL	3-TL CI SM	5-GA NN CI TL SM	1-GA	2-GA SM	3-GA CI SM	2-GA TL	3-GA TL SM CI	4-GA TL CI SM
								[p]	3-TL CI SM	1-TL	3-GA NN TL	3-GA CI SM	2-GA CI	1-GA	4-GA TL CI SM	3-GA TL CI	2-GA TL

Features:
Vocalic - V
Consonantal - C
Grave - GA
Compact - CD
Strident - SM
Nasal - NN
Continuant - CI
Voiced - TL

(continued)

[ʃ]	[tʃ]	[k]	[ʒ]	[dʒ]	[g]	[m]	[f]	[p]	[v]	[b]	[n]	[s]	[θ]	[t]	[z]	[ð]	[d]
									[v]	2-CI SM	4-GA NN CI SM	2-GA TL	3-TL SM	4-GA TL CI SM	1-GA	2-GA SM	2-GA CI
										[b]	2-GA NN	4-GA TL CI SM	3-GA TL CI	2-GA TL	3-GA CI SM	2-GA CI	1-GA
											[n]	4-NN TL CI SM	3-NN TL CI	2-NN TL	3-NN CI SM	2-NN CI	1-NN
												[s]	1-SM	2-CI SM	1-TL	2-TL SM	3-TL CI SM
													[θ]	1-CI	2-TL SM	1-TL	2-TL CI
														[t]	3-TL CI SM	2-TL CI	1-TL
															[z]	1-SM	2-CI SM
																[ð]	1-CI
																	[d]

Features:

Feature	
Vocalic	- V
Consonantal	- C
Grave	- GA
Compact	- CD
Strident	- SM
Nasal	- NN
Continuant	- CI
Voiced	- TL

appendix C:

Chomsky and Halle

Feature matrix (columns read left to right): (r) (l) (p) (b) (f) (v) (m) (t) (d) (θ) (δ) (n) (s) (z) (c) (č) (j) (š) (ž) (k) (g) (x) (ɣ) (h) (k") (g") (x")

Features:
- Vocalic - Vo
- Consonantal - Co
- High - H
- Back - B
- Low - L
- Anterior - A
- Coronal - Cĭ
- Round - R
- Voice - V
- Continuant - Cl
- Nasal - N
- Strident - S

(continued)

(continued)

Features:
Vocalic – Vo
Consonantal – Co
High – H
Back – B
Low – L
Anterior – A
Coronal – Cr
Round – R
Voice – V
Continuant – Ct
Nasal – N
Strident – S

appendix C (continued)

Features:

Vocalic	- Vo
Consonantal	- Co
High	- H
Back	- B
Low	- L
Anterior	- A
Coronal	- Cl
Round	- R
Voice	- V
Continuant	- Ct
Nasal	- N
Strident	- S

appendix D:

Voiers

	(h)	(k)	(t)	(p)	(t3)	(ʃ)	(s)	(θ)	(f)	(j)	(l)	(r)	(w)	(g)	(d)	(b)	(d3)	(3)	(z)	(δ)	(v)	(n)	(m)
(h)	1-Ss	1-Ss	1-Ss	1-Ss	2-Ss Sb	1-Sb	1-Sb	*0	*0	2-V Vl	2-V Vl	2-V Vl	2-V Vl	2-V Ss	2-V Ss	2-V Ss	3-V Ss Sb	2-V Sb	2-V Sb	1-V	1-V	3-V N Ss	3-V N Ss
(k)		(k)	1-C	1-C	1-Sb	3-Ss Sb C	3-Ss Sb C	2-Ss C	2-Ss C	3-V Ss Vl	3-V Vl Ss	4-V Vl Ss	5-C G V Vl Sb	3-V Sb Ss	4-V Sb Ss	5-C V Sb Ss	4-C G V Sb	5-C V Sb Ss Sb	4-G V Sb Ss	4-C V Sb Ss	4-C V Sb Ss	5-C V N Sb Ss	5-C G N V Sb Ss
(t)			(t)	1-G	2-C Sb	3-C Sb Ss	2-C Ss	2-C Sb	3-C G Sb	4-C V Vl Ss	3-V Vl Ss	3-V Vl Ss	4-G V Vl Ss	2-C V	2-G V	4-C G V	3-C G V Sb	4-C V Sb Ss	3-V Sb Ss	3-V C Sb	4-C V Sb	5-C G N V Sb	6-C G N V Sb
(p)				(p)	3-C G Sb	4-C Sb Ss	3-G Sb Ss	2-G Ss	1-Ss	4-C V Vl Ss	3-V Vl Ss	4-V Vl Sb Ss	4-G V Vl Ss Sb	4-C Sb Ss	4-C V Sb Ss	5-C V Sb Ss	4-C G V Sb	5-C V Sb Ss	4-G V Sb Ss	3-V C Sb	4-C V Sb	5-C V N Sb	5-G N V Sb Ss
(t3)					(t3)	1-Ss	2-C Ss	3-C Sb Ss	4-C G Sb Ss	4-C V Vl Ss	3-V Vl Ss	4-G V Vl Sb Ss	5-C G V Vl Sb Ss	3-V Sb Ss	4-V Sb Ss	5-C V Sb Ss	3-C G Sb	4-C V Sb Ss	3-C V Sb Ss	4-C V Sb Ss	4-C V Sb Ss	5-C V N Sb Ss	5-G N V Sb Ss
(ʃ)						(ʃ)	1-C	2-C Sb	3-C G Sb	3-V Vl Sb	3-V Vl Sb	3-V Vl Sb	4-G V Vl Sb	3-V Sb Ss	3-V Sb Ss	4-G V Sb Ss	2-V Ss	1-V	2-C V	3-V C Sb	4-C V Sb	5-C V N Sb Ss	5-C G N V Sb
(s)							(s)	1-Sb	2-G Sb	4-C V Vl Sb	3-V Vl Sb	3-V Vl Sb Ss	4-G V Vl Sb Ss	4-C Sb Ss	3-V Sb Ss	4-G V Sb Ss	3-C V Sb Ss	2-C V	1-V	2-V Sb	3-G V Sb	4-N V Sb Ss	5-G N V Sb Ss

Features:
- Compact — C
- Grave — G
- Nasal — N
- Sibilation — Sb
- Sustention — Ss
- Voicing — V
- Vowel-like — Vl
- Error — *0

(continued)

appendix D (continued)

	(h)	(k)	(t)	(p)	(tʃ)	(ʃ)	(s)	(θ)	(f)	(j)	(l)	(r)	(w)	(g)	(d)	(b)	(dʒ)	(ʒ)	(z)	(ð)	(v)	(n)	(m)
(h)	1-Ss							(θ)	1-G	3-C/V/Vl	2-V/Vl	2-V/Vl	3-G/V/Vl	3-C/V/Ss	2-V/Ss	3-G/V/Ss	4-C/Sb/Ss	3-C/V/Sb	2-V/Sb	1-V	2-G/V	3-N/V/Ss	4-G/N/V/Ss
(k)		1-C							(f)	3-C/V/Vl	2-V/Vl	3-G/V/Vl	2-V/Vl	3-C/V/Ss	3-C/V/Ss	2-V/Ss	5-C/G/V/Ss	4-C/G/V/Sb	3-G/V/Sb	2-G/V	1-V	4-C/N/V	3-N/V/Ss
(t)	1-Ss	1-C	(t)							3-C/V/Vl	2-V/Vl	2-V/Vl	3-G/V/Vl	2-Vl/Ss	2-Ss/Vl	3-G/Ss/Vl	3-Sb/Ss	2-Sb/Vl	2-Sb/Vl	1-Sb	2-G/Ss	3-N/Ss/Vl	4-G/N/Ss/Vl
(j)									(j)	*0	*0	1-C	1-C	3-C/V/Ss	3-G/V/Ss	3-Sb/Ss	4-C/Sb/Ss	3-C/Sb/Vl	2-Sb/Vl	1-Vl	2-G/Vl	3-N/Ss/Vl	4-G/N/Ss/Vl
(l)									(l)		*0	*0	1-G	3-C/Ss/Vl	2-Ss/Vl	3-G/Ss/Vl	4-C/Sb/Ss	3-C/Sb/Vl	2-Sb/Vl	1-Vl	2-G/Vl	3-N/Ss/Vl	4-G/N/Ss/Vl
(r)									(r)			*0	1-G	3-C/Ss/Vl	2-Ss/Vl	3-G/Ss/Vl	4-C/Sb/Ss	3-C/Sb/Vl	2-Sb/Vl	1-Vl	2-G/Vl	3-N/Ss/Vl	4-G/N/Ss/Vl
(w)									(w)					3-C/Ss/Vl	3-G/Ss/Vl	2-Ss/Vl	4-C/Sb/Ss/Vl	3-C/Sb/Vl	2-Sb/Vl	2-G/Vl	1-Vl	3-N/Ss/Vl	4-G/N/Ss/Vl
(g)									(g)						3-C/Ss/Vl	2-Ss/Vl	4-C/Sb/Ss/Vl	3-C/Sb/Ss/Vl	3-C/Sb/Ss/Vl	3-C/Ss/Vl	3-C/Ss/Vl	3-C/N/Ss/Vl	3-N/Ss/Vl
(d)									(d)							1-G	2-C/Sb	3-C/Sb/Ss	2-Sb/Ss	1-Ss	2-G/Ss	1-N	2-G/N

(continued)

Features:
- Compact — C
- Grave — G
- Nasal — N
- Sibilation — Sb
- Sustention — Ss
- Voicing — V
- Vowel-like — Vl
- Error — *0

306

	(h)	(k)	(t)	(p)	(tʃ)	(ʃ)	(s)	(θ)	(f)	(j)	(l)	(r)	(w)	(g)	(d)	(b)	(dʒ)	(ʒ)	(z)	(ð)	(v)	(n)	(m)
																(b)	3-C G Sb	4-C G Sb Ss	3-G Sb Ss	2-G Sb Ss	1-Ss	2-G N	1-N
																	(dʒ)	1-Ss	2-C Ss	3-C Sb Ss	4-C G Sb Ss	3-C N Sb	4-C G N Sb
																		(ʒ)	1-C	2-C Sb	3-C G Sb	4-C N Sb Ss	5-C G N Sb Ss
																			(z)	1-Sb	2-G Sb	3-N Sb Ss	4-G N Sb Ss
																				(δ)	1-G	2-N Ss	3-G N Ss
																					(v)	3-G N Ss	2-N Ss
																						(n)	1-G
																							(m)

Features:
- Compact - C
- Grave - G
- Nasal - N
- Sibilation - Sb
- Sustention - Ss
- Voicing - V
- Vowel-like - Vl
- Error - *0

appendix E:

Miller and Nicely

	n	m	3	z	ð	v	g	d	b	ʃ	s	θ	f	k	t	p
n	n	1-P1	4-N A D P1	3-N A D	2-N A	3-N A P1	2-N P1	1-N	2-N P1	5-V N A P1	4-V N A	3-V N A	4-V N A	3-V N P1	2-V N	3-V N P1
m		m	5-N A D P2	4-N A D P1	3-N A P1	2-N A	3-N P2	2-N P1	1-N	6-V N A D P2	5-V N A D P1	4-V N A P1	3-V N A	4-V N P2	3-V N P1	2-V N
3			3	1-P1	2-D P1	3-D P2	2-A D	3-A D P1	4-A D P2	1-V	2-V P1	3-V D P1	4-V D P2	3-V A D	4-V A D P1	5-V A D P2
z				z	1-D	2-D P1	3-A D P1	2-A D	3-A D P1	2-V P1	1-V	2-V D	3-V D P1	4-V A D P1	3-V A D	4-V A D P2
ð					ð	1-P1	2-A P1	1-A	2-A P1	3-V D P1	2-V D	1-V	2-V P1	3-V A P1	2-V A	3-V A P1

Features:
Nasality   - N
Affrication - A
Duration - D
Voicing   - V
Place: 1 or 2 - P1/P2

(continued)

308

	n	m	ʒ	z	ð	v	g	d	b	ʃ	s	θ	f	k	t	p
v						v	3-A P2	2-A P1	1-A	4-V D P2	3-V D P1	2-V P1	1-V	4-V P2	3-V P1	2-V A
g							g	1-P1	2-P2	3-V A D	4-V A D P1	3-V A P1	4-V A P2	1-V	2-V P1	3-V P2
d								d	1-P1	4-V A D P1	3-V A D	2-V A	3-V A P1	2-V P1	1-V	2-V P1
b									b	5-V A D P2	4-V A D P1	3-V A P1	2-V A	3-V P2	2-V P1	1-V
ʃ										ʃ	1-P1	2-D P1	3-D P2	2-A D	3-A D P1	4-A D P2
s											s	1-D	2-D P1	3-A D P1	2-A D	3-A D P1
θ												θ	1-P1	2-A P1	1-A	2-A P1
f													f	3-A P2	2-A P1	1-A
k														k	1-P1	2-P2
t															t	1-P1

Features:
Nasality   - N
Affrication - A
Duration   - D
Voicing   - V
Place: 1 or 2 - P1/P2

309

appendix F:

Singh; Singh and Black

	(p)	(b)	(t)	(d)	(tʃ)	(dʒ)	(k)	(g)	(f)	(v)	(θ)	(ð)	(s)	(z)	(ʃ)	(ʒ)	(w)	(r)	(l)	(j)	(h)	(w)	(m)	(n)
(p)	1-P	1-V	1-P	2-V/P	3-F/P2	4-V/F/P2	3-P	4-V/P3	1-F	2-V/F	2-F/P	3-V/F/P	3-F/D/P	4-V/F/D/P	4-F/D/P2	5-V/F/D/P2	2-V/G	4-V/L/R/P	3-V/L/P	4-V/G/P2	5-F/A/P3	2-F/G	2-V/N	3-V/N/P
(b)	1-V	(b)	2-P/V	1-P	4-V/F/P2	3-F/P2	4-V/P3	3-P	2-V/F	1-F	3-V/F/P	2-F/V	4-V/F/D/P	3-F/D/P	5-V/F/D/P2	4-F/D/P2	1-G	3-L/R/P	2-L/P	3-G/P2	6-V/F/A/P3	3-V/F/G	1-N	2-N/P
(t)	1-P	2-P/V	(t)	1-V	2-F/P	3-V/F/P	2-P	3-V/P2	2-F/P	3-V/F/P2	1-F	2-V/F	1-D	2-V/D	2-F/D/P	3-V/F/D/P	3-F/G/P	5-V/L/R/P	4-V/L/P	3-F/G/P2	4-F/A/P	3-F/G	3-F/N/P	2-F/N
(d)	2-V/P	1-P	1-V	(d)	3-V/F/P	2-F/P	3-V/P2	2-P	3-V/F/P	2-F/P	2-V/F	1-F	2-V/D	1-D	3-V/F/D/P	2-F/D/P	2-G/P	2-L/R	1-L	2-G/P2	5-V/F/A/P	3-V/F/G/P	2-N/P	1-N
(tʃ)	3-F/P2	4-V/F/P2	2-F/P	3-V/F/P	(tʃ)	1-V	2-F/P	3-V/F/P2	2-V/F	3-V/F/P2	3-V/F/P	4-V/F/P	1-D	2-V/D	1-D/P	2-V/D/P	4-F/G/P	4-F/L/R/P2	3-F/L/P2	2-F/G	2-F/A	3-G/P2	4-F/N/P2	3-N/P2
(dʒ)	4-V/F/P2	3-F/P2	3-V/F/P	2-F/P	1-V	(dʒ)	3-V/F/P2	2-F/P	3-V/F/P2	2-V/F/P2	4-V/F/P	3-V/F/P	2-V/D	1-D	2-V/D/P	1-D/P	2-G/P2	2-L/R/P2	1-L/P2	1-G	3-F/A/P2	5-F/G/P3	4-G/P3	3-N/P2
(k)	3-P	4-V/P3	2-P	3-V/P2	2-F/P	3-V/F/P2	(k)	1-V	...								1-G							
(g)	4-V/P3	3-P	3-V/P2	2-P	3-V/F/P2	2-F/P	1-V	(g)	...															

Features:
- Voicing – V
- Nasality – N
- Frication – F
- Duration – D
- Liquid – L
- Glide – G
- Retroflex – R
- Aspiration – A
- Place – P

(continued)

Feature-comparison matrix (upper triangle). Rows and columns are phoneme symbols; each cell gives a numeric value followed by the differing feature labels (see legend).

	(p)	(b)	(t)	(d)	(tʃ)	(dʒ)	(k)	(g)	(f)	(v)	(θ)	(ð)	(s)	(z)	(ʃ)	(ʒ)	(w)	(r)	(l)	(j)	(h)	(w)	(m)	(n)
(f)										1-V	1-P	2-V P	2-D P	3-V D P	3-D P2	4-V D P2	3-V F G	5-V F L R P	4-V F L P	5-V F G P2	4-A P3	1-G	3-V N F	4-V N F P
(v)											2-V P	1-P	3-V D P	2-D P	4-V D P2	3-D P2	2-F G	4-F L R P	3-F L P	4-F G P2	5-V A P3	2-V G	2-F N	3-N F
(θ)												1-V	1-D	2-V D	2-D P	3-V D P	4-V F G P	4-V F L R P	3-V F L	4-V F G P	3-A P2	2-G P	4-V N F P	3-V N F
(ð)													2-V D	1-D	3-V D P	2-D P	3-F G P	3-F L R P	2-F L	3-F G P	4-V A P2	3-V G P	3-N F P	2-N F
(s)														1-V	1-P	2-V P	5-V F G P	5-V F L R P	4-V F L P	5-V F G P	4-D A P2	3-D G P	5-V N F D P2	4-V N F D
(z)															2-V P	1-P	4-V F D G P	4-F D L R P	3-F D L	4-V F D G	3-D A P	4-V D G P	4-N F D P	3-N F D
(ʃ)																1-V	6-V F D G P2	6-V F D L R P	5-V F D L P	5-V F D G P	5-V D A P2	4-D G P2	6-V N F D P2	5-V N F D P2
(ʒ)																	5-F D G P2	5-F D L R P	4-F D L P	3-F D G	4-V D A P	5-V D G P2	5-N F D P2	4-N F D P2

Features:

Voicing - V
Nasality - N
Frication - F
Duration - D
Liquid - L
Glide - G
Retroflex - R
Aspiration - A
Place - P

(continued)

311

appendix F (continued)

(p)	(b)	(t)	(d)	(tʃ)	(dʒ)	(k)	(g)	(f)	(v)	(θ)	(ð)	(s)	(z)	(ʃ)	(ʒ)	(w)	(r)	(l)	(j)	(h)	(ʍ)	(m)	(n)
																(w)	4-L G R P	3-L G P	2-P	7-V G A P3	2-V F	2-G N	3-N G P
																	(r)	1-R	4-L G R P	7-V F L R A P2	6-V F L G R P	4-N L R P	3-N L R
																		(l)	3-L G P	6-V F L A P2	5-V F L G P	3-N L P	2-N L
																			(j)	5-V F G A P	4-V F P2	4-N G P2	3-N G P
																				(h)	5-G A P3	7-V N F A P3	6-V N F A P2
																					(ʍ)	4-V N F G	5-V N F G P
																						(m)	1-P

Features:
Voicing — V
Nasality — N
Frication — F
Duration — D
Liquid — L
Glide — G
Retroflex — R
Aspiration — A
Place — P

appendix G:

Wickelgren

	(h)	(j)	(l)	(r)	(w)	(ʒ)	(ʃ)	(z)	(s)	(ð)	(θ)	(v)	(f)	(g)	(k)	(dʒ)	(tʃ)	(n)	(d)	(t)	(m)	(b)	(p)
(h)	X	2-V P1	3-V P2	4-V P3	5-V P4	3-V 01 P1	2-01 P1	4-V 01 P2	3-01 P2	5-V 01 P3	4-01 P3	6-V 01 P4	5-01 P4	3-V 02	2-02	4-V 02 P1	3-02 P1	7-V N 02 P3	6-V 02 P3	5-02 P3	8-V N 02 P4	7-V 02 P4	6-02 P4
(j)		X	1-P1	2-P2	3-P3	1-01	2-V 01	2-01 P1	3-V 01 P1	3-01 P1	4-V 01 P2	4-01 P3	5-V 01 P3	3-02 P1	4-V 02 P1	2-02	3-V 02	5-N 02 P2	4-02 P2	5-V 02 P2	6-N 02 P3	5-02 P3	6-V 02 P3
(l)			X	1-P1	2-P2			1-01				3-01 P2											
(r)				X	1-P1			2-01 P1		1-01		2-01 P1							2-02				
(w)					X			3-01 P2		2-01 P1		1-01	2-V 01										
(ʒ)						X	1-V	1-P1	2-V P1			3-P3				1-01							
(ʃ)							X	2-V P1	1-V			2-P2					1-01						
(z)								X	1-P1	1-P1	2-V P1	1-P1	2-V P1										
(s)									X	2-V P1	1-V	2-V P1	1-P1										
(ð)										X	1-V	1-P1	2-V P1										
(θ)											X	1-V	1-V										

Features:
Openness - O
Place - P
Voicing - V
Nasality - N

(continued)

313

appendix G (continued)

	(h)	(j)	(l)	(r)	(w)	(ʒ)	(ʃ)	(z)	(s)	(ð)	(θ)	(v)	(f)	(g)	(k)	(dʒ)	(tʃ)	(n)	(d)	(t)	(m)	(b)	(p)
(θ)											X	2-V P1	1-P1	5-V O1 P3	4-O1 P3	4-V O1 P2	3-O1 P2	3-V N O1	2-V O1	1-O1	4-V N O1 P1	3-V O1 P1	2-O1 P1
(v)												X	1-V	5-O1 P4	6-V O1 P4	4-O1 P3	5-V O1 P3	3-N O1 P1	2-O1 P1	3-V O1 P1	2-N O1	1-O1	2-V O1
(f)													X	6-V O1 P4	5-O1 P4	5-V O1 P3	4-O1 P3	4-V N O1 P1	3-V O1 P1	2-O1 P1	3-V N O1	2-V O1	1-O1
(g)														X	1-V	1-P1	2-V P1	4-N P3	3-P3	4-V P3	5-N P4	4-P4	5-V P4
(k)															X	2-V P1	1-P1	5-V N P3	4-V P3	3-P3	6-V N P4	5-V P4	4-P4
(dʒ)																X	1-V	3-N P2	2-P2	3-V P2	4-N P3	3-P3	4-V P3
(tʃ)																	X	4-V N P2	3-V P2	2-P2	5-V N P3	4-V P3	3-P3
(n)																		X	1-N	2-V N	1-P1	2-N P1	3-V N P1
(d)																			X	1-V	2-N P1	1-P1	2-V P1
(t)																				X	3-V N P1	2-V P1	1-P1
(m)																					X	1-N	2-V N P1
(b)																						X	1-V
(p)																							X

Features:
Openness - O
Place - P
Voicing - V
Nasality - N

Structural Analysis of Syntagmatic Rules (from Smith, 1973)*

1. ↓ / ( ): REGRESSIVE POSITIONAL RULES
   V̲F̲↓ ( ) if F is unstressed.   An *initial* or postconsonantal unstressed vowel is deleted. Rule 14 [p.18].

2. ( ) / ↓ PROGRESSIVE POSITIONAL RULES
   ( ) C̲F̲↕ if F is alveolar.   Alveolar consonants are optionally deleted in *final* position. Rule 23 [p.21].

   ( ) P̲↓ if P is /l/.   /l/ is deleted *finally* and preconsonantally. Rule 6 [p.15].

   ( ) P̲ if P is /z/.   /z/ is deleted *finally*. Rule 11 [p.17].

3. ↓ / (C): REGRESSIVE CONSONANTAL RULES
   P̲↓ (C) if P is /l/.   /l/ is deleted finally and *preconsonantally*. Rule 6 [p.15].

   P̲↓ (C) if P is /s/.   /s/ is deleted *preconsonantally*. Rule 7 [p.15].

4. (C) / ↓: PROGRESSIVE CONSONANTAL RULES
   (C) C̲F̲↓ if F is alveolar.   *Postconsonantal* alveolar consonants are deleted. Rule 21 [p.21].

   (C) P̲₍ ₎↓ if P is a sonorant.   *Postconsonantal* sonorants /l,r,w,j/ are deleted. Rule 16 [p.18].

   (C) V̲F̲↓ if F is unstressed.   An initial or *postconsonantal* unstressed vowel is deleted. Rule 14 [p.18].

5. ↓ / (V): REGRESSIVE VOCALIC RULES
   P̲₍ ₎ (V) --- P if P is /f,v/.   /f,v/ become [w] *prevocalically*. Rule 20 [p.20].

6. (V) / ↓: PROGRESSIVE VOCALIC RULES
   No examples.

7. ↓ / CF: REGRESSIVE CONSONANTAL FEATURE RULES
   C̲F̲↓(CF) if F_1 = nasal and F_2 = voiceless.
       Nasal consonant is deleted before *voiceless consonants*. Rule 1 [p.13].
   C̲F̲ [ ] (CF) if F_1 = alveolar and palato-alveolar; $F_2 = F_1$
       if F_2 = velar relationship is obligatory.
       if F_2 = labial relationship is optional. Rule 19 [p.20].

8. CF / ↓: PROGRESSIVE CONSONANTAL FEATURE RULES
   (CF) C̲F̲ ↓ if F_1 = nasal and F_2 = voiced.
       Voiced consonant is deleted after a *nasal consonant*. Rule 2 [p.14].
   (CF) CF̲F̲ [ ] if F_1 = velar and F_2 = non-nasal; $F_3 = F_1$ if F_3 = alveolar or palatal.
       Non-nasal alveolar and palatal consonants harmonize to the point of articulation of a preceding velar. Rule 17 [p.19].

---

*Page numbers refer to pages in Smith.   *(continued)*

9. $\downarrow$ / VF: REGRESSIVE VOCALIC FEATURE RULES
   No examples.

10. VF / $\downarrow$: PROGRESSIVE VOCALIC FEATURE RULES
    (VF) $\underline{CF}$ --- P if F_1 = unstressed and F_2 = nasal.

    A nasal consonant following unstressed vowel becomes alveolar [n]. Rule 12 [p.17].

11. $\downarrow$ / P: REGRESSIVE PHONEME RULES
    $\underline{CF}$ (P) --- (CF) if F_1 = alveolar F_2 = velar.

    Alveolar consonants /n/ & /t,d/ become velars, [ŋ] and [g] before syllabic [l]. Rule 3 [p.14].

    $P_{<>} \, \phi$ (P) if P is /r/.

    /t/ and /d/ are optionally deleted before /r/. Rule 15. [p.18].

12. $\underline{P}$ / $\downarrow$: REGRESSIVE PHONEME RULES
    No examples.

13. 3 ELEMENT RULES
    $\underline{P}\phi$ (VCF) if P = /s/ and F = labial or alveolar. Rule 9 [p.16].
    if P = /ʃ/ and F = labial or velar. Rule 10 [p.16].
    (V)$\underline{P}_{<>}$(V) --- P if P_1 = /l,r,j/, P_2 = /w/.

14. 4 ELEMENT RULES
    (CP)$\underline{C}$(V) --- C_2F F = bilabial. Rule 8 [pp.15–16].

15. SIMPLE RULES
    $\underline{C}$ -- F

    All consonants are voiced. Rule 25 [p.21].

    $\underline{P}\downarrow$ if P is /h/.

    /h/ is deleted everywhere. Rule 13 [p.18].

    $\underline{P}$ -- P if P_1 = /l/

    Syllabic [l] vocalizes to [u]. Rule 4 [p.15].

    $\underline{P}_{<>}$ --- $P_{<>}$

    All alveolar and palato-alveolar consonants fall together as alveolars. /ʃ,ʒ,tʃ,dʒ,j,r/ neutralize as ultimately /d/, with allophones [t],[d], and [d]. Rule 23 [p.21].

    $\underline{P}_{<>}$ -- P

    /l,r,j/ are subject to neutralization as /l/ where /l,r,j/ are the only consonants. Rule 18a [p.19].

    $\underline{P}_{<>}$ -- P

    all nonsonorants are noncontinuant, nonstrident, nonaffricated, and nonlateral = /d/. Rule 24 [p.21].

    $\underline{P}_{<>}$ -- P

    /l,r,j/ are subject to behaving like other alveolar consonants elsewhere, i.e., are neutralized as /d/. Rule 18c [p.19].

    $\sim$V = C

    All non-vowels are true consonants. Rule 26 [p.22].

SYMBOLS

( ) = agent of action
___ = element affected by agent

(continued)

↓ = deletion
ɸ = deletion (optional)
C = consonant
V = vowel
F = feature
< > = sound class
[ ] = harmonization
P = phoneme
-- = becomes, is transformed to, etc.
~ = negative aspect
1,2,3 = element type

OPERATIONS
  1. REGRESSIVE or PROGRESSIVE (syntagmatic direction)
  2. DELETION, TRANSFORMATION, HARMONIZATION (optional or
     obligatory)
AGENTS
  ( ), C,V,F,< >,P
AFFECTED ELEMENT
  As above
TYPES OF RULES
  Paradigmatic or syntagmatic

Expansion Model of the Proportion of Sounds Under Each Subset (based on Dewey, 1926)

appendix I (continued)

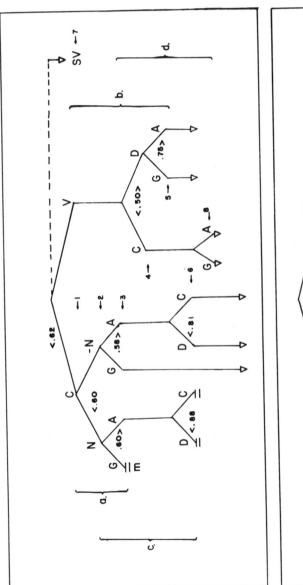

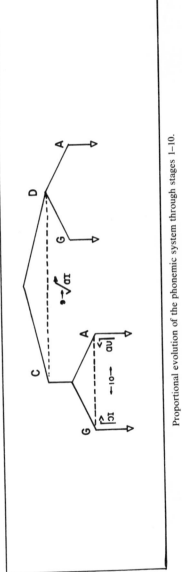

Proportional evolution of the phonemic system through stages 1–10.

(continued)

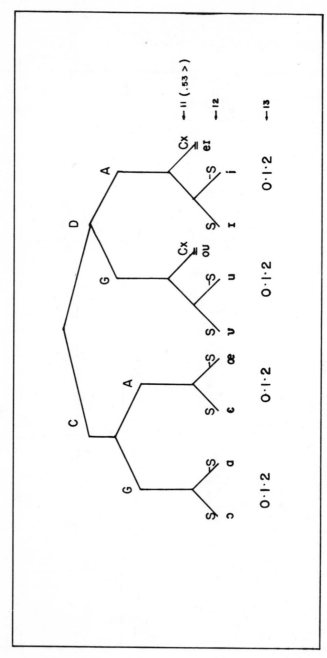

Proportional evolution of the phonemic system through stages 11–13.

(continued)

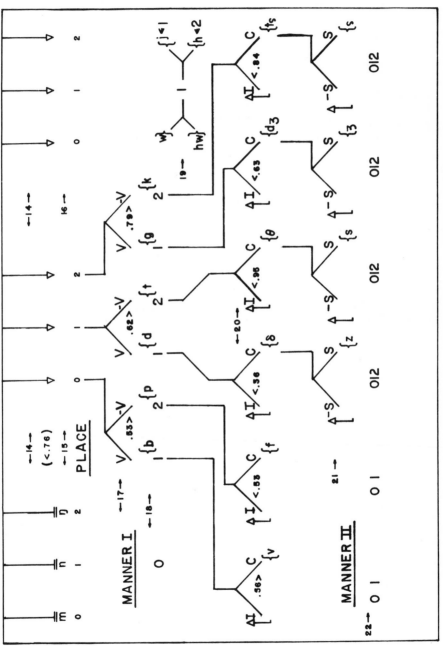

Proportional evolution of the phonemic system through stages 14–22.

Stimulus Word List*

1. MONKEY	[m-]	46. TOOTHBRUSH	[-θ-]
2. HAMMER	[-m-]	47. MOUTH	[-θ]
3. COMB	[-m]	48. THIS/THAT	[ð-]
4. KNIFE	[n-]	49. FEATHERS	[-ð-]
5. PENNY	[-n-]	50. SMOOTH	[-ð]
6. MOON	[-n]	51. CHAIR	[tʃ-]
7. FINGER	[-ŋ-]	52. MATCHES	[-tʃ-]
8. RING	[-ŋ]	53. WATCH	[-tʃ]
9. PIG	[p-]	54. JUMPING	[dʒ-]
10. PAPER	[-p-]	55. PAJAMAS	[-dʒ-]
11. CUP	[-p]	56. ORANGE	[-dʒ]
12. TABLE	[t-]	57. SUN	[s-]
13. POTATO	[-t-]	58. GLASSES	[-s-]
14. BOAT	[-t]	59. HOUSE	[-s]
15. CAT	[k-]	60. ZEBRA	[z-]
16. COOKIE	[-k-]	61. SCISSORS	[-z-]
17. DUCK	[-k]	62. EYES	[-z]
18. BICYCLE	[b-]	63. SHOE	[ʃ-]
19. BABY	[-b-]	64. DISHES	[-ʃ-]
20. BATHTUB	[-b]	65. FISH	[-ʃ]
21. DOG	[d-]	66. MEASURE	[-ʒ-]
22. LADDER	[-d-]	67. BEIGE	[-ʒ]
23. BED	[-d]	68. TEETH	[-i-]
24. GUN	[g-]	69. WITCH	[-ɪ-]
25. WAGON	[-g-]	70. TRAIN	[-eɪ-]
26. EGG	[-g]	71. BELL	[-ɛ-]
27. WHISTLE	[ʌ-]	72. HAT	[-æ-]
28. WINDOW	[w-]	73. BLOCKS	[-ɑ-]
29. FLOWERS	[-w-]	74. GUM	[-ʌ-]
30. LAMP	[l-]	75. BANANAS	[-ə-]
31. BALLOON	[-l-]	76. SAW	[-ɔ]
32. BALL	[-l]	77. CONE	[-OU-]
33. RABBIT	[r-]	78. BOOK	[-U-]
34. CARROT	[-r-]	79. TWO	[-u]
35. CAR	[-r]	80. PIPE	[-aɪ-]
36. YELLOW	[j-]	81. BOY	[-ɔɪ]
37. YOYO	[-j-]	82. COW	[-aU]
38. HORSE	[h-]	83. YOU	[IU]
39. FAN	[f-]	84. BIRD	[-ɛ-]
40. TELEPHONE	[-f-]	85. CRACKER	[-ɚ-]
41. LEAF	[-f]	86. DEER	[ɪr]
42. VACUUM	[v-]	87. BEAR	[-ɛr-]
43. TELEVISION	[-v-]	88. JAR	[-ɑr-]
44. STOVE	[-v]	89. FORK	[-or-]
45. THUMB	[θ-]		

*Note: To use this stimulus list only the phonemes indicated by the position markers are scored. Errors made in other positions are ignored or the percentile scores of Table 1, Chapter 20, do not apply.

Children who are not familiar with the words are told the desired words with normal articulation and no attempt is made to determine stimulability.

appendix K:

Type of Distinctive Features in Error*

	m	n	ŋ	p	t	k	b	d	g	f	v	θ	ð	tʃ	dʒ	s	z	ʃ	ʒ
m		F	FB	NV	NFV	NFB V	V	VF	NFB	NVC	NVC NC	NFV C	NFC	NFV CB	NFC B	NFV CS	NFC S	NFV CSB	NFC SB
n	F		B	NFV	NV	NVB NF	NF	N	NB	NVC F	NFC	NVC NV	NV	NVC B	NCB	NVC S	NCS B	NVC SB	NCS S
ŋ	FB	B		FBN V	BNV	NV	BFN	BN	N	FBN VC	FBN C	BNV C	BNC	NVC B	NC	CFS CS	NCS B	NVC S	NCS
p	NV	VNF B	FBN V		F	FB	V	VF	FBV	C	CV	CF	CFV	CFB V	CFB V	CFS	CFS V	CFS B	CFS BV
t	VFN	VN	VNB F	F		B	FV	V	BV	CF	CFV	C	CV	CB	CBV	CS	CSV	CSB	CSB V
k	FBN V	BNV	NV	FB	B		FBV	BV	V	FBC	FBC V	BC	BCV	C	CV	CSB	CSV B	CS	CSV
b	N	NF	FBN	V	FV	FBV		F	FB	VC	C	CFV	CF	CFB V	CFB V	CFS V	CFS	CFV SB	CFS B
d	FN	N	BN	FV	V	VB	F		B	CFV	CF	CV	C	VCB CB	CB	CSV	CS	CSV SB B	CSB B

*Key: N, nasality; V, voicing; F, front place; S, stridency; C, continuation; B, back place.

(continued)

325

appendix K (continued)

	m	n	ŋ	p	t	k	b	d	g	f	v	θ	ð	tʃ	dʒ	s	z	ʃ	ʒ
g	NFB	BN	N	FBV	BV	V	FB	B		FBC/V	FBC	BVC	CB	CV	C	CSV/B	CSB	CSV	CS
f	NVC/V	FCN/VN	FCB/VN	C	CF	FBC	CV	FCV/V	FBC/V		V	F	FV	FB	FBV	FS	FSV	FBS	FBS/V
v	CN	CFN/N	CFB/N	CV	VCF/V	FBV/V	C	CF	FBC	V		FV	F	FBV	FB	FSV	FS	FBS/V	FBS
θ	CVN/F	CVN/B	CVN/B	FC	C	CB	CVF	CV	CVB	F	VF		V	B	BV	S	SV	BS	BSV
ð	CNF	CN	CBN	FCV	CV	CVB	CF	C	BC	VF	F	V		BV	B	VS	S	SVB	SB
tʃ	CVN/FB	CVN/B	CVN	CFB	CB	C	CVF/B	CVB	CV	FB	FBV	B	BV		V	BS	BSV	S	SV
dʒ	CNB/F	CNB/V	CN/V	CBF	CBV	CV	CBF	CB	C	BFV	BF	VB	B	V		SBV	SB	SV	S
s	CSV/NF	CSV/N	CSV/NB	CSF	CS	CSB	CSV/F	CSV	CSV/B	SF	SFV	S	SV	BS	SBV		V	B	BV
z	CSN/F	CSN/B	CSN/B	CSF/V	CSF	CSV/B	CSF	CS	CSB	SFV	SF	SV	S	BSV	BS	V		BS	B
ʃ	CSV/NFB	CSV/NB	CSV/N	CSF/BV	CSB	CS	CSF/BV	CSB/V	CSB	SFB/V	SFB/V	BS	BSV	S	SV	B	BS		V
ʒ	CSF/BN	CSB/N	CSN/FB	CSV/B	CSV	CSV/B	CSB	CSB	CS	SFB/V	SFB/V	SB	SB	SV	S	BV	B	V	

326

appendix L:

Minimal-Pairs Sequence

Stage	Feature	Sound pair	Sample words
"Primitive system"			
2	Nasality	[m-p]	Two features in adult model, proceed to next step
3	Front place	[m-n]	mitt - knit, mail - nail, mine - nine, map - nap, moat - note, moose - noose, Tim - tin, cone - comb
		[p-t]	pin - tin, pool - tool, pie - tie, pier - tear, pen - ten, pot - tot, sip - sit, lip - lit
	Nasality	[n-t]	Two features in adult model, proceed to next step
"Vowel system"			
4	Compact	[i-ɑ]	peep - pop, team - Tom, neat - not, beetle - bottle, Pete - pot, Eeeeh! - Aaaah!
5	Grave	[i-u]	knee - new, teen - tune, beet - boot, seat - suit, heat - hoot, mean - moon
6	Stumpf's triangle	—	Proceed to discrimination phase of stage 15 if the vowel system is complete
7	Recoding stage	—	Proceed to next step
8	Grave	[æ-ɑ]	pat - pot, map - mop, hat - hot, gnat - not, cat - cot, Ann - on
9–10	Transitional stages	—	Proceed to next step
11	Complex	[i-eɪ]	see - say, bee - bay, key - Kay, he - hay, team - tame, Gene - Jane
		[u-oʊ]	new - no!, moo! - mow, boo! - bow, soup - soap, toot - tote, flute - float
		[æ-aɪ]	bat - bite, cat - kite, gnat - night, man - mine, sand - signed, pan - pine
		[i-aɪ]	beet - bite, neat - night, mean - mine, feet - fight, team - time, seed - side

(continued)

appendix L (continued)

Stage	Feature	Sound pair	Sample words
		[ɑ-ɔɪ]	baah! - boy, Raah! - Roy, aisle - oil, dolly - doily, John - join, Aaaah! - [ɔɪ:]
		[æ-ɔɪ]	baah! - boy, can - coin, Al - oil, Jan - join, [nonsense words with pictures]
		[ɑ-aʊ]	baah! - bow, Nah! - now, pa - pow!, Wah! - Wow!, [nonsense words with pictures]
		[æ-aʊ]	baah! - bow, Naah! - now, pat - pout, math - mouth, [nonsense words with pictures]
12	Short	[ɑ-ɔ]	cot - caught, knotty - naughty, odd - awed, Don - dawn, [nonsense words with pictures]
		[i-ɪ]	Pete - pit, eat - it, meat - mitt, neat - knit, beet - bit, seat - sit
		[u-ʊ]	pull - pool, look - Luke, soot - suit, [nonsense words with pictures]
		[æ-ɛ]	man - men, band - bend, sat - set, lad - led, land - lend, can - Ken
	Compact	[ɪ-ɛ]	pit - pet, lit - let, mitt - met, knit - net, tin - ten, pin - pen
		[ɔ-ʊ]	pull - Paul, soot - sought, balk - book, [nonsense words with pictures]
	Grave	[ɪ-ʊ]	pill - pull, sit - soot, Bic - book, Nick - nook, fit - foot, pit - put
		[ɛ-ɔ]	bell - ball, bet - bought, set - sought, pen - pawn, tell - tall, sell - Saul
13 "Back-nine system"	Recoding stage	—	Proceed to next step
14	Stumpf's triangle	—	Proceed to discrimination phase of stage 15
15	Back place	[t-k]	tea - key, tape - cape, table - cable, top - cop, ten - Ken, told - cold, bat - back, not - knock
		[n-ŋ]	win - wing, fan - fang,

(continued)

Stage	Feature	Sound pair	Sample words
			tan - Tang, sun - sung, run - rung, ton - tongue
"Semivowel system"			
16	Front place	[w-l]	wet - let, wed - led, weed - lead, wine - line, wait - late, Wes - less, win - Lynn, wok - lock
	Back place	[l-j]	let - yet, Lou - you, yes - less, lay - Yeah!, lack - yak, [nonsense words with pictures]
"Back-nine system"			
17	Voicing	[p-b]	pea - bee, pig - big, peach - beach, pear - bear, pat - bat, pier - beer, cap - cab, tap - tab
		[t-d]	toe - dough, time - dime, tear - deer, tot - dot, town - down, tore - door, lit - lid, kit - kid
		[k-g]	curl - girl, cave - gave, cap - gap, coat - goat, back - bag, sack - sag, rag - rack, dig - Dick
	Nasality	[b-m]	beet - meat, belt - melt, bat - mat, bike - Mike, bunny - money, bear - mare, Bob - bomb, robe - roam
		[d-n]	'D' - knee, deer - near, deck - neck, dot - not, dots - knots, name - dame, Lynn - lid, ten - Ted
		[g-ŋ]	wig - wing, rig - ring, bag - bang, rug - rung, log - long, sag - sang
	Front place	[b-d]	big - dig, bark - dark, bow - doe, door - boar, deer - beer, nob - nod, rib - rid, cob - cod
	Back place	[d-g]	deer - gear, date - gate, done - gun, dough - go, get - debt, dot - got, Ed - egg, bed - beg
18	Recoding stage	—	Proceed to next step

(continued)

appendix L (continued)

Stage	Feature	Sound pair	Sample words
"Semivowel system"			
19	Voicing	[w-hw]	[This contrast is of little linguistic importance.] Weee! - we
		[j-h]	you - Who?, yen - hen, Yah! - hay, yellow - hello, Ho!Ho! - yoyo, hack - yak
20	Continuation	[p-f]	pin - fin, pan - fan, pour - four, pull - full, pine - fine, pat - fat, lap - laugh, cap - calf
		[t-θ]	tree - three, tie - thigh, torn - thorn, bat - bath, [nonsense words with pictures]
		[b-v]	bee - 'V', base - vase, bat - vat, boat - vote, Ban - van, 'B' - 'V', bail - veil
		[d-ð]	doze - those, ladder - lather, [nonsense words with pictures]
	Front place	[f-θ]	free - three, fin - thin, fought - thought, [nonsense words with pictures]
		[v-ð]	'V's - these, van - than, vat - that, [nonsense words with pictures]
	Voicing	[f-v]	fat - vat, fan - van, face - vase, fine - vine, fees - 'V's, have - half, save - safe, five - fife
		[θ-ð]	teeth - teethe, [nonsense words with pictures]
	Continuation	[k-tʃ]	keys - cheese, kick - chick, case - chase, cane - chain, chop - cop, core - chore, hack - hatch, back - batch
		[g-dʒ]	Gail - jail, goose - juice, ghoul - jewel, jobs - gobs, bag - badge, egg - edge, [nonsense words with pictures]
20	Back place	[θ-tʃ]	thief - chief, thick - chick, thin - chin, thumb - chumb, bath - batch
		[ð-dʒ]	[nonsense words with pictures]
	Voicing	[tʃ-dʒ]	cello - jello, cherry - Jerry, chunk - junk, char - jar,

(continued)

appendix L (continued)

Stage	Feature	Sound pair	Sample words
"Sibilant system"			chess - Jess, Chet - jet, batch - badge, match - Madge
21	Stridency	[θ-s]	think - sink, thick - sick, thumb - some, sum - thumb, theme - seem, sin - thin, thank - sank, Beth - Bess
		[tʃ-ʃ]	chip - ship, chin - shin, chair - share, chop - shop, chew - shoe, cheek - sheik, mash - match, leash - leech
		[ð-z]	tease - teethe, [nonsense words with pictures]
		[dʒ-ʒ]	legion - lesion, [nonsense words with pictures]
	Back place	[s-ʃ]	sip - ship, seat - sheet, sell - shell, save - shave, sack - shack, sign - shine, mess - mesh, Cass - cash
		[z-ʒ]	Caesar - seizure, [nonsense words with pictures]
	Voicing	[s-z]	sip - zip, Sue - zoo, buzz - bus, eyes - ice, lacy - lazy, race - raise, 'Z' - see, sorrow - Zorro
		[ʃ-ʒ]	[nonsense words with pictures]
22	Recoding stage	—	The consonantal system should be complete

index